Nutrition, Physical Activity, and Health in Early Life

Jana Pařízková

CRC Press

Boca Raton   New York   London   Tokyo

Library of Congress Cataloging-in-Publication Data

Pařízková, Jana.
    Nutrition, physical activity, and health in early life: studies
in preschool children / Jana Pařízková.
       p. cm. -- (Nutrition in exercise and sport)
    Includes bibliographical references and index.
    ISBN 0-8493-7919-9 (alk. paper)
    1. Children--Nutrition.   2. Child development.   3. Exercise for
children--Health aspects.   4. Preschool children--Health and
hygiene. I. Title. II. Series.
RJ206.P34   1996
618.92--dc20
                                       95-41134
                                          CIP

© 1996 by CRC Press, Inc.

No claim to original U.S. Government works
International Standard Book Number 0-8493-7919-9
Library of Congress Card Number 95-41134
Printed in the United States of America 1 2 3 4 5 6 7 8 9 0
Printed on acid-free paper

NUTRITION in EXERCISE and SPORT

Editors, Ira Wolinsky and James F. Hickson, Jr.

Published Titles

Nutrients as Ergogenic Aids for Sports and Exercise
Luke Bucci

Nutrition in Exercise and Sport, 2nd Edition
Ira Wolinsky and James F. Hickson, Jr.

Exercise and Disease
Ronald R. Watson and Marianne Eisinger

Nutrition Applied to Injury Rehabilitation and Sports Medicine
Luke Bucci

Nutrition for the Recreational Athlete
Catherine G.R. Jackson

NUTRITION in EXERCISE and SPORT

Editor, Ira Wolinsky

Published Titles

Nutrition, Physical Activity, and Health in Early Life
Jana Pařízková

Exercise and Immune Function
Laurie Hoffman-Goetz

Sports Nutrition: Minerals and Electrolytes
Constance Kies and Judy Driskell

Forthcoming Titles

Nutrition and the Female Athlete
Jaime S. Rudd

Body Fluid Balance: Exercise and Sport
E.R. Buskirk and S. Puhl

Biochemical Methods for Exercise Assessment
Jon Karl Linderman

Handbook of Sports Nutrition: Vitamins and Trace Minerals
Ira Wolinsky and Judy Driskell

SERIES PREFACE

The CRC Series on Nutrition in Exercise and Sport provides a setting for in-depth exploration of the many and varied aspects of nutrition and exercise, including sports. The topic of exercise and sports nutrition has been a focus of research among scientists since the 1960s, and the healthful benefits of good nutrition and exercise have been appreciated. As our knowledge expands, it will be necessary to remember that there must be a range of diets and exercise regimes that will support excellent physical condition and performance. There is not a single diet-exercise treatment that can be the common denominator, or the single formula for health, or panacea for performance.

This series is dedicated to providing a stage to explore these issues. Each volume provides a detailed and scholarly examination of some aspect of the topic.

I welcome the volume *Nutrition, Physical Activity, and Health in Early Life*, a monograph by Dr. Jana Pařízková, who has made so many significant contributions in the field.

Ira Wolinsky
Series Editor

"Childhood is surely the time of sowing: later life produces the harvest. It is clear therefore that the most salutary thing that can happen to young people is to be wisely taught from their earliest years at every possible opportunity. In a word, ever-lasting happiness depends on good health, good death, good life on good training habits formed by practice in well-doing, but this begins with foundations well laid in childhood .... Therefore, the most important nurturing of the human race occurs in our cradles."

J.A. Comenius* (1592–1670): Panpaedia[59]

The health of children is the key to the health of the adult population, and thus to the prosperity of the whole society. The factors that not only limit pathological situations, but that also develop and promote above average health should be defined and developed for the benefit of children.

During the last few years, more attention has been focused on the early stages of life, starting with the fetal period, even though the principle that diet during the early stages of life might influence the rate of growth and development was formulated more than 20 years ago.[212] Some of the most dangerous diseases have fetal and infant origins,[17,18,165] some of which may depend on early diet and general lifestyle.

Until recently, the majority of data on morphological, nutritional, functional, and metabolic development concerned either infants or school children and adolescents.[16,347] *The period of early and preschool age has been studied considerably less*,[113,142–143] but some new data have recently appeared.[76–77,141]

Relatively much more have been known about the influence of negative and/or pathological factors than about natural, favorable factors such as nutrition and physical activity in promoting adequate and/or optimal development of the human being. In those studies, *the actual consequences were investigated the most, but the delayed effects* of certain influences that affect the organism at the very beginning of life were studied much less. This applies both to experimental models and to studies in humans, where this problem was only tackled marginally.

Human growth and development was followed and analyzed extensively. The majority of data focuses on the morphological changes in the growing

---

* J. A. Comenius (1592–1670) was a Czech philosopher and theologist, a theoretician of education, a social reformer, and the founder of pedagogy. Born in Southern Moravia, Comenius studied in Germany and was active as a Protestant preacher and teacher in the Moravian Church (Unitas Fratum). He was forced into exile at the beginning of the Thirty Years Wars, and he worked in Poland, England, Sweden, and Hungary. He died in Amsterdam and was buried in Naarden in Holland.

organism, as well as on the psychological, social, and nutritional parameters. Less attention was given to the studies of the functional, motor, and biochemical characteristics of growth in normal, healthy young children. Comprehensive studies which simultaneously cover several aspects are rare, because most growth studies focus on one particular or very few of the above mentioned issues.

This volume aims to report on the results of comprehensive studies of development during the preschool years, as it relates to environmental conditions, including nutrition, with special attention to physical activity and performance. Some of the problems, e.g., the influence of the composition of the maternal diet during pregnancy on the newborn, could only be dealt with marginally, as few studies of this sort exist. Therefore, select ontogenetical problems could only be followed in experiments using laboratory animals, as many observations could not be made in humans for ethical reasons and with regard to time. The conclusions on the influence of dietary and physical activity manipulations in laboratory animals, however, cannot be transferred directly to other species and/or to humans. This could provide, though, some general ideas on how to promote health in preschoolers using adequate diet and physical regimes, starting at the beginning of life. This could also eventually point up how to use these simple natural factors to promote health in humans.

Under present conditions, nutrition and physical activity reveal two extremes: malnutrition and/or overeating, on the one hand, and excess work load and/or hypokinesia, on the other. The right amount of dietary intake and physical work load — so as to achieve optimal results — has not yet been exactly defined and implemented. Contrasting examples from the industrially developed and/or developing countries give a vivid picture of this fact. Of course, research cannot provide an answer to all of these problems because the causes must be solved using different means; scientific data, however, can be useful as a guideline.

This book cannot offer complete information on the rather broad topic of nutrition and physical activity, but it may cite certain examples from experimental models, as well as from human studies. The material presented is not homogeneous, but it does have one common denominator: ***motion***, it relationship to ***diet***, and its influence on the ***development*** of the organism. Selected examples should serve as motivation for early intervention, especially using adequate diet, along with motor stimulation and exercise from the very beginning of life.

THE AUTHOR

Dr. Jana Pařízková, M.D., Ph.D., D. Sc., is a Senior Scientist and Associate Professor in the Laboratory of Health Promotion (4th Department of Internal Medicine/1st Medical Faculty) at Charles University in The Czech Republic, Prague.

Dr. Pařízková received her medical degree in 1956 at Charles University, where she graduated summa cum laude. She then pursued her doctorate degree in medical physiology at the Institute of Physiology in the Czechoslovak Academy of Sciences, graduating in 1960. She also continued on at the Academy to receive her doctorate of science degree in nutrition and metabolism (ibidem) in 1977. She also had a fellowship at the Laboratoire de Nutrition Humaine, Hôpital Bichat in Paris, France from 1965–1966.

Dr. Pařízková is a member of the Czech Medical Association J.E. Purkyné (CzME JEP), the Czech Association for Nutrition, the Czech Anthropological Society, the Czech Association on the Study of Obesity, and the Advisory Committee for Nutrition with the Czech Ministry of Health. In addition, she also has memberships in the following organizations: the European Academy of Nutritional Sciences (EANS), the European Association of the Study of Obesity and the International Commission for Anthropology of Food (ICAF) for Europe through the International Union of Anthropological and Ethnological Sciences (IUAES). She served as Chairperson of the "Nutrition and Physical Performance" committee through the International Union of Nutritional Science (IUNS); as a member of the Executive of the International Society for the Advancement of Kinanthropometry (ISAK); as a member of both the Scientific Committee of the International Council for Sport and Physical Education (ICSPE) through UNESCO and the American Association of Physical Education. She was also elected a member of the New York Academy of Sciences and has been conferred with an honorary appointment to the Research Board of Advisors of the American Biographic Institute.

Dr. Pařízková is the author of several monographs including "Development of lean body mass and depot fat in children" (1962); "Body composition and lipid metabolism under conditions of various physical activity" (1974), which is in Czech with updated translations by Martinus Nijhoff, B.V. Medical Division (The Hague, 1977) and by Editora Guanabara Dois (Rio de Janeiro, 1982) entitled "Body fat and physical fitness"; in addition, she has edited and co-authored eight other monographs. She is also the author of more than 450 scientific articles in international and national journals and from many proceedings, including the International Congresses. She has also been an invited speaker at more than 100 international scientific congresses and symposia, especially the IUNS, where she was also the Chairperson and organizer in 1975, 1978, 1981, and 1989.

Her appointments include: the World Health Organization as a Visiting Professor, the International Course on Nutrition and Hygiene,

Hydarabad—SEARO 1977; consultant to the World Health Organization, Geneva, 1978; member of the panel of experts, Food and Agricultural Organization/World Health Organization/United Nations University, FAO, Rome, 1981 on "Energy and protein requirements", published by the World Health Organization, Geneva, 1985; and a member of the consultation group "Epidemiology of Obesity", Warsaw, 1987 (Regional Office of the World Health Organization, Europe). Dr. Pařízková has also served as the President of the Institute Danone, The Czech Republic.

Dr. Pařízková's main research interests include body composition, physical fitness and performance, dietary intake and nutritional status, motor and sensomotor development, lipid metabolism variables, and physical activity regimes during growth and development, as related to the development of obesity and cardiovascular risk later in life. In addition, she emphasizes the topics of health promotion and the reduction of health risks through early and/or later nutritional and physical activity interventions. Another main area of research is obesity with joined metabolic and clinical problems as related to actual diet and physical activity in all age categories.

Among other awards, she has received the Memorial Medal from Charles University and The Philip Noel Baker Research Prize, ICSPE, by UNESCO.

ACKNOWLEDGMENT

Special thanks to Ing. Z. Roth, head of the Statistical Department of the State Health Institute in Prague, for advice and statistical evaluation of research data during our long-lasting professional relationship.

TABLE OF CONTENTS

Chapter 6

Chapter 7

Chapter 13

DEDICATION

To my husband, Jiří Pařízek

Chapter 1

INTRODUCTION: FIRST STEPS TO OPTIMAL HEALTH AND FITNESS THROUGHOUT LIFE

"Give me a child until he is seven and I will give you a man"

Seventeenth century Jesuit maxim

I. POTENTIAL FOR HEALTH

The human being is born with great potential which may or may not be actualized later in life. Select stimuli may enhance and/or suppress the development of this potential, thus resulting in either adequate, optimal health or in a deteriorated, inferior form.

According to the World Health Organization, *health is the status of full mental, physical, and social well-being, and not the mere absence of illness and/or infirmity.*[393,394] It is, therefore, necessary to apply substantial effort to assure the full realization of the potential of all children, in order to develop them further using all available means. Moreover, "*positive health*" is also defined as *an above average status regarding the physiological, mental, and social abilities of the humans.*

The World Health Organization, the Food and Agricultural Organization, and the United Nations University, along with other organizations, pay great attention to growth and development in various populations in relation to nutrition. Numerous documents exist concerning these problems.[379] Among the most important are documents dealing with energy and protein requirements,[393] Prevention of adult cardiovascular diseases in early childhood,[395] as well as many others.[395]

Practical experience and theoretical studies allow for the evaluation of the factors that negatively influence growth and development — malnutrition, lack of social and mental stimulation, and physical overloading. On the other hand, excess food intake and a lack of physical and overall activity can also be harmful. To achieve positive health, then, it is necessary to define the optimal range of both nutrition and physical activity.

II. HISTORICAL ASPECTS: PEDAGOGY AND EDUCATION

In his philosophy on the formation of man ("formatio hominis"), J.A. Comenius (1592–1670),[57–59] the founder of pedagogics and "the teacher of nations", stressed the importance of education in early childhood. From his monographs, we can deduce that *education of the child starts in the womb of the mother*. This Czech philosopher, theologist, and scientist was already ahead of his time in recognizing that the condition of the expectant mother and the various stimuli influencing her during pregnancy, i.e., both her physical and mental status, may be later reflected in the development of the child.

J.A. Comenius considered the period of childhood as an important stage of open possibilities regarding development during subsequent life. As in nature, he recognized *motion as a basic principle*. For the human world, *this activity includes the activity of the body and the spirit in mutual harmony*. This physical and spiritual activity was considered an important contribution in any educational effort. J.A. Comenius also appreciated children's games as an essential means for natural development and education, just as important as nutrition and sleep.[58]

In the development of the overall system of education and the perfection of man, physical education had a firm position as one of the components in the process of the perfection of the human being. These ideas appear in School of Infancy (Schola Infantiae[58]). J.A. Comenius also stressed the importance of the early development of the abilities and skills of the hand in order "to make people active beings, diligent and skilful. Human nature is full of life, likes motion and activity and does not need anything, except wise direction." He also defined three principles of early development: starting to exercise early, being active, and gaining mobility which will not be lost when developed by repetition. In addition, he emphasizes that "… it is necessary to allow boys to play, to run, and always to do something." All of this should be executed with enthusiasm, not with reluctance, always keeping some goal in mind.

"The more the child is employed in something, runs about, is occupied, is doing something, the sweeter is its sleep, the more easily it digests, the more richly it grows, becomes vigorous and flourishing both in body and mind …" (J.A. Comenius, Schola Infantiae, 1650–1654).[58]

Numerous pedagogues followed the ideas of J.A. Comenius because these concepts were so advanced for his period. In some respects, these ideas have not been fulfilled, even in the present time.

III. PHYSIOLOGY OF CHILDREN

In 1867, E. Allix published "Étude sur la physiologie de la première enfance",[9] material which covers the first 2 years of life. A more detailed analysis was presented by K. Vierordt (1877)[366] in his textbook on "Physiology of Childhood" in which he compared the absolute and the relative development of body weight during different stages of development, as well as the composition of the organism (changes of individual organs) in newborn and adult (Tables 1.1 and 1.2).

TABLE 1.1 Weight of the Individual Organs as Percentage of Total Body Weight

Organs	Newborn	Adult
Skeleton	16.7	15.35
Muscles	23.4	43.09
Skin	11.3	6.3
Brain	14.34	2.32
Spinal chord	0.20	0.067
Eyes	0.28	0.023
Salivary glands	0.24	0.12
Thyroid gland	0.24	0.05
Lungs	2.15	2.01
Heart	0.89	0.52
Thymus	0.54	0.0086
Stomach and intestines	2.53	2.34
Pancreas	0.12	0.15
Liver	4.39	2.77
Spleen	0.41	0.346
Adrenals	0.31	0.014
Kidneys	0.88	0.48
Testicles	0.037	0.08

Modified from Vierordt, K., *Physiologie des Kinesalters,* Verlag der H. Laupp'schen Buchhandlung, Tübingen, 1877.

Then, he analyzed the change in several body segments during different growth periods, which also enabled the evaluation of their function. His results are interesting with respect to the description of the character of growth in different stages of development and as data on growth of children and youth in the second half of the 19th century.

Vierordt[366] also examined the relationship of body height and pulse rate, deriving a formula for the calculation of pulse rate from body length, which gives close to exact results.[366] The changes of nutrition and function in the gastrointestinal system were also described as well as respiration, metabolic changes, vegetative functions, chemical reactions during breathing and voiding, neuromuscular function, and thermoregulation. For the first time, this book analyzed the development of function during growth from the time of birth.

Many other textbooks followed the writings of Vierordt. Among them are "Auxology" by DeToni et al.,[79] covering both fetal and postnatal ontogeny; "Human Growth" by Falkner and Tanner;[98] "Clinical and Paediatric Physiol-

TABLE 1.2 The Development of Body Weight (BoW) After Quetelet, Expressed as Percentage of Birth Weight (BiW), and the Changes of Weight Increments Expressed in Absolute (WI-A) and Relative Values (WI-R)

Age (years)	Boys				Girls			
	BoW (kg)	% BiW	WI-A	WI-R	BoW (kg)	% BiW	WI-A	WI-R
0	3.20	100	—	—	2.90	100	—	—
1	9.45	295.3	6.25	1.960	8.79	302.1	5.88	2.020
2	11.4	354.4	1.89	0.200	10.67	366.7	1.88	0.214
3	12.47	389.7	1.13	0.099	11.79	405.2	1.12	0.105
4	14.23	444.7	1.74	0.141	13.00	446.7	1.21	0.103
5	15.77	492.8	1.54	0.108	14.36	403.5	1.36	0.105
6	17.24	538.8	1.47	0.093	16.00	549.8	1.64	0.115
7	19.10	569.9	1.86	0.108	17.54	602.8	1.54	0.096
10	24.52	766.3	5.42	0.086	23.52	808.3	5.98	0.102
15	43.62	1363	19.1	0.122	40.37	1387	16.85	0.114
18	57.85	1807	14.3	0.099	51.03	1753	10.66	0.080
25	62.93	1966	—	0.08	53.28	1831	—	0.019

Modified from Vierordt, K., *Physiologie des Kindesaltes,* Verlag der H. Laupp'schen Buchhandlung, Tübingen.

ogy" by Godfrey and Baum;[129] and many others. Monographs of the time mostly covered the whole period of growth or certain growth periods such as adolescence.[347] The period of preschool age, i.e., from 3 to 6 years old, was usually not analyzed in great detail or in all of its complexity.

IV. SECULAR TREND: ACCELERATION OF GROWTH

Along with the environmental changes during this century, many of the conditions of life changed. The growth acceleration mainly related to morphological parameters, sexual maturation, etc. A comparison of the height and weight of Czech children measured by Matiegka[209] in 1895 and recently by Hainiš shows a significant increase in height and weight of 6- to 7-year-old children. Boys of this age in the Czech republic are by now 11.5 cm and girls are 13.5 cm taller than in 1895.[209] Similar changes also occurred in body weight and in the body mass index (BMI) of children of the same age. These numbers are higher nowadays.

Changes in the development of the individual systems, in organs, and in tissues have not been described in detail. The same applies to the *development of functional capacity of the whole organism* as well as to various functions, especially of *the cardiovascular system*.[233]

Some studies[327] indicate that *the acceleration of physical growth and the increase in body size was not always paralleled with accelerated functional development*. This happened in, for example, Canadian Inuits who changed their lifestyle and adopted a westernized diet and who consequently now have increased body size along with an increased fat ratio. Simultaneously, the levels of functional capacity and fitness deteriorated.[327] Therefore, extending the potential for body size does not automatically parallel the extension of the functional potential.

A similar phenomenon is also described in other populations; e.g., Guminskyi et al.[144] compared body size and aerobic power (characterized by oxygen uptake during a maximal work load as related to body weight in kilograms) in Russian children and adolescents shortly after World War II and then approximately 15 years later. The height and weight of children increased, but *aerobic power declined*. In the diet of both compared samples, the food intake was much worse just after the war than later on: *both energy and protein intake were on a lower level then.* Increased energy intake, along with all other dietary components including high quality protein, resulted in increased body size but not in an improved aerobic power, i.e., higher level of cardiovascular fitness, which applies mainly to dynamic performance.

In the *Czech population,* there were *higher average values of body mass index (BMI, correlating with depot fat*[243]) as compared to other populations, e.g., the French.[294] Recommended dietary allowances for the Czech population were higher[171] than those in Western Europe (i.e., the European Community[398]) and the U.S.[397] Most often the real intake was even higher. The prevalence of cardiovascular diseases and death rate were also higher in The Czech population compared to other countries.[360] The practice of prevention has, therefore, become an essential issue in Central and Eastern Europe.

V. THE INFLUENCE OF ENVIRONMENTAL FACTORS

In infants 3 to 5 months old, it was already possible to elaborate conditioned reflexes for the turning of the head in response to a sound signal. An infant was lying in the cot, and from the direction of his/her feet, a soft sound signal was given. After 5 seconds an illuminated moving toy appeared in a small window at the side of the infant. At the beginning of these experiments, the infant reacted by turning its head toward the window with the toy only after it was illuminated (unconditioned, orientation reflex). When this situation was repeated several times, the infant began to turn its head to the window after just the sound (conditioned reflex). For elaboration of this reflex, though, it was always necessary to illuminate the window. When this was not done, the reflex disappeared.[182,183,224–226] This example confirms the *possibility tof elaborating certain reflexes and habits much earlier than was originally assumed; the consequences of this may be manifested in some developmental changes of the child later in life or even in adulthood.*

The influence of motor stimulation on the infant is demonstrated by Koch,[182–183] who showed that stimulated children were advanced in their development in certain respects. This principle has been adopted in some systems of childhood education and has proven to be beneficial for the actual and future development of children (see Chapter 10).

The influence of an inadequate diet during fetal and postnatal ontogeny can also have *negative consequences, persisting possibly throughout life*. This condition could not be followed up most of the time in the same subjects. The influence of an adverse diet concerns many aspects of *later development of the individual*.

Different environment may have a significant influence on the development of children, both positive and negative. Air and water pollution can have an influence on the outcome of pregnancy and on the subsequent development of the child.[402] For example, a lower birth weight in newborns of smoking mothers was observed.[361] Air pollution and noise can also reduce birth weight, thus affecting the future development of the child, who may remain smaller, may become more frequently sick, and may show other handicaps. The negative impact of some medicines and/or drugs ingested by mothers during pregnancy was also proven.

The growth and development of children may be negatively influenced at any period of growth, but during **certain periods** (called **"critical"**, e.g., the weaning period), *more serious delayed consequences can occur later in life*. **Preschool age** was also defined as a "critical period" for the predisposition of later **obesity**.[80] Sensitive critical periods exist for learning about food, i.e., the first 2 to 3 years.[48] The same applies to **motor development** and **physical activity**.[233,254–256]

VI. WHAT ARE THE AIMS?

We know much about the influence of negative factors on the development of children and eventually on the impact of their elimination. However, the impact of the opposite situation, i.e., when the conditions during earliest periods of life are optimal in all necessary aspects, has not been analyzed sufficiently. This includes the influence of natural factors in affecting young children i.e., what happens when infants, toddlers, and preschool children live under various conditions of physical activity, dietary intake, and other environmental factors which vary but which may still remain within normal limits. This situation is understandable because many more urgent and actual problems exist concerning negative conditions of the development of children. Unfortunately, many of these problems could be avoided without scientific knowledge. However, under any circumstances and adverse conditions it is always worthwhile to develop a creative approach to positive health for the overall optimal evolution of human beings.

Chapter 2

THEORETICAL CONSIDERATIONS: WHAT CAN WE LEARN FROM THE NATURAL AND EXPERIMENTAL MODELS?

I. INFLUENCE OF DIET EARLY IN LIFE AND ITS DELAYED EFFECTS

A. GROWTH, BODY COMPOSITION, AND PHYSICAL ACTIVITY

"Early diet, later consequences"[60] was the topic of the 13th British Nutrition Foundation Annual Conference in 1991. It was shown that animals from large litters[323] grew more slowly than animals from small litters who got more mother's milk. This difference was evident long after birth. Classical observations of Widdowson and McCance[388,389] showed in greater detail the impact of early nutrition on the later somatic development of rats. When 2 litters of rats born on the same day were combined and 3 were taken at random and returned to one mother to suckle, those in the small group grew much more rapidly than those in the larger group compared to the remaining 15 to 20 of the others.

When these animals were weaned at 3 weeks, each individual from the small group weighed two to three times as much as those in the large nest because they got more milk.[60] The mother with the large number to suckle produced a greater total volume of milk, but not the five to six times as much that would be necessary for all of the animals in the small nest. Thus, the sucklings from the large nest grew more slowly. These animals never caught up in body size, even later when they had access to food intake *ad libitum,* and they still ate less. This results because of a later maturation of the appetite centers in the hypothalamus which can only fully develop 10 days after birth.

Realimented children are usually able to catch up in growth after a period of malnutrition because in the human infant the appetite centers are fully developed at birth. The consequences of malnutrition depend significantly on its degree and duration; marginal malnutrition (which mainly reduces body weight and fat ratio, but not the size of vital organs, and essential muscle groups) is easier to compensate and does not always have a deteriorating impact functionally. The realimentation and "catch-up" growth of malnourished children is further accelerated with certain levels of physical activity[367–368] which can have a natural anabolic effect, especially in the development of lean body mass.

In two series of our experiments with **rats breastfed** and weaned in nests with different numbers of litters, i.e., in **small nests** with less than 6 (Group A) and in **large nests** with more than 12 animals (Group B) up to the 28th day of life, it was shown that animals from the largest nests were not only smaller (Figure 2.1a) but also leaner with smaller epididymal fat pads and a *lower percentage of total body fat*. In this experiment, the body weight of the animals from Group B was significantly lower at certain periods of growth, and this difference disappeared gradually. The intake of food as related to body weight tended to be temporarily higher (Figure 2.1b).[272,273]

The size of **vital organs**, such as the **heart** and **adrenal glands** and/or the soleus **muscle**, were not influenced, but the weight of the epididymal fat pads (which correlates significantly with total body fat assessed gravimetrically[233,275]) was significantly reduced in Group B.

There are other consequences resulting from different dietary intakes in early life: the level of **spontaneous physical activity**, measured in rotation activity cages (which enable the measurement of distance run in m/day), was *significantly higher* in rats from large litters (Group B), i.e., *with lower intake of mothers' milk and with lower final body weight* (Figure 2.1c). The average distance covered during one day in the rotation cages was more than 6 km, indicating a *satisfactory level of functional development of these animals*. This was also confirmed in other experiments.[272,273]

Thus, it seems that more modest food intake at the beginning of life and smaller body dimensions, along with lower percentage of body fat, may not be deleterious in all respects, even though it was generally believed that the reduced implementation of the potential for developing maximal body size is highly undesirable. However, achieving the maximum growth potential does not seem ideal when also other potentials are considered, e.g., the level of spontaneous physical activity and capacity for running, which is obviously linked with a higher level of functional capacity of the organism and better functioning of vital organs and systems. This factor is also suggested by their unchanged size.

On the other hand, in her experiments on laboratory rats, Fraňková[114–117] demonstrated that early overnutrition was not beneficial for later exploratory behavior, learning ability, and resistance to pharmacological or nutritional stress.

B. INFLUENCE OF TEMPORARY DIET WITH LOWER ENERGY AND PROTEIN

The influence of food intake with reduced energy and proteins was studied in another series of experiments.[272–274] During the lactation period, rat mothers were fed a diet with reduced content of proteins (10%) up to weaning. The

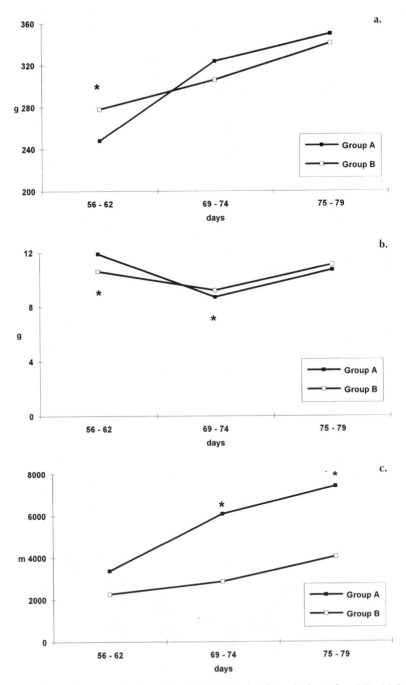

FIGURE 2.1 Changes in body weight **(a)**, food intake **(b)** and physical activity **(c)** in rotation wheels in groups of male rats suckled in different-sized litters (A < 12, B > 6). * means statistically significant difference between groups.

offspring (males) had a diet with 5% of protein up to the 49th day of life, and their intake of this diet was spontaneously reduced (i.e., the intake of protein and energy was reduced in these animals — Group REP). These animals were then fed a normal laboratory diet similar to that of the control group (20% casein — Group C) since weaning. The overall dietary intake in absolute values (g/day) of the REP group was lower than those in the group of control animals. The growth of the animals in Group REP was significantly reduced compared to control animals, up until the end of experiment, i.e., 125 days of age.[274]

Moreover, the development of spontaneous physical activity in rotation, activity cages was followed up in both groups (REPA and CA). *REPA animals* gradually developed a *significantly higher level of spontaneous physical activity than CA animals*. The energy cost of growth increments in the REPA subgroup (expressed as g food/1 g of weight increment) was significantly lower than that in CA animals. *The energy economy of growth and development was thus more effective*, especially when we also consider the increased energy output necessary for running as much as 9 km/day. Such an increase of spontaneous physical activity in rotation cages was observed in several subsequent and similarly arranged experiments.[261,262,272–274]

C. LIPID METABOLISM

Selected parameters of the lipid metabolism were also influenced by the dietary change at the beginning of life (REPA), which might be related to the modified physical activity level in the rotation cages. The concentration of lipids in the liver was significantly increased, and the synthesis of lipids was decreased in REPA male rats as compared with CA rats[272,274] (Figure 2.2).

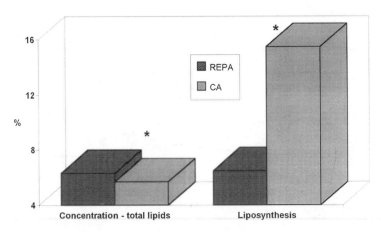

FIGURE 2.2 Changes in lipid metabolism in the liver of male rats with different diet at the beginning of life (REPA — reduced energy and protein, CA — control diet) living in rotation activity cages. * means statistically significant difference between groups.

Similar changes were also found in male rats breast fed in large (A) and small nests (B), which developed different physical activity level as mentioned above. The lipid concentration in small intestine was significantly higher in the females of Group A (Figure 2.3a[233,272–274]). The synthesis of lipids in the small intestine was significantly higher in both sexes of group A (Figure 2.3b). The concentration of fatty acids in the liver and in the small intestines was significantly greater in both males and females from group A (Figure 2.3c). The synthesis of fatty acids was significantly increased in both sexes of Group A in the small intestine (Figure 2.3d) and significantly lower in the liver. Cholesterol concentration in the liver and carcass was the same in all groups; however, synthesis of cholesterol in the liver was significantly lower in males of group A (Figure 2.3e) and in the whole carcass in both sexes (Figure 2.3f[272,273]).

The impact of early diet and resulting development of the level of spontaneous physical activity were closely interrelated, and their interaction had, in many respects, a *significant delayed effect on lipid metabolism in various organs.* The mechanisms and importance of such changes have not been fully elucidated yet; however, the impact of early nutritional manipulations seems to be important.

D. OTHER CONSEQUENCES OF EARLY DIETARY MANIPULATIONS

Manipulation of diet after weaning may also influence the spontaneous selection of foodstuffs.[228] In another experiment, groups of male rats were followed from birth up to the age of 230 days. The animals were weaned at the age of 18 days and fed ad libitum a high fat diet up to the 30th day (FI) and/or the 42nd day (FII). Then, both groups had a free selection of pure foodstuffs — starch, fat, casein, water, vitamin B complex, and KCl and NaCl solution *ad libitum.* The third group was fed the self-selected foodstuffs mentioned above immediately after weaning, i.e. from the 18th day of life (S), without any intermediate diet. The last (fourth) group had the usual laboratory diet (C).

Both groups with the temporary high fat diet (I, II) grew similarly to the control group (C). The group with the self-selection of pure foodstuffs from the 18th day (S) was retarded in growth and remained the smallest and leanest of the groups (i.e., with lowest percentage of depot fat) until the end of the experiment.

Both groups with the temporary high fat diet (FI, FII) had an altered self-selection of foods, i.e., they consumed significantly more fat during certain periods of growth (days 41–91) and then they consumed significantly more casein (days 101–111) than Group S. The consumption of starch was the same in all three groups. Apparently, *the introduction of a certain diet very early in life may have a delayed effect with regard to the self-selection of foodstuffs later on* during ontogeny along with **growth** and **body composition changes.**[228]

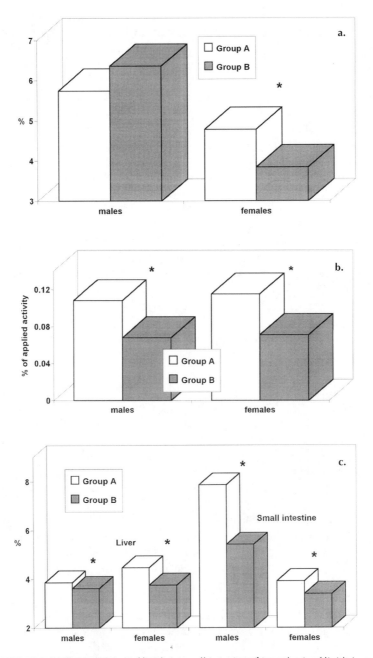

FIGURE 2.3   **(a)** Concentration of lipids in small intestine, **(b)** synthesis of lipids in small intestine, concentration of fatty acids in the liver **(c)**, synthesis of fatty acids in the liver and small intestine **(d)**, synthesis of cholesterol in the liver **(e)**, synthesis of cholesterol in the carcass **(f)** in groups of male rats suckled in different-sized litters (A < 12, B > 6). * means statistically significant difference between groups.[272–274]

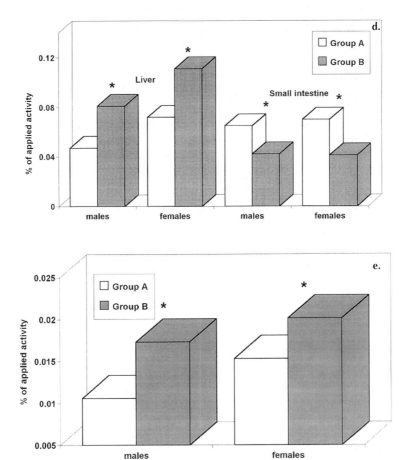

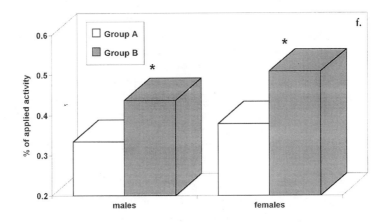

FIGURE 2.3 (continued)

II. INFLUENCE OF INCREASED PHYSICAL ACTIVITY DURING PREGNANCY ON THE LATER DEVELOPMENT OF OFFSPRING

A. METABOLIC REACTIONS DURING PREGNANCY

The impact of various stimuli on the pregnant organism results in certain metabolic reactions. Certain characteristic changes may appear, reflected not only in the maternal organism, but may be also manifested in the organism of the offspring, either immediately or later on. This applies to the dietary intake and physical activity of the pregnant mother. The maternal free fatty acid level is related to the adipose tissue development of the offspring.[345] Metabolic changes in the maternal organism during pregnancy may be transmitted to the fetus.[70]

Increased physical activity has a significant impact on the energy output and turnover as well as on a number of metabolic parameters in the blood (glycemia, free fatty acids, lactate, etc.) during all periods of life. This also applies to pregnancy. Physical activity of pregnant rabbits increased the frequency of movement in the fetus. This was explained by an increased lactic acid level in the blood of the mother.[12]

B. LIPID METABOLISM

Changes in selected indicators of lipid metabolism in the liver of female and male offspring of *rat mothers exercised during pregnancy* were measured. Exercise started 2 to 3 days after mating for 1 hour/day at a speed of 14 to 16 m/minute, which is mild exercise of an aerobic character (Group E) and of inactive control, were followed up. Male offspring of exercised mothers (Group E) were heavier at the age of 35 days and lighter at the age of 90, 100, and 108 days, respectively. The concentration of total lipids and fatty acids in the liver was raised in female offspring at the age of 35 and 90 days, and they did not differ nor did they lower in male offspring of exercised mothers (Group E) compared to controls (C). The cholesterol concentration in the liver was increased in both female and male offspring of exercised mothers (E).

Liposynthesis, studied *in vivo* after injection of Na-acetate-1-^{14}C, tended to be lower in female offspring and varied in male offspring of exercised mothers (E). In a subsequent *in vitro* study in which liver slices were incubated with Na-acetate-1-^{14}C, a lower total lipid and fatty acid concentration in the liver of 108-day-old male offspring of exercised mothers was also found along with a higher level of free fatty acid serum level and unchanged liposynthesis.[272,273]

Finally, a higher cholesterol concentration, lower cholesterogenesis, and higher fatty acid synthesis in the small intestine of a 100-day-old male offspring of exercised mothers, compared to those of control mothers, was seen (Figures 2.4a, 2.4b, and 2.4c). These data seem to indicate that a *daily aerobic work load of the mother during pregnancy results in significant changes of lipid metabolism in the liver and small intestines of the offspring during their later ontogenesis.*[273]

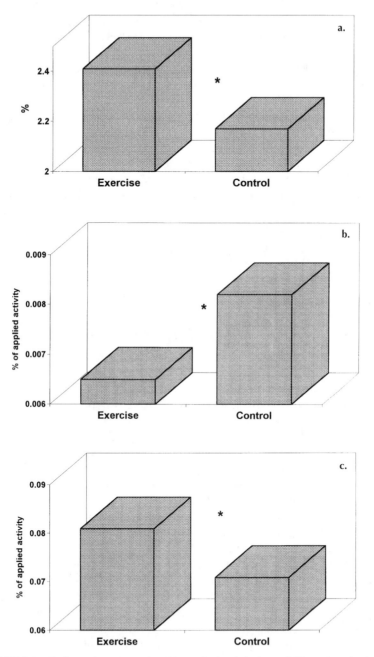

FIGURE 2.4 Cholesterol concentration **(a)**, synthesis of cholesterol **(b)**, and synthesis of fatty acids **(c)** in small intestine in the offspring of rat mothers exercised during pregnancy and in the offspring of control rats.[273]

On the basis of all the above experimental data, it is difficult to explain the mechanisms and the impact of these delayed changes. This especially applies given the possible participation of these delayed effects concerning lipid metabolism in the pathogenesis of some metabolic and/or cardiovascular diseases, e.g., atherosclerosis. As mentioned above, Szabo et al.[345] showed that the free fatty acid level of the mother has an important impact on the development of adipose tissue of the fetus. Fluctuations of the free fatty acid level (and also of other metabolites) in the blood of pregnant rats exercising daily may also occur in other organs and may apply to other characteristics of the offspring. Moreover, further changes (hormonal, neurohumoral, biochemical, etc.) occurring during a work load in the mother's *milieu intérieur* may be transmitted to the fetus and may cause some changes that may appear immediately and/or as delayed effects later in life. There are no data in the available literature on the impact of exercise during pregnancy and the resulting metabolic changes in the offspring of laboratory animals.

III. INFLUENCE OF OTHER FACTORS DURING PREGNANCY

The placenta is considered to be a barrier through which not all metabolites can be transported; however, some studies showed changes in the fetus due to the change in maternal metabolic status. *The effect of **maternal fasting** on the fetal and placental lipid metabolism* in pigs was investigated by Ruwe et al.[312] Fasting caused maternal free fatty acid (FFA) levels to increase 2.5-fold, beta-hydroxybutyric acid levels 4.8-fold, and triglyceride levels to decrease 1.8-fold, while no change in the plasma glucose concentration (compared to controls) was found. Fasted fetuses had a 1.3-fold increase in FFA, a 1.9-fold decrease in triglycerides, a 1.5-fold decrease in glucose, and no change in beta-hydroxybutyric acid levels compared with controls. Distribution of FFA in fetal plasma was different from distribution of FFA in maternal plasma. Esterification of ^{14}C-palmitate by maternal placenta and fetal adipose tissue was reduced by fasting; other parameters of fatty acid metabolism were unaffected. Fasting decreased lipoprotein lipase activity by 35% in the placenta and by 44% in fetal adipose tissue. These data suggest that fasting mobilizes maternal fuel stores, but that these stores are not effectively used by the placenta and/or used by the fetus for storage, as carcass lipids were not changed. Changes in other organs or tissues were not investigated. However, *changes in plasma levels of the fetus,* which *run parallel with those of the fasting mother, were found.*

Studies of the effects of altering the **umbilical blood flow** and **umbilical free fatty acid (FFA)** concentration on the transfer of FFA across the rabbit placenta showed that placental FFA clearance from the maternal circulation was not significantly affected by the umbilical blood flow rate. It was shown, though, that maternal-fetal FFA concentration gradient varied between +1.58 mmol/1 and –2.81 mmol/l, and that there was a *significant relationship between the increment of the maternal-fetal gradient and the increasing transfer of FFA across the placenta.* Moreover, net transfer of FFA into the umbilical circulation was observed even with a zero concentration gradient.[342]

Placental transfer of essential and non-essential fatty acids was studied in **diabetic rats**. Results indicate that increasing maternal glycaemia is associated with a decrease in unidirectional transfer of both essential and non-essential fatty acids. This reduced transfer of both essential and non-essential fatty acids depends upon the uteroplacental blood flow, which is compromised in diabetic animals. The transfer of essential fatty acids was always twice as high as that of non-essential fatty acids, regardless of the total amount of lipids transferred, indicating a selective mechanism in the transfer of these moieties.[160]

The *transfer of metabolites across the placenta*[70] in various physiological and pathological situations was recently studied.[282] However, the *impact of work load of the pregnant mother* with regard to possible changes of this transfer was *not studied*. The above mentioned experiments show that FFAs move across the placenta to the fetus, and that the changes in the maternal organism could be transmitted to the fetus, mainly without any apparent actual metabolic effect. The energy contribution may be relatively small.[37,69,160,351,353] In addition, the situation varies markedly in different species.

The transfer of metabolites may be influenced by an excess intake by the mother; however, the fetus *seems to be protected against an increased intake of dietary lipids by the pregnant mother.*[153] This situation, though, was *not studied in great detail with respect to delayed effects.* More discrete changes may not be immediately apparent in the offspring, but may manifest later only in certain respects and only in selected tissues and organs. Even on the basis of our limited actual knowledge about delayed effects, it does not seem probable that great excesses in food intake before and during pregnancy and early after delivery (especially an unbalanced diet with too much protein, sugar, saturated fat, etc.) could be completely indifferent for the actual and later development of the offspring, from both the physiological and pathological point of view.

IV. EXERCISE DURING PRE- AND POSTNATAL ONTOGENY AND THE CARDIAC MICROSTRUCTURE OF THE OFFSPRING

The impact of exercise during pregnancy was also studied with respect to delayed changes in the cardiac muscle. In two series of experiments, body weight and the microstructure of the cardiac muscle in the male offspring of exercised and inactive control mothers were investigated. In a 50-day-old male offspring, total body weight and heart weight did not differ. In a 100-day-old offspring, the heart weight was significantly higher in those from mothers exercising throughout pregnancy (Group E), i.e., similar to the previous experiment, for 1 hour, 5 times per week, 14 to 16 m/min; this work load was again of a mild, aerobic character as compared to offspring of control mothers (C).

With regard to the microstructure of the cardiac muscle (contrasted with PAS reaction[234,237]), the differences were significant, both in younger and older animals. *The number of muscle fibers and capillaries per mm² in the heart was significantly higher in male offspring of exercised mothers.* The *capillary to fiber ratio was significantly higher*, and the *diffusion distance* (i.e., the distance between the center of a capillary and the center of a muscle fiber) was significantly *shorter in male offspring of exercised mothers.* During the prenatal period, a favorable effect of work load for the offspring could be induced more easily, even with mild aerobic and short daily exercise, than later during postnatal life.[232] Exercise after weaning also had a significant impact on the microstructure of the cardiac muscle, (but the changes were relatively smaller[234,237]) as did the changes in the excitability of the central nervous system.[233,269]

Our later experimental study focused on the *combined effect of aerobic exercise during pregnancy and on exercise during postnatal ontogeny of the offspring*. In this experiment, male rats were again used (in females the analysis of the impact of running activity is more complicated due to marked changes of spontaneous physical activity during the estrous cycle). The same aerobic work load on a treadmill (1 hour) was used in pregnant rats. Some male offspring, selected at random after weaning, from both exercised and control mothers did/did not start to exercise on the treadmill at the age of 28 days, and the work load was practically the same as that of the pregnant mother rats.

After weaning, the animals were divided into *four subgroups*:

Exercised offspring of exercised mothers (EE)
Exercised offspring of control mothers without exercise (EC)
Exercised offspring of control mothers (CE)
Control offspring of inactive, control mothers without exercise (CC).

All animals were sacrificed at the age of 110 days.[234]

The results confirmed the conclusions of the previous experiments. Mild aerobic exercise during pregnancy significantly increased the number of capillaries and fibers, increased the value of the capillary to fiber ratio, and decreased the diffusion distance, especially in subgroup EE.[234] Such a microstructure of the cardiac muscle is considered favorable from a functional point of view and as a characteristic of a higher level of functional capacity and physical fitness. Similar characteristics were found in wild animal species, as compared to domesticated ones, as shown for wild and laboratory rats by Wachtlová et al.[372]

There seems to be evidence that *aerobic exercise during pregnancy is more effective than a much more intensive and longer daily work load during later periods of life.*[237] During the fetal period the organism may be more sensitive to various stimuli than later during postnatal ontogenesis; this also includes the impact of work loads of the pregnant mother. This was also apparent in this experiment from the significant differences in the number of fibers and capillaries, the capillary to fiber ratio, and the diffusion distance between subgroups EC and CE. These parameters were always better in subgroup EC male rats.[234]

No significant differences appeared in the number of capillaries per mm^2 between subgroups EC and EE, even when subgroup EE had more favorable results. However, these differences were significant between subgroups CC and CE. The same situation was found in the capillary to fiber ratio and the diffusion distance. Exercise during postnatal ontogenesis results in a significant difference in the offspring of inactive control mothers, i.e., a significant increase in the number of capillaries and fibers per mm^2 in the heart, a significant increase in the capillary to fiber ratio, and a significant decrease in the diffusion distance. Even when there is some other change due to exercise during postnatal ontogenesis of the offspring of exercised mothers, the difference is not significant, indicating the *relatively greater importance of maternal exercise during pregnancy.*

Extreme differences in all characteristics of heart microstructure were apparent between groups of exercised offspring of exercised mothers (EE) and inactive control offspring of control mothers.[234] As follows from our data, the *positive effect of a regular, optimal work load can be transmitted to the offspring when work is performed during pregnancy, and subsequent exercise of the offspring potentiates this effect even more.*

This experiment also shows that the changes in the microstructure of the heart are not necessarily accompanied by changes in total body weight or heart size. Moreover, these changes in heart size and body weight are also not always apparent after regular and more intensive aerobic exercise performed by rats during postnatal ontogenesis.[233,277]

Finally, the same experiment was repeated in both males and females subdivided in the same way (CC, CE, EC, EE male and female subgroups, Figures 2.5a and 2.5b). As the animals were followed up during longer period, i.e., until 120 days of life, the possible effect of the fluctuation of spontaneous physical activity during the estrous cycles can be reduced. No remarkable differences occurred in the reaction of female and male offspring, caused by prenatal and postnatal exercise[237], i.e., both in males and females there were changes in cardiac microstructure considered favorable from the functional point of view (Figures 2.5a and 2.5b). According to the available experimental evidence, the mechanisms of these changes have not been elucidated yet.

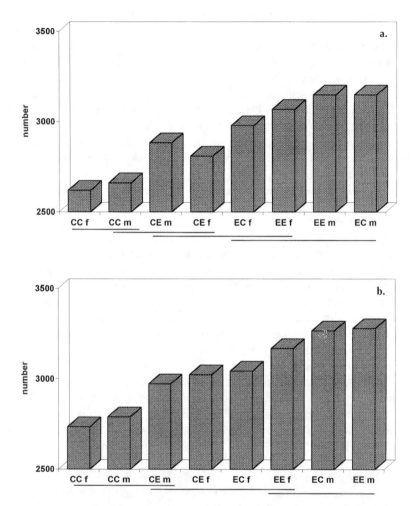

FIGURE 2.5 Number of capillaries **(a)** and fibers/mm^2 **(b)** in heart muscle in male (m) and female (f) offspring of exercised (E) and control, inactive rat mothers (E,C — first capital letter) which exercised or were inactive during their postnatal life (E,C — second capital letter). Differences among groups were evaluated statistically using the Duncan test; underlined groups do not differ significantly.[237]

V. INFLUENCE OF PHYSICAL ACTIVITY ON THE DEVELOPMENT OF EXPERIMENTAL CARDIAC NECROSIS

A. EXERCISE DURING POSTNATAL LIFE

Previous experiments showed that adaptation to aerobic exercise during postnatal ontogenesis may reduce the risk of the development of experimental cardiac necrosis induced by the administration of isoprenaline.[99–101,233] Various levels of physical activity, started at different ages, were tested. Male rats started to run on a treadmill at the age of 21, 32, and 55 days, respectively, and continued until 90, 100, 125, and 205 days, respectively (E). Simultaneously, other groups of the animals of the same age were placed in small spaces (8.75 × 21.25 cm) with wire net walls (limitation of isolation stress, six animals in a subdivided normal laboratory cage, LA). Control groups of animals living in usual laboratory cages were always followed up simultaneously (C).

With regard to *body weight*, only the group of the 205-day-old animals showed significant differences from the E and LA groups. The weight of the soleus muscle always varied according to the intensity of physical activity (i.e., was highest in Group E), except for in the oldest group. The *percentage of body fat* (estimated gravimetrically, using a chloroform extract of the carcass saponified in a mixture of 30% KOH in 50% ethanol) was always lowest in Groups E. As a rule, the heart weight was not affected.

Myocardial necrosis was induced with the administration of two doses of *isoprenaline* given subcutaneously at an interval of 24 hours to each rat at the end of the experimental period. Rats who did not die were decapitated 24 hours after the second injection. The heart was removed and the degree of cardiac damage was estimated, using the scale described by Rona et al. (1, no damage; 5, spontaneous death[233,260]).

Isoprenaline produced less cardiac damage in the exercised rats (E) than in controls (C) and rats with limited activity (LA). Animals who died following the injection of isoprenaline had a higher percentage of body fat than animals with minimal cardiac damage. It was not possible to compare the results of separate experiments, as the doses of isoprenaline were always set individually for a particular group of animals followed at different periods of time.[99–101,233,260–264]

Exercised animals with a lower percentage of body fat were more resistant to the impact of isoprenaline compared to control or inactive animals, similar to young animals compared to older ones. The same difference was found in animals weaned in large (14) or small (3) nests who also differed in fatness and weight: light and lean animals, i.e., young animals or those with a reduced food intake at the beginning of life, were more resistant to the cardiotoxic impact of isoprenaline.[99,233] (The same differences were also found between genetically lean strains of rats, i.e., Lewis, and Wistar rats[99]). These results seem to indicate that an organism with a certain metabolic stereotype, characterized *inter alia* by higher ratio of depot fat, is more prone to develop cardiac damage under the same conditions of the exposure to noxious factors.

With regard to the influence of exercise, after 3 weeks of induced running on the treadmill (2 to 4 hours), the cardiotoxic effect of isoprenaline was reduced. The adequate daily dose of exercise depended on both the distance run per day and the rate and intensity at which the animals ran. If the training regimen continued for another few weeks with the same daily dose of exercise, there was no significant increase in its protective effect. In the animals less than 3 months old, myocardial resistance changed only after much higher daily doses of running than those needed for the same effect, i.e., the ame difference between Group E and Group C, in older animals, similarly as body composition (percentage of fat), metabolic activity of adipose tissue, etc. This may be explained by a high level of spontaneous motor activity in all growing animals.[233] The cardioprotective effect of increased motor activity was not conditioned by an increase in the weight of the heart.[101]

B. SPONTANEOUS ACTIVITY AND CARDIAC DAMAGE

The impact of the motor activity level was also followed up using rotation cages, rendering possible the evaluation of the level of 24-hour spontaneous physical activity. In one of our experiments, it was shown that the level of spontaneous physical activity increased with age until the end of puberty and young adulthood (6562 m/day at the age of 3 months). Then, the level of spontaneous physical activity in rotation cages decreased.[100] At the age of 10 months, the activity was, on the average, only 561 m/day. In all experimental groups in which spontaneous activity was higher than this limit, a decrease in the cardiotoxic effect of isoprenaline was found after 2 to 3 weeks in rotation cages.

The extent of heart lesions in the individual animals was not proportional to the degree of their motor activity. The slightest myocardial damage was not found in animals that ran the longest distance and *vice versa*. A marked decrease in the extent of cardiac lesions occurred when the motor regimen was prolonged to 70 days.[233,260–261] *The condition of the positive effect of running was at a certain level* (i.e., certain intensity and duration) of running and *with a permanent regular impact of work load.*[100]

C. DELAYED CONSEQUENCES OF TEMPORARY EXERCISE

There was a question as to how long the protective effect of increased motor activity in the rotation cages would persist when the animals were transferred to normal laboratory cages and when they did not have the opportunity to run any longer. After a 3 day break, reduction of the cardiotoxic effect of isoprenaline still persisted. The extent of heart lesions after a 2 week interruption of exercise corresponded to the values found in animals not allowed access to rotation cages.[100] The condition for the protection of the heart was thus an uninterrupted physical activity regimen or only with brief pauses of decreased activity.

In conjunction with studies on the impact of exercise during postnatal ontogenesis, *the influence of exercise throughout pregnancy on the cardiotoxic effect of isoprenaline in the offspring* was investigated. The same protocol, as mentioned above, was used regarding the aerobic work load of pregnant rats and the evaluation of cardiac damage after isoprenaline administration.

Male offspring of exercised mothers showed lower damage of the heart after isoprenaline administration compared to offspring of inactive control mothers.[235] Thus, aerobic exercise of pregnant mother rats was manifested in a positive way regarding delayed effects in their offspring.[235] This may be related to the above mentioned changes in cardiac microstructure, as well as to changes in lipid and cholesterol metabolism, or others which were not yet investigated.

VI. IMPACT OF THE INTERACTIONS BETWEEN EARLY DIET AND PHYSICAL ACTIVITY ON EXPERIMENTAL CARDIAC NECROSIS

Previous experiments seem to indicate that *the possibility for spontaneous physical activity is a more favorable and more important stimulus than induced running on a treadmill.* This was also proven by Suzuki[344] who demonstrated a significant decrease of systolic blood pressure in genetically hypertensive rats that had access to rotation cages. In contrast to that group, a similar group of rats with induced exercise of similar intensity on a motor driven treadmill exhibited an increase in blood pressure.

As mentioned above, physical activity is highest during the growth and development period, decreasing later in life. Thus, this is a feature that characterizes the young organism in addition to many other morphological and other parameters: a lower proportion of adipose tissue, which is metabolically more active (i.e., it releases *in vitro,* spontaneously or after adrenaline, more free fatty acids, FFA) and a higher activity of lipid metabolism in skeletal muscles along with higher food intake especially when related to body weight. In many respects, physically active organism have characteristics similar to younger ones.[233]

The opportunity for spontaneous exercise in the rotation wheels also decreased the cardiotoxicity of isoprenaline, which was lower in exercising animals. This difference was similar to that between younger and leaner and older and fatter animals. The former were always more resistant to the cardiotoxic effect of isoprenaline.[233]

A. IMPACT OF EARLY DIET

Increasing or reducing the number of animals in one nest, which results in decreased and/or increased fatness and weight, can change the heart's resistance to noxious factors. When we compared the cardiotoxicity of isoprenaline in smaller and leaner animals from large nests (14 litters) with heavier and fatter animals from small nests (3 litters), it was significantly higher in the latter.[233] As mentioned above, the level of spontaneous physical activity was also different in these groups with different food intake early in life.[262,272-274] This means that *changes in early nutrition,* with all its consequences, may also *change the sensitivity of the cardiac muscle to isoprenaline.*

B. SPONTANEOUS PHYSICAL ACTIVITY INFLUENCED BY EARLY DIET AND CARDIAC RESISTANCE TO ISOPRENALINE

Some of the above mentioned experiments also show that animals with a *decreased food intake at the beginning of life develop a higher level of spontaneous physical activity in the rotation cages. This concerned not only male rats weaned in large (A) and small nests (B)*[272,274]; *the introduction of a diet with reduced protein content in lactating rats and later in their offspring up to 7 weeks of age also increased the level of spontaneous physical activity in rotation cages (REPA), resulted in a lower body weight and fatness.* We also used this experimental model to examine the impact of this interactive situation regarding the cardiotoxicity of isoprenaline.

The groups of rats with reduced protein and energy (REP) intake during lactation and up to the age of 49 days, along with a group of control animals with the usual laboratory diet (C), were investigated. Half of the animals from both groups were always placed individually in rotation cages. Thus, the four subgroups of animals could be compared: those from mothers with REP who continued with the same diet until puberty, starting with the C diet later, were put in rotation cages where they could be active (REPA) or were placed in the normal laboratory cages, where they were relatively inactive (REPI). Then, we simultaneously followed the animals from C mothers, which were either put in rotation cages (CA) or placed in normal cages (CI).

REPA animals developed higher levels of spontaneous physical activity, were lighter and leaner than controls (Figure 2.6a), and also showed higher levels of energy economy because the food intake per 1 gram of body weight during the period of realimentation after the 49th day of life was significantly lower. In this experiment, we also found significant changes in the relative weight of the heart (Figure 2.6b), the right ventricles (Figure 2.6c), and the left ventricles (Figure 2.6d); animals with the opportunity for spontaneous exercise in this experiment developed relatively larger hearts.[261]

In this experiment, we were also able to test the resistance of the cardiac muscle to the impact of isoprenaline using $^{203}HgCl_2$ administration to show the increased permeability of the membranes of the necrotic cardiac muscle cells.[161] This comparison (Figure 2.6e) showed the best situation in REPA animals and the worst in CI animals.

Therefore, *modest food intake with less protein until puberty, resulting in a significantly lower body weight and less body fat and higher levels of spontaneous physical activity, was related to a greater resistance of the cardiac muscle.*

Animals with a higher level of energy turnover were more protected from the impact of isoprenaline, shown by a lower degree of cardiac damage which was demonstrated in REPA animals by significantly lower values of cpm/mg heart tissue (Figure 2.6e[261]).

The differences in cardiac resistance to isoprenaline were again similar to those between groups of young and old animals[99,233,261] or to animals of

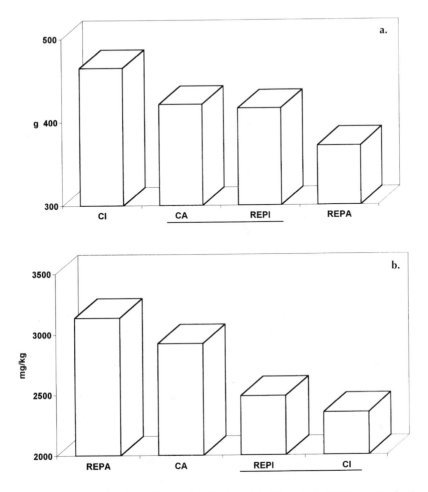

FIGURE 2.6 Body weight **(a)**, heart weight/body weight **(b)**, weight of right ventricle/body weight **(c)**, weight of left ventricle/body weight **(d)**, and counts per minute/mg heart tissue **(e)**, after application of $^{203}HgCl_2$, characterizing the degree of cardiac damage in male rats with reduced energy and protein diet at the beginning of life (REP) and control diet (C) living in rotation, in activity cages (REPA, CA) or in normal laboratory cages (REPI, CI). Differences among groups were measured using the Duncan test; underlined groups do not differ significantly.[261]

mothers exercised during pregnancy and/or during a much longer period of time during postnatal ontogenesis.

However, it is necessary to mention that *the level of motor activity, result-ing spontaneously from a changed diet at the beginning of life, was markedly higher when the animals had access to rotation cages reflecting a free choice* either *to run* (more than 9 km per day) or *to remain inactive.* Such a work load and performance was impossible to achieve when inducing daily running

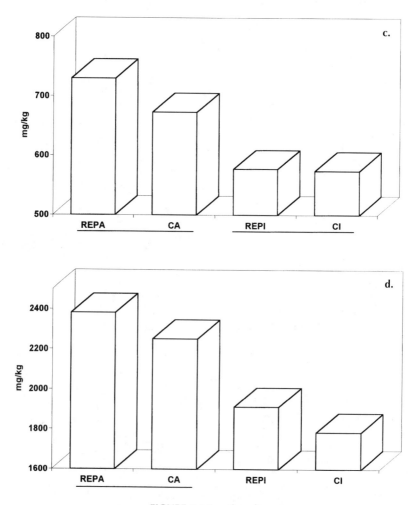

FIGURE 2.6 (continued)

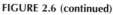

on a motor driven treadmill. Thus, *the best results were achieved by influencing the level of spontaneous physical activity with an early diet, reduced in protein and energy.* On the other hand, the worst results regarding cardiotoxicity were always found in rats fed *ad libitum* which were restricted in spontaneous activity by placing them in small spaces after weaning. These conditions resulted in larger body size and a higher body fat ratio.[233]

VII. GENERAL CONSIDERATIONS

Obviously, results from experimental models using laboratory animals may only suggest the possibility that certain early manipulations may have

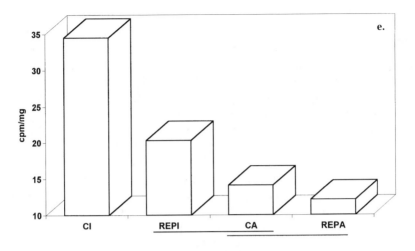

FIGURE 2.6 (continued)

some meaningful effects later in life. Even when different degrees of maturity are achieved with different species at the time of birth, all these studies seem to indicate that *influencing the organism during the fetal period, the subsequent period of lactation, and early growth may be of utmost importance for a better prognosis in later development.* More detailed information was therefore presented to demonstrate this phenomenon in spite of an actual lack of explanation.

The impact of simple natural stimuli such as food and motor activity may substantially affect, in both positive and negative ways, the actual and later ontogenetical development, thus resulting in a different health status, size of the body, and of its compartments.

It was shown that the long-term effects of feeding the high carbohydrate (HC) diet of rat pups in the pre-weaning period by gastrostomy resulted in the development of obesity later in life, even though there was no change in the body weight of this group compared to normally breast fed pups (MF) during the actual weaning period. HC rats were hyperinsulinemic, and their growth rates were greater than MF rats. The lipogenic capacity of the liver, as well as adipose tissue, was also higher in HC rats. Adipose cell size of HC rats in adulthood was greater.[158] This experiment can serve as an enhancement model of adult obesity by practicing early overfeeding with a high carbohydrate diet, which did not correspond to the composition of mother's milk; this did not happen with a high fat diet, which mimics mother's milk.[158] Early diets had later consequences, significant only after a period of delay.

The significant consequences of the early manipulations of both diet and exercise may appear at different levels of functional capacity in different systems, in higher and/or lower sensitivity and reactivity to positive and negative stimuli, and also in changes of the resistance of the cardiac muscle to noxious factors.

There seems to be evidence that various individual variations explained by inborn, genetic factors may be often elicited more naturally by using various manipulations of the organism during the period before and around birth and during the first stages of life. The rate of growth and mature weight has an important relationship to lifespan.[384] Ross et al.[308,309] showed that longevity correlates with both the amount and type of diet an animal elects to consume before mid-life. Dietary practices during early life are particularly important. The quantity and composition of food determines, in large part, the weight changes during a lifespan. Growth rate and other body weight related expressions may also correlate with lifespan: *rats that grew slowly (especially between 50 and 150 days of age) were shown to have, in general, an extended lifespan.* Chronic underfeeding of complete diets was shown to be the only means known for increasing the length of life in homoiothermic laboratory animals beyond the limits characteristic for the species; chronic overfeeding and other excesses or imbalances curtailed lifespan.

None of these changes were considered in relation to energy output; however, they did show that *slower weight increase during growth periods was a favorable prerequisite for longer lifespan,* and that this may be related to the factors that *regulate the susceptibility to some age-related diseases.*[308,309]

It should be stressed, however, that the results mentioned above are not a basis for advocating and recommending malnutrition or an excessive work load at the beginning of life. Rather that it is indispensable to reevaluate and define more precisely, on a physiological basis, the adequate energy balance and turnover, which result from an optimum diet, desirable physical activity work load level, and stimulating exercise from the beginning of life.

In conjunction with all the results mentioned above, it should be emphasized that the goal of these experiments was not to develop maximal performance but, mainly, *to promote health and the early prevention of diseases,* especially those of the cardiovascular system.

Some reduction of the contemporary recommended dietary allowances, along with the elimination of hypokinesia, so common nowadays, would be highly desirable.[289] The actual trend for increasing body weight and fatness, e.g., in the U.S. population,[188] seems to be another reason to consider prevention early in life.

The effort "to achieve the maximal growth potential", which is too often identified with achieving a maximal body size, is not the best way to promote health and optimal life expectancy.[214,308,309]

Chapter 3

NUTRITION OF MOTHERS DURING PREGNANCY AND ITS INFLUENCE ON THEIR CHILDREN: HUMAN STUDIES

"... the mother should be careful not to indulge in excessive sleep, indolence, or torpor, but perform with all agility her usual employment, with all the promptitude, and celerity of which she is capable; for as she then is, such will be the nature of her offspring ..."

J.A. Comenius (1592–1670), School of Infancy

I. VARIABILITY OF THE PRACTICES DURING PREGNANCY AND LACTATION IN DIFFERENT SOCIETIES

All that happens in the maternal organism during pregnancy can have a decisive impact on the future of the child. Many diseases that cause premature death originate during the fetal and infant period.[17,18] Up until now, it has been generally believed that genetic and possibly pathological factors determine most of the characteristics of the offspring. Less attention was paid to natural factors within physiological conditions, namely diet and physical activity during pregnancy and their influence on the offspring.

In industrially developed countries, it is not easy to spot the delayed consequences of early nutritional and/or other practices because of their great variability and the interference of a number of other factors influencing a child's development. This includes body composition, the amount as well as distribution of fat, and the functional and metabolic characteristics of maternal and child organism.

In more *traditional societies*, where the conditions were simpler and much more homogeneous for generations, some interesting phenomena can be observed. It would be difficult to repeat such experiences at the present time; this information, though, can focus on selected issues, such as *early diet, weaning practices, and the handling of the infant and their possible delayed consequences*: e.g., the oldest Sioux boy was nursed the longest, with the average nursing period at about 3 years. Today, this period is much shorter although instances of prolonged nursing persist. A teacher reported that an Indian mother recently had come to school during recess to nurse her 8-year-old boy, who had a bad cold. He was nursed with the same worried devotion with which we ply our sniffing children with vitamin pills.[96]

Among the Sioux, there was no systematic weaning at all. The children were weaned by the mother with gradual introduction of other foods. Before finally abandoning the breast altogether, the infant may have fed himself for many months on other food, allowing time for his mother to give birth to the next child and to restore her milk supply.

The privilege of this practically unlimited access to the mother's breast had some limitations. To be permitted to suckle, the infant had to learn not to bite the breast. The biting child was "thumped", and he would fly in wild rage. Sioux mothers used to say what our mothers say earlier in their babies' lives: let him cry, it will make him strong. (Crying is also one of the most important exercises for the infant, who is able to move only in a very limited way.) Good future hunters especially could be recognized by the strength of their infantile fury.

The Sioux baby, when filled with rage, was strapped up to his neck in the cradleboard. He could not express his rage with the usual violent motion of the limbs. This was not meant as a punishment; on the contrary, at first they are undoubtedly comfortable in firm, womblike compartments in which they are wrapped and rocked and bundled for the mother to carry around while working.[96] However, it may be assumed that the particular construction of the board, its customary placement in the household, and the duration of its use are variable elements used by different cultures as amplifiers of the basic experiences and the principal traits that they develop in their young.

Generosity and fortitude were the main virtues of Sioux life. First impressions suggest that the cultural demand for generosity had its early foundation in the privilege of enjoying the nourishment and reassurance emanating from the unlimited breastfeeding, while the necessity of suppressing the biting rage contributed to the tribe's ferocity in that this rage was stored up, channelled, and diverted toward prey and enemy. Naturally, *certain ways of handling the child do not guarantee a definite and fixed predisposition;* rather, their *early start, reinforced in later development with the continuing support of these characteristics* by public opinion, has *lasted for generations.* However, these traits are presumably anchored in *early childhood training.*[96]

In contrast to the Sioux way of handling babies and the resulting traits of character, Yurok child training is very different. Yuroks are shy, polite, and timid. Many attempts are made to accelerate the autonomy of the child, beginning *in utero;* the pregnant mother eats little, carries much wood, and preferably, does work that forces her to bend forward, so that the fetus "will not rest against her spine", i.e., relax and recline. She rubs her abdomen often, especially when daylight is waning, in order to keep the fetus awake and to forestall an early tendency to regress to the state of prehistory which, as Western culture says, is the origin of all neuroses. The newborn Yurok is not breastfed for 10 days, but is given a nut soup from a tiny shell. The breastfeeding begins with Indian generosity and frequency. However, unlike the Sioux the Yurok have a definite weaning time of around the sixth month, i.e., around the teething period, a minimal breastfeeding period for American Indians. Weaning is called "forgetting the mother" and, if necessary, is enforced toward the end of the first year by the mother's going away for a few days.[96]

The child's first solid food is salmon or deer meat well salted with seaweed. Salty foods are the Yurok "sweets". The child is admonished never to grab food in haste, never to take without asking, always to eat slowly, and never to ask for a second helping — an oral puritanism hardly equaled among other tribes. Later, not only does early weaning further require him to release his mother, *the baby's legs are often uncovered* in the Yurok version of the cradleboard and, from the 20th day on, they are *massaged* by the grandmother *to encourage early creeping.* The cooperation of the parents in this matter is assured by the fact that they may resume intercourse when the baby makes vigorous strides in creeping. The baby is also kept from sleeping in the late afternoon and early evening, lest dusk close his eyes for the whole night.

The first postnatal crisis, therefore, has quite a different quality for the Yurok child than the one experienced by the little Sioux. It is characterized by a close proximity in the time of teething, enforced weaning, encouraged creeping, and the mother's early return to former sexual practices and eventually new children. Yurok children are discouraged by a number of devices from feeling comfortable in, with, and around his mother. He is trained to be a fisherman, "one who has his nets ready for a prey" which (only if he behaves nicely and says "please") must come to him. The good Yurok is characterized by an ability to cry while he prays, thus gaining influence over the food-sending powers beyond the visible world.[96]

A number of other observations in the late consequences of behavior and physical traits of Sioux and Yurok people were explained by early nutritional and other manipulations. At the present time, it would be difficult to validate this information with experiments using humans in other populations; these have been mentioned here in more detail because it would be difficult to find other data of a similar character. However, some general conclusions on a profound impact of early manipulations — dietary and behavioral — may be derived. If possible, it would be desirable to verify them with further observations.

II. POSITION IN INDUSTRIALLY DEVELOPED COUNTRIES

Even under physiological conditions, nutritional events that take place in a woman's body in the industrially developed societies are subject to a wide range of variations. This concerns nutritional, health, environmental, psychological, and social factors. Their qualitative and quantitative assessment have not been completed yet although several studies were carried out. The nutritional behavior of the mother, her psychic and emotional status, and many of her habits before and during pregnancy including the level of physical activity can affect the final output of this system.[4-7] This applies to any population group, even at the present time.

Due to the influence of environmental and organism-related stressors, pre- and postnatally, the attention and effort to develop "positive health" and to reduce the risk of the "diseases of civilization", mainly cardiovascular and metabolic diseases, have also focused on the earliest periods of life.

III. THE INFLUENCE OF HEREDITY ON HEALTH RISK FACTORS IN OFFSPRING

Many studies have examined blood lipid levels in neonates and infants in relation to the blood lipid levels of their parents (e.g., Bogalusa heart study[67]), thus screening possible familial hypercholesterolemia.[34] Children of parents with high levels of beta and/or pre-beta cholesterol, caused by any factor, were considered individuals with an enhanced risk of cardiovascular diseases because they reflect their parents' lipoprotein cholesterol levels.[67]

When the energy homeostasis was followed in infants at the age of 3 months, those who later became obese had an energy output 20% lower than the other infants that maintained normal body weight.[108] There is a question as to whether later obesity was the consequence of low energy output early in life or whether there were some genetic traits conditioning both of these phenomena. Genetic predisposition for developing obesity was also identified in humans.[38-40]

Thus, genetic endowment may be manifested very early in life. Blood lipid values at the beginning of life may predict the later development of atherosclerosis.[219] Children who have a high serum level of cholesterol at birth still have elevated values at the age of 3 years.[369-371] The interaction of genetic factors, dietary habits, nutrient intake, and other lifestyle-associated factors were scrutinized from early childhood in longitudinal studies,[371] and the importance of early intervention was stressed. *Increased intake of protein early in life has been recently considered as a factor that enhances the risk for later obesity.*[307] Therefore, it is recommendable to gain information on these risk factors as early as possible and to introduce measures to rectify such a situation.

IV. THE IMPACT OF MATERNAL STATUS ON THE OFFSPRING

Even during completely normal, physiological pregnancies, a great variability in anthropometric, nutritional, metabolic, and biochemical characteristics has always been demonstrated.[85] There is a significant relationship between birth weight and maternal lipoprotein, fuels, hormones, and body weight at 36 weeks of gestation in normal healthy women, reported by Knopp et al.[181]

A. THE INFLUENCE OF MATERNAL DIET AND NUTRITIONAL STATUS

Many of the above mentioned variables (i.e., body weight, fatness etc.) are influenced significantly by dietary intake and energy balance. The impact of malnutrition and supplementation has been defined in a number of studies.[177,193,311] Thus, supplemented African women gained more weight and body fat during pregnancy and gave birth to heavier children.[192] The impact of increased food intake was most evident, however, when compensating for previous malnutrition or starvation.

Nutritional influences under conditions in which most mothers in developed countries live, with an energy margin large enough to ensure the needs of the fetus and/or the maternal organism, are less clear and may seem less important. Such influences depend on a number of additional factors, especially the initial, pregestational nutritional status (characterized by body composition, biochemical parameters in the blood and tissues, and so forth).

In developed countries women with an adequate nutritional status who gain too much fat during pregnancy still may not have bigger children; surplus energy normally results in more ample fat deposition in the mother.[191] Increased food intake during pregnancy (i.e., the proverbial "eating for two") with the intention of providing enough food for the nutritional requirements of mother and fetus is advocated by a number of experts.[285,386] However, it is very difficult to define such a dietary intake and a proper energy balance, especially when also considering the energy output of the mother.

It was also shown that *in an industrialized country the mother's dietary intake correlates very weakly with the birth weight of the child, or there is no relationship at all.*[191] Such a relationship between the dietary intake of the mother and birth weight, as well as body composition of the full term child, only appears when extreme differences exist, i.e., when comparing malnutrition and deficient intake on the one hand and excessive dietary intake of the mother on the other. Within the range of the usual dietary intake, even if it is wide, it is practically impossible to find significant relationships between actual food intake and weight. This applies not only to the mothers during pregnancy, but also to all individuals during their postnatal ontogeny, in all age categories, including children.[304]

B. THE INFLUENCE OF EXERCISE

The impact of an increased energy output caused, e.g., through hard physical work and/or athletic activities during pregnancy, was also considered. ***Pregnant women*** who continued, e.g., in ***endurance exercise,*** gave birth to children with a significantly *lower birth weight, lower ponderal index, smaller fetoplacental weight ratio, and lower skinfold thickness.* However, crown-heel length and head circumference were not influenced.[55] Other parameters were not investigated (e.g., blood lipids), and later measurements of the above mentioned anthropometric characteristics were not reported. Studies of this type are still quite rare. Important data were gained mainly in animal studies.[384,385]

However, it would be interesting to know whether some functional parameters of the offspring were modified by the work load of the mother during pregnancy. In this connection, we have in mind not only later development of the functional capacity of the offspring, but also the morbidity and mortality from cardiovascular, etc. diseases in individuals with an identical genetic and hereditary background and social and economic conditions with a different dietary and physical activity regimen at the very beginning of life. The same question arose regarding delayed consequences of restricted dietary intake of the mother during pregnancy and lactation (marginal malnutrition), and there is a theoretical possibility of a similar situation with regard to the impact of marked work load. But such long-term studies are too demanding and too difficult to interpret, mainly due to the interference of economic, social, and nutritional factors which occur simultaneously in groups of pregnant women who have to work hard during their pregnancy. To our knowledge, there is no such data available in the literature.

V. RELATIONSHIPS BETWEEN ANTHROPOMETRIC, DIETARY, AND SERUM LIPID VARIABLES OF THE MOTHER AND NEWBORN

Alberti et al.[6,7] executed a study to show how selected ***nutritional variables of the mother*** during pregnancy are related to similar variables in the newborn. Attention was focused on selected indicators that have also been assumed to be possible markers of some pathological conditions, i.e., fat pattern.

Seventy Italian women were followed up longitudinally during the first, second, and third trimester of pregnancy.[6,7] The average age of the mothers in the beginning of pregnancy was 26.3 ± 4.6 years; their height was 160.5 ± 5.9 cm; the average weight at the time was 57.6 ± 9.2 kg; the body mass index (BMI) was 22.5 ± 3.8. These characteristics did not differ significantly from the characteristics of women in other populations. Anthropometric variables and blood lipid levels of the newborns were assessed after birth.

The mothers were mostly sedentary, with a generally low level of physical activity and a light work load. Only women with more than one child displayed a slightly higher activity level than primipara.[6,7]

Significant variations from the first trimester to 5 days post partum for abdomen, thigh, and calf circumferences, body weight, and BMI were shown by ANOVA analysis in this survey by Alberti et al.[6,7] Arm circumference did not change. The thickness of seven skinfolds was assessed, and the suprailiac

TABLE 3.1　Changes of Anthropometric Variables During Various Trimesters of Pregnancy and 5 Days Post Partum

Trimester	1st		2nd		3rd		5 days pp	
	$\bar{x}$	SD	$\bar{x}$	SD	$\bar{x}$	SD	$\bar{x}$	SD
Weight (kg)	59.1	10.1	65.6	10.1	71.2	9.9	64.8	9.4
BMI (kg/m²)	23.0	4.0	25.6	3.9	27.7	3.8	25.2	3.6
Circumference								
Thigh (cm)	55.0	4.9	57.0	4.6	57.8	4.6	54.6	10.8
Abdomen (cm)	86.0	11.6	96.3	9.2	104.3	7.7	95.6	8.8
Skinfolds								
Suprailiac (mm)	12.2	6.6	18.1	6.1	18.0	6.3	15.2	5.9
Thigh (mm)	30.8	7.0	35.1	6.0	37.0	6.7	35.4	6.5
Sum of 7 (mm)	114.6	35.5	133.2	31.3	135.0	30.0	125.7	30.7
Indices								
1	0.96	0.36	1.00	0.33	1.02	0.35	1.05	0.35
2	0.63	0.21	0.66	0.19	0.68	0.23	0.69	0.22
3	1.26	0.42	1.31	0.38	1.37	0.46	1.39	0.43
4	0.38	0.13	0.45	0.11	0.44	0.12	0.42	0.12
5	0.67	0.21	0.80	0.20	0.81	0.22	0.77	0.21

Note: pp, post partum; SD, standard deviation; BMI, body mass index. Indices: 1, subscapular/triceps; 2, subscapular/triceps + biceps; 3, subscapular/(triceps + biceps) × 0.5; 4, subscapular + suprailiac/triceps + biceps + thigh + calf; 5, subscapular + suprailiac/triceps + biceps + thigh.

Adapted from Alberti-Fidanza, A., et al., *Eur. J. Clin. Nutr.,* 49, 289, 1995 and from Alberti-Fidanza, A., et al., Changes in anthropometric variables and fat pattern during pregnancy and their relationship to newborn values, in press.

and thigh skinfolds, as well as the sum of all skinfolds, increased significantly from the first to the third trimester. After delivery, they decreased again. The changes were similar to those in other studies.[346] The indices of fat distribution also varied significantly (Table 3.1). Hand grip strength did not vary during pregnancy, decreasing slightly after delivery.[6,7]

Food intake analysis revealed a low intake of milk, cheese, fish, eggs, and legumes with an increased intake of meat. There were no significant differences regarding dietary intake during pregnancy[106] except for a significant increase in carbohydrate intake between the second and third trimester (Table 3.2). The highest food intake was observed during the second trimester, but the differences between trimesters did not differ significantly. The energy content and composition of the diet did not differ significantly from the diets of pregnant women in other industrially developed countries.[285] The paired *t* test showed significant differences for the relative intake of protein, fat, and polyunsaturated fatty acids between the second and third trimesters. Blood lipids during pregnancy also increased significantly; the most relevant changes were observed for total triglycerides and total cholesterol.[6,7]

Anthropometric variables and *blood lipids of the newborn* are given in Table 3.3. After 24 hours the usual decrease of body weight and BMI was observed. Cord blood lipids did not differ significantly in newborn boys and girls, but indices 1 and 3 did not.

TABLE 3.2   Dietary Intake of the Macrocomponents of Diet of the Mothers Before (0) and at Different Trimesters of Pregnancy Ranging from 1 to 3 (Intake of Individual Nutrients Expressed as Percentage of Total Energy Intake) and of Cholesterol

	0		1		2		3	
	$\bar{x}$	SD	$\bar{x}$	SD	$\bar{x}$	SD	$\bar{x}$	SD
Energy (MJ)	9.0	2.6	8.9	3.0	9.5	2.4	9.0	2.4
Protein (%)	16.0	2.3	15.9	3.4	15.8	2.5	16.3	2.7
Fat (%)	34.4	4.8	33.8	4.5	33.7	5.0	35.2	5.3
CHO (%)	47.5	6.7	47.6	5.4	47.0	6.4	45.1	7.1
Chol (mg)	287	111	275	138	280	139	265	98

Note: CHO, carbohydrates; Chol, Total cholesterol.

Compiled from Alberti-Fidanza, A., et al., *Eur. J. Clin. Nutr.,* 49, 289, 1995.

TABLE 3.3   Birth Weight and Cord Blood Lipids of Boys (n = 23, Girls n = 19)

	Boys		Girls	
	$\bar{x}$	SD	$\bar{x}$	SD
Age (weeks)	39.5	1.6	40.0	1.3
Birth weight (g)	3223	455	3274	398
TChol (mmol/l)	1.74	0.64	1.70	0.3
HDL (mmol/l)	0.85	0.30	0.72	0.11
HDL/T (Chol)	0.50	0.10	0.4	0.1
TGI (mmol/l)	0.46	0.33	0.64	0.22
Index 1	0.8	0.1	1.0	0.1
Index 2	0.5	0.1	0.5	0.1
Index 3	0.9	0.1	1.1	0.1

Note: TChol, total cholesterol; HDL, high density lipoprotein; HDL/T, total high density lipoproteins; Chol, cholesterol; TGI, triacylglycerols. Index 1 = subscapular/triceps, Index 2 = subscapular/triceps + biceps, Index 3 = subscapular/(triceps + biceps × 0.5).

Modified from Alberti-Fidanza, A., et al., *Eur. J. Clin. Nutr.,* 49, 289, 1995 and from Alberti-Fidanza, A., et al., Changes in anthropometric variables and fat pattern during pregnancy and their relationship to newborn values, in press.

Significant **correlations** were found most often in the mothers for BMI and sum of seven skinfolds and indices 4 and 5, which were present in all trimesters. No relationship between anthropometric variables and blood lipids was found in the mothers in any trimester of their pregnancy.[6,7]

Anthropometric variables of the mother during pregnancy were also correlated with her dietary intake. Very few significant relationships were found between the percentage of energy from protein and anthropometric variables. *The percentage of energy from fat was significantly related to the characteristics of body composition and fat distribution* (sum of skinfolds at first trimester, indices 4 and 5 during first and third trimester, and BMI during third trimester). Similar correlations with the percentage of energy from carbohydrates were significantly negative. No significant correlation between anthropometric variables and absolute intake of energy and protein, fat, and carbohydrates (grams) during various trimesters of pregnancy was found.[6,7]

Maternal blood lipids, i.e., **total cholesterol** and **triglycerides**, were most often *related to total energy intake* and/or *to the percentage of energy derived from individual nutrients* during various trimesters. During the first trimester, significant correlations were found between total energy intake and total cholesterol (a negative correlation). A positive correlation was found between the energy from protein and triglycerides.[6,7] During the second trimester, triglycerides were correlated negatively with the percentage of energy from fat and polyunsaturated fatty acids (PUFA) and positively with the energy from carbohydrates. During the third trimester, triglycerides were correlated negatively with energy from PUFA and with the P/S ratio (polyunsaturated/saturated fatty acids). This ratio correlated positively with total cholesterol. HDL-cholesterol correlated negatively with the percentage of energy from carbohydrates.[6]

In newborns, only a *significant relationship between triglycerides and index 2 of fat distribution* (r = 0.4027, p = 0.0414) *was found.*

Regarding *the relationships between the variables of the pregnant mother* and those of *the newborn*, a significant relationship between birth weight and maternal weight during the first, second, and third trimester was only found in boys. The mother's BMI during the first and second trimester correlated with the birth weight of boys.[6,7] Individual skinfolds of the mother correlated in different trimesters with similar variables of the newborn. *Mother-son correlations were more frequent than mother-daughter correlations.*[6]

The maternal subcutaneous fat distribution, as characterized by indices (Table 3.4), only correlated significantly in a few cases in the group of all newborns. *Significant correlations were found most often for mother's fat distribution during the second and third trimester of pregnancy and that of their newborn sons.* No significant correlations were found for girls.[6]

Some relationships exist between *weight gain during pregnancy* (calculated in absolute values and as a percentage of the prepregnant value) and the anthropometric variables in the newborn. Negative correlations were found between maternal weight gain and biceps and triceps skinfolds and BMIs of their sons. Positive correlations were found between maternal weight gain and birth weight, subscapular skinfold, and BMIs of their daughters. Similar correlations were also found for mothers and preschool children (see below).

TABLE 3.4 Relationships Between the Indices of Subcutaneous Fat Distribution of Mothers During Different Trimesters of Pregnancy and Similar Indices in Newborns (Evaluated Always for the Maximum Number of Pairs)[6,7]

Mothers	Trimester	Newborns (all)		Boys		Girls	
		r	p	r	p	r	p
INDEX 1		INDEX 2	INDEX 2				
	1st	0.30	0.050	—	—	—	—
		INDEX 1	INDEX 1	INDEX 1	INDEX 1		
	2nd	0.32	0.037	0.71	0.0001	—	—
		INDEX 2	INDEX 2	INDEX 2	INDEX 2		
		0.33	0.032	0.58	0.0039	—	—
		INDEX 1	INDEX 1	INDEX 1	INDEX 1		
	3rd	0.37	0.016	0.73	0.0001	—	—
		INDEX 2	INDEX 2	INDEX 2	INDEX 2		
		0.42	0.006	0.62	0.0039	—	—
INDEX 2		—	—	INDEX 1	INDEX 1		
	1st			0.50	0.0148	—	—
				INDEX 2	INDEX 2		
				0.44	0.0334	—	—
		—	—	INDEX 1	INDEX 1		
	2nd			0.70	0.0002	—	—
				INDEX 2	INDEX 2		
				0.61	0.0018	—	—
		INDEX 1	INDEX 1	INDEX 1	INDEX 1		
	3rd	0.31	0.043	0.73	0.0001	—	—
		INDEX 2	INDEX 2	INDEX 2	INDEX 2		
		0.37	0.018	0.64	0.0013	—	—
INDEX 4		—	—	INDEX 1	INDEX 1		
	2nd			0.52	0.0103	—	—
				INDEX 2	INDEX 2		
				0.47	0.0236	—	—
		INDEX 2	INDEX 2	INDEX 1	INDEX 1		
	3rd	0.31 0.046	0.046	0.42	0.0503	—	—
				INDEX 2	INDEX 2		
				0.44	0.0401	—	—

Adapted from Alberti-Fidanza, A., et al., *Eur. J. Clin. Nutr.*, 49, 289, 1995 and from Alberti-Fidanza, A., et al., Changes in anthropometric variables and fat patterns during pregnancy and their relationship to new born values, in press.

In relationships between *prepregnant body weight* and anthropometric variables at birth, significant correlations with body weight ($r = 0.5943, p = 0.022$) and recumbent length ($r = 0.5675, p = 0.038$) were found only in boys.[6,7]

Anthropometric variables in boys were generally correlated negatively with the absolute nutrient intake of their mothers, while the correlation coefficients for girls were mostly positive.[6,7]

Some correlations between the relative intake of nutrients (percentage of energy intake) of the mother and a combined group of newborns was, however, found; the *correlations were mostly frequent between the maternal dietary intake during the second and third trimesters of pregnancy and the anthropometric variables of boys.* Correlations were usually positive for proteins and fats and negative for carbohydrates. Significant correlations for girls were rare.[6,7]

The maternal diet was also significantly related to cord blood lipids. Most relationships were established for carbohydrate intake, total cholesterol, and HDL-cholesterol, which were significantly negative in the group of boys and then in the combined group of all newborns, while no significant correlations were found in newborn girls.[16]

A significantly negative correlation between the mother's energy intake and total cholesterol in boys was revealed. The same was established between energy from *carbohydrates and HDL-cholesterol. The percentage of energy from protein was positively correlated with total cholesterol in boys* (Table 3.5). *The energy from fat and carbohydrates correlated with HDL-cholesterol in newborn boys,* positively for fat and negatively for carbohydrates.[7]

TABLE 3.5   Relationships Between Daily Energy and Nutrient Intake (as % of Energy) of Mothers During Different Trimesters of Pregnancy and Cord Blood Lipids (Only Significant Values Given)

Maternal diet	Trimester	Newborns (all)		Boys		Girls	
		r	p	r	p	r	p
		TChol	TChol	TChol	TChol		
Energy	1st	−0.44	0.023	−0.56	−0.56	— —	— —
	2nd	−0.48	0.011	−0.56	−0.56	— —	— —
Proteins	1st	0.43	0.024	0.53	0.027	— —	— —
(% of energy)	2nd	0.51	0.006	0.51	0.036	— —	— —
Fat	1st	— —	— —	— —	— —	−0.75	0.017
(% of energy)		HDL	HDL	HDL	HDL	— —	— —
	2nd	0.44	0.020	0.63	0.007		
	3rd	0.55	0.003	0.78	0.0002	— —	— —
CHO	2nd	−0.46	0.015	−0.52	0.0323	— —	— —
(% of energy)	3rd	−0.59	0.001	−0.74	0.0007	— —	— —
				TChol	TChol		
				−0.49	0.048	— —	— —

Note: TChol, total cholesterol; HDL, high density lipoproteins; CHO, carbohydrates.

Adapted from Alberti-Fidanza, A., et al., *Eur. J. Clin. Nutr.,* 49, 289, 1995 and from Alberti-Fidanza, A., et al., Changes in anthropometric variables and fat pattern during pregnancy and their relationship to newborn values, in press.

Very few relationships were found between maternal and neonatal blood lipids. Maternal triglycerides correlated negatively with cord blood HDL-cholesterol, and total maternal cholesterol and HDL-cholesterol were correlated in the combined group of newborn boys and girls and/or only in girls, i.e., the total maternal cholesterol level and HDL cholesterol correlated positively with triglycerides and with HDL-cholesterol/total cholesterol ratios in girls only.[7]

Studies by Kesteloot and Dodion-Fransen[176] and Vobecky and Vobecky[369–371] found similar relationships in larger groups of newborns. The correlation coefficients found in these studies were also low, i.e., for total cholesterol of the mother and that in cord blood (r = 0.30 measured in 556 pairs of mothers and newborns). Therefore, there surely exists a weak, nevertheless significant, relationship.

Relationships between maternal anthropometric variables, including fat distribution, were also found in another study of ***preschool children*** *2 to 5 years old.* Again there were significant relationships between the skinfolds of mothers and their children (chin, thigh, calf), which were significant for boys, with only one exception for thigh skinfolds in girls. *The relationships between the indices of the fat pattern were again significant for mothers and their sons only* (Table 3.6).[249]

VI. GENERAL CONSIDERATIONS

Theresults of Alberti et al.[4–7] presented here indicate that *maternal nutritional status* — body weight, fat, and its distribution during pregnancy — *are significantly related to a number of variables in newborns.* These relationships seem to be different in boys and girls; regarding investigated variables, the *relationships are more frequent in paired mothers and newborn sons* and much less frequent for daughters. These sex-linked relationships were weak, nevertheless significant, and occurred regularly. *In preschool boys, these relationships were closer,* as apparent from the higher values of correlation coefficients (Table 3.6).

TABLE 3.6   Relationships Between Anthropometric Variables and Indices of Fat Distribution of the Mothers and Preschool Children (2 to 5 Years of Age)

	Boys + Girls (n = 73)	Boys (n = 43)	Girls (n = 29)
Height	0.422**	0.571**	
Sitting height	0.614**	0.777**	
Biacromial breadth	0.412**	0.548**	
Thigh circumference			0.387*
BMI	0.686**		
Fat pattern Index I	0.669**	0.764**	
Fat pattern Index II	0.421**	0.534**	

Note: ** $p < 0.01$; * $p < 0.05$; Index I, subscapular/triceps skinfold; Index II, chest 1,2 + abdomen + suprailiac/cheek + chin + triceps + thigh + calf.[249]

The fat pattern is assumed to be related to metabolic and cardiovascular characteristics[38] and can serve as a marker for some health risks of cardiovascular diseases later in life. Therefore, it may be speculated that if the *fat pattern in sons is significantly related to the same indicator in the mothers,* the health risks manifested in mothers might also appear later in life of their sons. Even when correlations are weak, they exist and may indicate some sort of predisposition that may be more obvious in boys.

The maternal diet also has an influence on a number of parameters, including serum lipids, mainly in sons. It is, therefore, not inconsequential what the future mother eats during pregnancy. *It seems that under conditions of satisfactory energy intake, the composition of the diet, i.e., relative amounts of individual nutrients and their mutual relationships, is more important than absolute amounts in the diet.* However, the absolute amount of carbohydrates (g/day) correlates significantly with total cholesterol in boys only.

It would be difficult, on the basis of existing data, to explain the sex-linked relationships and their different characteristics in boys and girls. These peculiarities may be related to the effect of sex hormones from the earliest periods of life. As described before, sex-linked differences in subcutaneous fat amount and distribution are already apparent at birth; the suprailic skinfold is significantly larger in girls.[231,233] In this study, sex-linked differences were observed for indices 1 to 3 (Table 3.3).

Our results on the different relationships between mothers and newborn boys and girls may also be influenced by the different number of males and females in our study. However, this does not seem to be the case: when comparing the values of correlation coefficients for all and/or just male newborns, in most instances we found higher r values for males alone than for the combined group of males and females.

Girls seem to be more protected than boys against the possible negative impact of their mother's diet during pregnancy. This difference in the relationship of blood lipids of the newborn to mother's diet may be further related to other female characteristics that differ, such as depot fat ratio and distribution and the lower risk of deviations of lipid metabolism, which may less frequently result in the development of cardiovascular diseases later in life.

Obviously, it would be necessary to validate these findings in larger groups of mothers and newborns (which is extremely difficult to assure) while also following up longer on the children. The study continues, and it should bring further instructive data that either confirms or denies the above mentioned conclusions.

Because some relationship between subcutaneous fat in Italian newborns (i.e., significant relationship between serum level of triglycerides and fat distribution, Index 2) was found, we may speculate that the changes in blood lipids of mothers adapted to endurance exercise, which limit the deposition and distribution of fat in newborns, may also influence blood lipid levels in their offspring. However, no valid data are available on this issue as was the case with the other data mentioned above.

In preschool children, a significant relationship between total cholesterol and triglycerides and skinfold thicknesses and the percentage of fat was also found at the age of 4.6 years.[243] Further studies focusing on these relationships in mothers with different physical activity regimens are also needed.

Chapter 4

GROWTH AND SOMATIC DEVELOPMENT OF PRESCHOOL CHILDREN

Numerous growth grids were prepared and used for the evaluation of the growth level in children.[299,300,348,349,382] Most studies concern the whole growth period from birth to maturity, especially those focused on ontogenetical changes of height and weight. More detailed data on growth, including further anthropometric measurements such as length, breadth, circumferential, variables are less common, similar to studies assessing body composition, functional capacity, and gross and fine motorics.

Dietary intake and metabolic development as characterized by biochemical parameters were mostly studied separately. However, it is interesting to note how all these characteristics are interrelated and interdependent. All are related to the environment, which varies markedly not only in different parts of the world, but also within the same country. This was the topic of our previous monograph "Human Growth, Fitness and Nutrition",[245–327] which mainly included data on school children and adolescents. The continuation of these efforts was the symposium on "Human Growth, Dietary Intake and Other Environmental Influences", organized within the framework of the 13th International Congress of Anthropological and Ethnological Sciences[259] in Mexico City in 1993 (Proceedings, Institute Danone, Paris 1995). The main aim of both of these meetings was the integration of the results of research concerning numerous aspects of human growth and development, as related to environmental conditions in different parts of the world.

The period between infancy and school age has been relatively neglected regarding more comprehensive studies also including functional, motor, and nutritional evaluations.

Growth curves for ***body mass index (BMI)*** were developed for children and adolescents in France,[299–307] in former Czechoslovakia,[35,147,290–294] and in other countries.[149,329] This also made the evaluation of preschooler's growth possible and gave researchers the opportunity to define obesity (Table 4.1) because BMI correlates significantly with total body fat, not only in adults,[243] but also in children.[249]

The comparison of the values of BMI in the Czech Republic and France showed that Czech children after the age of 7 years are heavier, i.e., obviously

**TABLE 4.1   Body Mass Index (BMI, Weight
kg/Height cm²) Variations (mean ± SD)
in Czech Children Aged 3 to 7 Years**

Age	Boys		Girls	
(years)	x̄	SD	x̄	SD
3.0	16.0	1.4	15.7	1.5
3.5	15.7	1.4	15.5	1.5
4.0	15.7	1.4	15.4	1.6
5.0	15.5	1.4	15.4	1.6
6.0	15.9	3.0	15.6	1.8
7.0	15.9	1.7	15.9	1.9

Note: SD, standard deviation.

Adapted from Prokopec, M. and Bellisle, F., *Ann. Hum. Biol.,* 20, 517, 1993.

fatter, than French children. Regarding health, some data indicate that being overweight as an adult and other weight-related pathological conditions are more prevalent in the Czech Republic and other East European countries compared to most countries in Western Europe, the U.S., Japan, etc.[360] This comparison indicates that predisposition for being overweight and later health problems start at an early age.[248,250] Recommended dietary allowances (RDAs) for protein and fat in former Czechoslovakia were always much higher, including those for children,[171] compared to the U.S.[397] or European Community RDAs;[398] for the most part, the real intake was even higher (see Chapter 5).

The BMI values of 90th percentile are higher in Czech children compared to French children at the age of 5 and 6 years;[294] this applies both to boys and girls. After the age of 7 years, Czech children are heavier in all percentiles of the BMI distribution than French children. *The adiposity rebound, i.e., the increase in adiposity* (as indicated by an increase of BMI), *occurred earlier in fat rather than in thin children, a confirmation of the French observation.*[303,306] As shown by Roland-Cachera et al.,[301,303] early adiposity rebound can predict obesity in adolescence and in adulthood.

A comparison of the changes in BMI in Czech children spanning nearly a hundred years calculated from the values of height and weight measured by Matiegka in 1895[209] and similar values measured by Hainiš[147] in 1988–1989 showed an increase in the average values from 14.87 to 15.88 in boys aged 6 to 7 years (values of height and weight for younger children in 1895 were not available) and from 15.09 to 15.71 in girls of the same age. Changes of BMI in older age categories are even more obvious.

A cross-sectional study of BMIs in adults in former Czechoslovakia revealed that a high (over 25%) proportion of individuals have, at the present time, BMIs higher than 25 kg/m², which is generally accepted as the cut-off point defining Grade I obesity.[276] More recent measurements by Hainiš[147] show higher ratios of individuals with increased BMIs in the Czech population.

Although it could be argued that body frame or even muscular mass could account for some of the differences of BMI between subjects from former Czechoslovakia and other countries such as England, Finland, France, the Netherlands, and the U.S.,[305] it is likely that the *high BMIs reflect a high adiposity level, the origin of which lies in a combination of bad eating habits and lifestyle from early childhood.* High intake of protein and fats in Czech Republic seems to be responsible: early rebound and higher average BMI values during growth, as well as in adulthood, run parallel to a greater prevalence of obesity, higher morbidity, and mortality from cardiovascular diseases in the Czech population.[360] High intake of protein during childhood is considered one of the main causes of later obesity.[299] However, the prevalence of subjects with higher BMIs in the U.S. increased considerably too.[188] Increased BMI values during growth can predict whether a child will be overweight at the age of 35.[145]

Therefore, high BMI values do not seem to be, under present living conditions in the industrially developed countries, an advantage for the child. However, at the same time, it is necessary to check not only the amount of fat as an important indicator of obesity (being overweight does not always imply high depot fat ratio), but also the level of functional capacity and physical fitness.

I. CROSS-SECTIONAL SURVEYS OF ANTHROPOMETRIC VARIABLES

Repeated cross-sectional and longitudinal measurements were compiled from representative samples in the Czech Republic. In these groups data on environmental, social, family, and health characteristics along with data on height, weight, and BMI[256] were assembled. More detailed measurements (anthropometric, body composition, functional capacity, gross and fine motorics, food intake, biochemical characteristics, body posture, and psychological evaluation) were repeatedly executed in smaller samples (Table 4.2).

In our first survey (A), 238 children from Prague kindergartens were followed up. (In late Czechoslovakia and/or now Czech Republic more than 80% of preschool children attend day care centers where they spend 7 to 8 hours per day). Day care centers were selected to represent different environ-. mental conditions in Prague, and those where our research team was given the opportunity to make the necessary measurements. The examinations were made always in the morning between 7:30 a.m. and 9:00 a.m. when the children play freely in the playroom and where our examinations generally did not interfere with their daily schedule (study A; n = 238; 142 characteristics assessed; Table 4.2). Day care centers are subordinated to the Ministry of Education. The teachers have to absolve special pedagogic high schools. The daily program is prepared by the Ministry of Education and includes free

TABLE 4.2   Individual Surveys of Preschool Children and Their
Program (A, B, C, D₁, D₂, G, H, I, J — Cross-sectional;
E, F — Longitudinal Follow-ups)

	Survey						
	A	B	C	D_1	D_2	E	F
n	238	5598	3712	9587	1005	58	764
Anthropometry 1	+	+	+	+	+	+	+
Anthropometry 2	+	-	-	-	-	+	-
Skinfolds	+	-	-	-	-	+	+
Somatotypes	+	-	-	-	-	+	+
Body posture	+	+	+	-	+	+	+
Step test	+	-	-	-	-	+	-
Performance	+	+	+	-	+	+	+
Skill	+	+	+	-	+	+	+
Sensomotor tests	+	+	+	-	+	+	+
Questionnaire 1	+	+	+	+	+	+	+
Questionnaire 2	+	+	+	+	+	+	+

Note: Anthropometry 1, simple program (see text and tables); Anthropometry 2, detailed
simple program (see text and tables); Questionnaire 1, family, social, environmental,
etc. characteristics; Questionnaire 2, participation, character of physical education.

In addition to the above mentioned assessments: dietary intake (food record forms) — surveys G, H, I, J; blood lipids (total, HDL, LDL cholesterol, triglycerides) — surveys H, I, J.

Compiled from Pařízková, J., unpublished data.

games, educational programs, physical education, walks and other activities
outside. Relaxation and sleep occur after lunch.

Another survey only included children 6.4 years of age from all over The
Czech Republic (study B, n = 5598, 42 indicators measured; see Table 4.2).
Study C included children of similar age groups (n = 3712) from the whole
country. Study D again comprised ***cross-sectional*** groups of children from 4
to 6 years old (n = 9587, subsample n = 1005) from different districts of our
country. Study E was ***longitudinal***, starting at 3 to 6 years of age (n = 58) and
including part of Prague children from study A who were available for repeated
measurements. Study F was again longitudinal, from 4 to 6 years, i.e., children
(n = 764) from the whole country were measured three times. All measurements were made at regular intervals from the beginning of the 1970s (1971)
until the end of the 1980s (1989). Surveys in smaller samples G and H also
included the ***dietary intake***, and surveys I and J included the assessment of
serum lipids (Table 4.2; see also Chapters 6, 9, and 10). Dietary intake was
also assessed longitudinally in a group of the children from survey E.

A questionnaire was given to the parents to assess data pertaining to age,
height, and body weight of the parents; their occupation; per capita income
in the family; the number of family members; the health status of the entire
family; the birth rank of the child; case-record of the child, including its birth
weight, period of breastfeeding, and motor development (i.e., at the age of the

beginning of sitting and independent walking); and sanitary standard of housing. These data helped to characterize the living conditions of the child outside of the day care centers.[256] The protocols and arrangements of our measurements varied in the individual surveys, depending on the given possibilities under various settings of our surveys. The formulas for the individual assessments are given in Appendices 1–4. Questionnaires concerning social, familial, economic etc. information were not included as these assessments are specific for individual countries.

The development of height, weight, and body mass index (BMI) corresponded to reference values[147] (Table 4.3a; Figures 4.1a and 4.1b). In comparison to the standards of Roland-Cachera et al.,[303] the average values of BMI of our children were slightly higher, especially after the age of 5 years. This corresponds to the findings of Prokopec and Bellisle,[294] who also found higher average BMI values in another group of Prague preschool children.

TABLE 4.3a   Height, Weight, Sitting Height and Body Mass Index (BMI) in 238 Children from 3 to 6 Years of Age in Prague (survey A)

AGE (years)		Height (cm)	Weight (kg)	Sitting Height (cm)	BMI (kg/m²)
3–4	Boys				
	x̄	101.6	16.62	57.8	16.0
	SD	4.5	1.97	2.8	1.6
	Girls				
	x̄	99.5	15.69	56.3	15.8
	SD	5.0	2.24	3.2	1.2
4–5	Boys				
	x̄	109.0	19.18	62.0	16.2
	SD	3.9	2.86	2.3	1.3
	Girls				
	x̄	107.7	18.34	60.0	15.8
	SD	5.9	3.48	2.4	1.3
5–6	Boys				
	x̄	113.5	20.85	63.8	16.2
	SD	5.8	2.76	2.7	1.4
	Girls				
	x̄	112.8	19.65	62.5	15.4
	SD	4.4	2.52	2.5	1.5
6–7	Boys				
	x̄	119.2	22.10	65.5	15.6
	SD	4.1	2.68	2.6	1.4
	Girls				
	x̄	118.6	21.59	64.7	15.3
	SD	4.9	2.81	2.8	1.3

Note: SD, standard deviation

Modified from Pařízková, J., et al., *Growth, Fitness and Nutrition in Preschool Children,* Charles University, Prague, 1984.

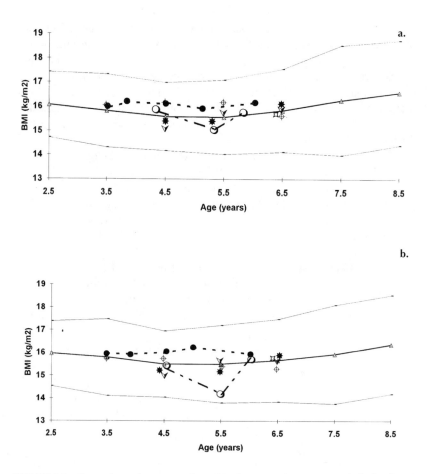

FIGURE 4.1 Comparison of average values of body mass index (BMI, weight kg/height m²) in boys **(a)** and girls **(b)** assessed in surveys A–J with national standards of Hainis ($\bar{x} \pm$ SD).[147]. Survey A, ⊕; B, ⊐; C, γ ; D, ＊; E, ●; F, ○.

Similar conclusions resulted from comparisons of other child groups (studies B, C, D; the values of height and weight see along with other characteristics in Tables 4.4, 4.5, 4.6a, and 4.6b). A longitudinal study of 58 boys and girls in Prague (E) which covered approximately the same age span (see Table 4.7a) also showed higher average BMI values (i.e., on the level of 55th to 70th percentiles of our standards) and even slightly higher at the age of 5 to 6 years when compared with French BMI standards.[303–306] Survey F (see Table 4.8) showed slightly lower values of BMI at the age of 4 to 5 years, which further declined at the occasion of the second measurement, but then increased at the occasion of the last measurement.

When we evaluated BMIs from representative samples of children measured in all of The Czech Republic (B and D), we found average values close to the 50th percentile,[35] but higher values when comparing the data with French

BMI standard values. However, these values were still within the normal range of the standards for height and weight. BMI values were usually higher in boys compared to girls, which also corresponds to other findings in our and other child populations.[293]

Further *anthropometric variables* such as **length, breadth, and circumferential measures** were assessed (see Table 4.3b, 4.3c, 4.3d, 4.3e, 4.3f) in cross-sectional study of 238 preschool children (A) and study E where some of the same children were followed up repeatedly (n = 58; see Table 4.7a, 4.7b, 4.7c, 4.7d). In studies B, C, and D only circumferential measurements were recorded. Measurements were made as recommended for the International Biological Programme.[97,240,328]

As detailed data on morphological development of preschool children are relatively rare, all variables measured in studies A and E are given. The following tables show the results of measurements in individual age categories from 3 to 4, 4 to 5, 5 to 6, and 6 to 7 years, separately for boys and girls (survey A). Also with *sex-linked differences*, the comparison of lengths reveals slightly higher values in boys (Table 4.3b), but rarely do these differences in this smaller Prague group reach the level of statistical significance.

With **breadth measures**, there is a trend toward higher values of shoulder width (biacromial breadth) in boys which again is not significant (Table 4.3c). The width of the chest is markedly greater in boys, and this difference is significant in older age groups. The same applies to the depth of the chest. The breadth of the pelvis (biiliocristal breadth) was smaller in girls. The differences in this case were significant at the age of 5 to 6 years (Table 4.3c).[256]

The robusticity of the skeleton was evaluated according to selected dimensions, i.e., breadth measurements on the upper and lower extremity (Table 4.3d). Boys had a more robust skeleton — the dimensions were significantly larger in the majority of age groups. This applied particularly to the breadth of the hand, humoral and femoral condyles and the breadth of the ankles. In the width of the wrist, a significant sex-linked difference was only found at the age of 6 to 7 years.

The comparison of *circumferential measurements* showed that the head circumference was significantly greater in boys of all age groups, the circumference of the neck in all except the 4- to 5-year-old ones. Sex-linked differences in the chest circumference were relatively smaller and significant only in 3- to 4- and 5- to 6-year-old children. Also, the waist (abdomen) circumference differed less, the difference only being significant in children aged 5 to 6 years old. Thus, sex-linked differences on the head were somewhat more marked than those of the trunk.[256]

The circumferences of the arm did not differ by sex, which was also manifested in the circumferences of the forearm (Table 4.3f). On the other hand, the circumferences of the thigh tended to be higher in girls. This was the only indicator of those used where it was the case. With the calf circumferences, there was a tendency toward higher values in 6- to 7-year-old girls. There were remarkable age-related changes in the *relative increase of different*

TABLE 4.3b   Length Measures on the Extremities in 238 Children Aged 3 to 6 Years in Prague (survey A)

Age (years)		1	2	3	4	5	6
3–4	Boys						
	x̄	42.5	17.2	13.6	56.8	26.0	21.6
	SD	2.0	1.0	1.0	2.8	1.5	1.7
	Girls						
	x̄	40.9	16.8	13.0	55.1	25.5	21.4
	SD	2.5	1.1	1.0	3.2	1.9	2.3
4–5	Boys						
	x̄	46.0	18.9	14.9	62.1	30.9	23.1
	SD	2.2	1.2	1.1	3.3	2.1	1.6
	Girls						
	x̄	44.9	18.8	14.6	61.7	30.3	22.6
	SD	2.4	1.3	1.3	3.3	2.4	1.2
5–6	Boys						
	x̄	48.9	20.0	16.1	65.5	32.6	24.3
	SD	3.2	1.1	1.0	3.9	2.4	1.7
	Girls						
	x̄	46.8	19.4	15.1	65.2	32.5	23.9
	SD	2.5	1.2	1.0	3.3	2.7	1.4
6–7	Boys						
	x̄	51.1	20.8	16.4	69.1	34.1	25.8
	SD	1.9	0.8	0.7	2.6	1.9	1.4
	Girls						
	x̄	50.0	20.4	16.4	69.1	34.1	25.8
	SD	2.4	1.1	0.9	3.1	2.5	2.1

Note: 1, total of upper extremities; 2, acromion-radiale; 3, radiale-stylion; 4, total of lower extremities; 5, iliospinale-tibiale; 6, tibiale-sphyrion.

Individual measures: total length of upper extremity, i.e., acromion-dactylion, acromion-radiale, radiale-stylion; total length of lower extremity, i.e., iliocristale-base, iliospinale-tibiale, tibiale-sphyrion.

Adapted from Pařízková, J., et al., *Growth, Fitness and Nutrition in Preschool Children,* Charles University, Prague, 1984.

morphological parameters during preschool age; some increased much more than others; e.g. the height of 6- to 7-year-old children was roughly by 17 to 19% higher than in 3- to 4-year-old children. In the increase in height the growth of the trunk participates less (increase of sitting height by 13 to 15%) than that of the lower extremities (by 21 to 22%). In the lower extremity, there is a relatively greater increase in the length of the thigh (increase of iliospinale-tibiale by 31 to 38%) than of the calf (increase of tibiale-sphyrion by 19 to 23%). The length of the upper extremities increases relatively less than the length of the lower extremities, i.e., by 20 to 22%. In this increase, the upper

TABLE 4.3c   Breadth Measures on the Trunk (cm) in Children Aged 3 to 6 Years in Prague (n = 238, Survey A)

Age (years)		Biacromiale	Chest breadth	Chest depth	Biiliocristale
3–4	Boys				
	$\bar{x}$	23.1	17.1	12.7	16.8
	SD	1.0	0.5	0.8	0.8
	Girls				
	$\bar{x}$	22.8	16.6	12.0	16.5
	SD	1.2	0.7	0.8	1.0
4–5	Boys				
	$\bar{x}$	24.6	18.1	13.2	18.0
	SD	1.0	0.8	0.9	1.2
	Girls				
	$\bar{x}$	24.3	17.8	12.5	17.7
	SD	1.4	1.2	0.7	1.1
5–6	Boys				
	$\bar{x}$	25.6	18.7	13.5	18.6
	SD	1.4	0.9	0.7	0.9
	Girls				
	$\bar{x}$	25.5	17.8	13.5	18.0
	SD	0.9	0.7	1.7	1.5
6–7	Boys				
	$\bar{x}$	26.2	19.2	13.7	19.4
	SD	1.0	0.8	0.6	0.9
	Girls				
	$\bar{x}$	26.1	18.6	13.2	19.2
	SD	1.1	1.2	0.9	1.1

Modified from Pařízková, J., et al., *Growth, Fitness and Nutrition in Preschool Children*, Charles University, Prague, 1984.

segment of the arm (acromion-radiale by 20 to 21%) as well as the lower segment of the arm (radiale-stylion by 20 to 26%; Table 4.3b) participates evenly.

The width of the trunk changes less than the length dimensions. The relatively greatest increase occurs in the pelvic dimensions (biiliocristal breadth, by about 15 to 16) and in the breadth of the shoulders (biacromial breadth) by about 13 to 14%. The breadth of the chest in 6- to 7-year-olds is about 12% greater than in 3- to 4-year-olds, while the depth of the chest changes relatively little during this period (see Table 4.3c).

The *robusticity of the skeleton* increased more on the upper extremity, i.e., the breadth of the hand increases by 11 to 12%, the breadth of the wrist by 8 to 10%, the breadth of the humeral condyles by about 9%. The breadth of the femoral condyles is, in the oldest group of 6- to 7 year-old children (compared to the youngest one), by about 4 to 5% greater. The breadth of the ankle is greater by 5 to 6% (Table 4.3d).

The circumferential measures change little during this age period (see Table 4.3e), compared to other indicators except for the thigh circumference.

**TABLE 4.3d Breadth Measures on the Extremities
(cm) in Children Aged 3 to 6 Years
(n = 238) in Prague (survey A)**

Age (years)		Hand	Wrist	Humeral condyle	Femoral condyle	Ankle
3–4	boys					
	$\overline{x}$	5.4	3.8	4.4	7.1	5.2
	SD	0.3	0.2	0.2	0.3	0.3
	girls					
	$\overline{x}$	5.2	3.7	4.2	6.6	4.9
	SD	0.4	0.2	0.4	0.4	0.3
4–5	boys					
	$\overline{x}$	5.9	3.9	4.7	7.3	5.4
	SD	0.5	0.2	0.3	0.4	0.3
	girls					
	$\overline{x}$	5.5	3.8	4.4	6.9	5.1
	SD	0.3	0.2	0.3	0.4	0.2
5–6	boys					
	$\overline{x}$	5.9	4.0	4.8	7.4	5.5
	SD	0.4	0.3	0.2	0.3	0.3
	girls					
	$\overline{x}$	5.6	3.9	4.5	7.0	5.1
	SD	0.3	0.2	0.2	0.3	0.3
6–7	boys					
	$\overline{x}$	6.1	4.2	4.8	7.5	5.5
	SD	0.5	0.2	0.3	0.3	0.3
	girls					
	$\overline{x}$	5.8	4.0	4.8	7.5	5.5
	SD	0.2	0.2	0.2	0.5	0.3

Compiled from Pařízková, J., et al., *Growth, Fitness and Nutrition in Preschool Children,* Charles University, Prague, 1984.

The head circumference in our oldest age group (6 to 7 years) is only by 3 to 4% greater than in the youngest age group of 3- to 4-year-old children. The neck circumference differs even less, i.e., by 2 to 4%. The chest circumference is 7 to 8% greater in the oldest age group, and the waist circumference 10 to 12%. The same applies to the calf.[256]

When comparing the relative increase of bodily dimensions in our groups of children, it was revealed that in girls this increase is somewhat more marked.

The increase in total body weight during this period is 32 to 37% greater than the relative increase in height. BMI decreased slightly both in boys and girls (see Figures 4.1a and 4.1b), which corresponds to general trends of development assessed in Czech children, as well as in other child populations.[294,302]

As apparent, individual bodily dimensions of preschool children change in a different way. *The greatest relative increase is that of total body mass, followed by the length of the thigh along with other longitudinal dimensions of the skeleton. The breadth of the trunk increases much less, and the same* applies to the robusticity of the skeleton and the circumferences of the lower

TABLE 4.3e Circumferential Measurements on the Head and Trunk (cm) in Children from Prague Aged 3 to 6 Years of Age (n = 238; Survey A)

Age (years)		Head	Neck	Chest	Waist
3–4	Boys				
	x̄	50.4	25.5	54.2	50.8
	SD	1.1	1.0	2.4	3.6
	Girls				
	x̄	49.3	24.3	52.6	49.7
	SD	1.7	1.0	2.6	3.3
4–5	Boys				
	x̄	51.3	25.9	57.0	53.0
	SD	1.3	1.3	3.5	3.5
	Girls				
	x̄	49.5	24.6	54.2	51.5
	SD	1.3	1.2	2.7	4.4
5–6	Boys				
	x̄	51.4	25.9	57.3	54.3
	SD	1.5	1.4	2.7	3.4
	Girls				
	x̄	50.4	24.9	55.3	51.8
	SD	1.2	1.1	2.6	2.8
6–7	Boys				
	x̄	52.3	26.2	58.1	54.0
	SD	1.5	0.9	3.1	3.5
	Girls				
	x̄	51.3	25.2	57.2	53.7
	SD	1.4	1.2	3.3	4.5

Modified from Pařízková, J., et al., *Growth, Fitness and Nutrition in Preschool Children*, Charles University, Prague, 1984.

extremities. *The relatively smallest increase is that of the head and neck circumferences.*

Proportionality also changes during preschool age. Young children have relatively shorter extremities than older ones. This was shown in our groups by examining the reduction of the values of the *index* (relative value which evaluates sitting height in relation to height; see Table 4.3g) and conversely by increasing the relative length of the lower extremities. The relatively smaller increase in the breadth of the trunk was also manifested by a decline in the relative shoulder breadth in relation to height (Table 4.3g). All these differences are statistically significant. The relative breadth of the pelvis in relation to height and shoulder breadth did not change markedly during the preschool period.[256]

When measuring groups of children, a markedly *different variability of individual morphological variables,* characterized by the coefficient of variation

**TABLE 4.3f Circumferential Measurements
on the Extremities (cm) in
Children Aged 3 to 6 Years in
Prague (n = 238; Survey A)**

Age (years)		Arm	Forearm	Thigh	Calf
3–4	Boys				
	$\bar{x}$	17.0	16.8	32.0	21.9
	SD	1.1	0.8	2.3	1.3
	Girls				
	$\bar{x}$	16.6	16.5	32.2	21.7
	SD	1.3	1.1	2.5	1.6
4–5	Boys				
	$\bar{x}$	17.2	17.2	33.5	23.4
	SD	1.2	0.9	3.4	1.2
	Girls				
	$\bar{x}$	16.9	16.7	34.1	22.9
	SD	1.4	1.2	3.2	2.2
5–6	Boys				
	$\bar{x}$	17.5	17.5	34.8	23.7
	SD	1.2	1.0	2.6	1.6
	Girls				
	$\bar{x}$	17.4	16.9	35.2	23.0
	SD	1.2	1.0	3.2	1.2
6–7	Boys				
	$\bar{x}$	17.7	17.6	35.4	24.1
	SD	1.1	0.8	2.5	1.1
	Girls				
	$\bar{x}$	17.7	17.4	36.3	24.5
	SD	1.2	0.9	2.5	1.6

Adapted from Pařízková, J., et al., Growth, Fitness and
Nutrition in Preschool Children, Charles University, 64

Prague, 1984.

(CV) was also found. The greatest variability was found in body weight where
the CV varies from 11 to 14% in different age groups. The longitudinal
dimensions, including height, have CV values of roughly 4 to 7%, breadths
on the trunk and indicators of skeletal robusticity of 4 to 6%. *The smallest
variability at that age is found for the head circumference* (2 to 3%); the
remaining circumferential measures have CVs within the range of 4 to 7%,
similar to longitudinal measures and breadths. Apparently, body weight is
mainly influenced by environmental factors, particularly dietary intake, which
applies to the earliest periods of life.

Some of these morphological variables were also measured in a representa-
tive sample of children (age 6.4 years; sample B) from the whole Czech
Republic. In this group of children only selected measurements could be made
(Table 4.4). Average values from this larger sample were also higher than those

**TABLE 4.3g   Indices of Body Build and Proportionality in Children Aged
3 to 6 Years in Prague (n = 238; Survey A)**

Age (years)		Sitt. ht × 100/HT	Lgth l. extr. × 100/HT	Biacr. × 100/HT	Bicr. × 100/HT	Bicr. × 100/biacr.
3–4	Boys					
	x̄	56.86	55.83	22.73	16.59	73.02
	SD	2.27	1.24	0.85	0.84	3.43
	Girls					
	x̄	56.53	52.28	22.95	16.2	72.53
	SD	1.65	1.15	1.08	0.9	.93
4–5	Boys					
	x̄	56.88	56.97	22.56	16.51	73.17
	SD	1.26	1.89	0.69	0.73	3.47
	Girls					
	x̄	55.56	56.68	22.58	16.39	72.67
	SD	1.52	1.64	1.13	0.86	3.62
5–6	Boys					
	x̄	56.34	57.70	22.62	16.39	72.56
	SD	1.82	2.04	1.04	0.65	3.70
	Girls					
	x̄	55.49	57.64	22.68	16.00	70.59
	SD	1.69	1.18	0.76	1.72	5.40
6–7	Boys					
	x̄	54.98	57.99	22.02	16.26	73.95
	SD	0.97	1.07	0.66	0.64	3.88
	Girls					
	x̄	54.52	58.12	22.02	16.20	73.64
	SD	1.08	1.80	0.68	0.67	3.41

Note: Sitt. ht., sitting height; Lgth l. extr., length of lower extremities; Biacr., biacromial
breadth; Bicrist., biiliocristal breadth.

Adapted from Pařízková, J., et al., *Growth, Fitness and Nutrition in Preschool Children,*
Charles University, Prague, 1984.

of the same age category (i.e., 6 to 7 years of age) mentioned above (survey
A), but the differences were mostly insignificant. This applied first of all to
the values of height and weight. BMIs tended to be higher in girls only. The
values of the waist (abdomen) circumference were higher in boys, and those
of the arm were higher in both sexes. Otherwise the values from survey A
were closer to the values of survey B, concerning 6.4-year-old children
(Table 4.4).

After a 5-year interval, cross-sectional measurements of the same morphological characteristics in 1848 boys and in 1864 girls at the age of 4 to 6
years (survey C) were repeated (Table 4.5). The BMI values and the other
parameters mentioned above did not differ markedly from the previous measurements (Figures 4.1a and 4.1b). Some variations were apparent, e.g., a
slight increase in the average values of height. Also, the circumferences of

TABLE 4.4   Somatic Development of Preschool Children in Czech Republic at the Age of 6.4 Years (All Regions: Boys n = 2587, Girls n = 2505; Survey B)

Measurement		$\bar{x}$	SD
Height	Boys	118.7	5.3
(cm)	Girls	117.8	5.2
Weight	Boys	22.24	3.24
(kg)	Girls	21.76	3.34
Body mass index (BMI)	Boys	15.8	1.2
(kg/m²)	Girls	15.7	1.3
Circumferences			
Chest (cm)			
rest	Boys	59.3	3.3
	Girls	58.0	3.3
inspiration	Boys	62.7	3.5
	Girls	61.3	3.7
expiration	Boys	58.7	3.4
	Girls	57.5	3.7
Abdomen (cm)	Boys	55.3	4.4
	Girls	54.8	5.0
Arm (cm)	Boys	18.2	1.7
	Girls	18.4	1.8
Thigh (cm)	Boys	35.5	3.5
	Girls	37.2	3.6

Modified from Pařízková, J., et al., *Growth, Fitness and Nutrition in Preschool Children,* Charles University, Prague, 1984.

chest, abdomen, and arm tended to be greater when larger population samples of boys and girls 6 to 7 years of age were compared after the mentioned period of time. However, the values of body weight and thigh circumference were practically the same. BMI varied insignificantly in boys and was slightly higher in girls measured later (survey C). The average values of BMI for the whole group measured in the Czech Republic (survey B) corresponded to that ascertained earlier in girls in Prague (survey A), where most of the measurements always revealed higher values.

The last cross-sectional measurements of similar parameters in the same age groups (4 to 6 years, survey D, Table 4.6a) in 1988 to 1989 were made in 9587 preschool children. A subsample of 1005 boys and girls was followed up in greater detail as in surveys A and E (see Table 4.6b). *Average values of height and weight from this measurement did not differ significantly compared to the average values of height ascertained in surveys A and B* (see Tables 4.3a, 4.3b, 4.3c, 4.3d, 4.3e, 4.3f, 4.3g, 4.4). During the 1970s and 1980s, the acceleration of growth in the Czech Republic was minimal,[147] which was also apparent in our group of preschoolers. Average BMI values in the last survey (D) were, in some cases, slightly lower than in previous surveys.[251]

TABLE 4.5   Somatic Development of Preschool Boys (n = 1848) and Girls (n = 1864) in Czech Republic (Height, Weight, Circumferential Measurements of the Chest, Abdomen, Arm and Thigh) (Survey C)

Age (years)	Height (cm)	Weight (kg)	BMI (kg/m^2)	Chest circumference (cm)	Waist (cm)	Arm (cm)	Thigh (cm)
4–5							
Boys, n = 630							
x̄	106.5	17.93	15.01	55.9	53.2	17.5	32.6
SD	4.9	2.15	1.6	2.9	3.8	1.4	2.8
Girls, n = 665							
x̄	105.6	17.63	15.01	57.9	54.5	16.2	33.9
SD	5.9	2.19	1.7	4.2	4.2	2.3	3.7
5–6							
Boys, n = 682							
x̄	113.5	20.20	15.68	57.9	54.5	16.2	33.9
SD	4.9	2.60	1.9	4.2	4.2	2.3	3.2
Girls, n = 653							
x̄	113.3	20.02	15.60	56.8	54.3	18.2	35.4
SD	4.6	2.60	2.0	3.7	4.2	1.1	3.3
6–7							
Boys, n = 536							
x̄	119.0	22.29	15.80	59.6	56.1	18.7	34.9
SD	4.6	2.63	1.8	3.6	5.2	2.4	3.5
Girls, n = 546							
x̄	118.3	21.83	15.60	58.3	55.4	18.8	36.6
SD	4.9	2.68	1.9	4.0	5.3	2.6	4.5

Modified from Pařízková, J., *Physical fitness assessment,* in *Principles, Practices and Applications,* R.J. Shephard and H. Lavallée, Eds., 1980.

TABLE 4.6a   Anthropometric Variables in Preschool Children (Survey D, n = 9587)

Age (years) n		4–5 Boys 1637	Girls 1607	5–6 Boys 2521	Girls 2514	6–7 Boys 665	Girls 643
Height	x̄	108.0	107.4	114.2	113.2	117.8	117.5
(cm)	SE	0.13	0.13	0.11	0.11	0.20	0.23
Weight	x̄	18.7	17.92	20.28	19.77	21.59	21.34
(kg)	SE	0.05	0.06	0.06	0.05	0.12	0.12
BMI	x̄	16.12	15.54	15.55	15.42	15.55	15.46
(kg/m^2)	SE	0.04	0.04	0.03	0.03	0.06	0.07
Birth weight	x̄	3412	3276	3399	3257	3354	3245
(g)	SE	12	12	10	9	20	18

Note: SE, unknown

Compiled from Pařízková, J., unpublished data.

TABLE 4.6b   Somatic Development of Preschool Children (n = 1005, Survey D)

Age (years)		4–5		5–6		6–7	
		Boys	Girls	Boys	Girls	Boys	Girls
n		138	158	301	267	67	74
Height	$\bar{x}$	107.6	107.1	114.1	113.1	118.2	116.6
(cm)	SD	5.7	5.0	5.8	5.1	4.8	4.4
Weight	$\bar{x}$	18.1	17.7	20.2	19.8	22.0	21.2
(kg)	SD	2.6	2.3	2.9	3.0	4.2	2.9
BMI	$\bar{x}$	14.6	15.43	15.52	15.48	15.74	15.6
(kg/m²)	SD	1.8	1.5	1.5	1.8	2.0	1.7
Circumference measures							
Chest	$\bar{x}$	56.0	55.2	57.7	56.6	59.2	57.4
(cm)	SD	4.1	3.4	3.0	3.8	4.9	3.3
Waist	$\bar{x}$	52.7	51.9	53.7	52.5	54.3	52.4
(cm)	SD	4.7	3.5	3.6	4.2	5.5	3.7
Hips	$\bar{x}$	58.4	58.6	60.4	60.9	62.0	62.7
(cm)	SD	4.5	3.7	4.1	4.2	5.0	3.9
Waist/Hip	$\bar{x}$	0.90	0.88	0.88	0.86	0.87	0.83
—	SD	0.18	0.15	0.20	0.18	0.14	0.21

Modified from Pařízková, J., *World-Wide Variation in Physical Fitness*, A.L. Classens, J. Lefevre, and B. Vanden Eynde, Eds., Institute of Physical Education, Katholieke Universiteit, Leuven, Belgium, 1993, 131 and from Pařízková, J., *Nutrition in Pregnancy and Growth*, in press.

II. LONGITUDINAL STUDIES OF CHILDREN FROM 3 TO 6 YEARS OLD

Growth trends during the preschool period were also followed-up in a longitudinal investigation of children (boys n = 36, girls n = 22, survey E) who were available for further measurements during the period from 3.5 up to 6.0 years (Tables 4.7a, 4.7b, 4.7c, 4.7d, Figures 4.1a and 4.1b). The children were measured first in the autumn when they started to visit two kindergartens in the surroundings of our laboratory. The characteristics of the children's family, age of parents, number of siblings, economic standard of the family, health record, etc. did not differ significantly from characteristics obtained in a cross-sectional sample of a larger number of children as described above (see Tables 4.3a, 4.3b, 4.3c, 4.3d, 4.3e, 4.3f, 4.3g).

In particular, attention was focused on the changes of body build and composition as related to the development of functional capacity and motor abilities. By investigating the same children we tried to confirm the conclusions of cross-sectional surveys, therefore reducing the impact of selection of certain somatic and functional types that may interfere with the evaluation of growth trends in different age groups in cross-sectional studies.

TABLE 4.7a Height, Weight, Body Mass Index (BMI), and Sitting Height in Preschool Boys (n = 36) and Girls (n = 22) Followed Longitudinally Five Times (1–5, Survey E)

Measurement		Age (years)	Height (cm)	Weight (kg)	BMI (kg/m²)	Sitting Height (cm)
1	Boys					
	$\bar{x}$	3.487	102.0	16.72	16.07	57.9
	SD	0.299	4.42	1.96	1.2	2.9
	Girls					
	$\bar{x}$	3.534	99.2	15.70	15.95	56.1
	SD	0.364	5.72	2.28	1.1	3.1
2	Boys					
	$\bar{x}$	3.934	104.5	17.70	16.20	59.3
	SD	0.349	4.65	2.34	1.4	2.0
	Girls					
	$\bar{x}$	3.928	101.7	16.4	15.8	57.7
	SD	0.358	5.14	1.90	1.4	2.5
3	Boys					
	$\bar{x}$	4.548	109.0	19.18	16.14	62.0
	SD	0.339	3.96	2.86	1.2	2.3
	Girls					
	$\bar{x}$	4.486	106.4	18.2	16.07	60.0
	SD	0.372	5.15	3.27	1.3	2.7
4	Boys					
	$\bar{x}$	5.102	112.7	20.13	15.85	63.4
	SD	0.348	4.32	2.90	1.3	2.6
	Girls					
	$\bar{x}$	5.021	109.8	19.53	16.19	61.8
	SD	0.351	5.29	3.71	1.2	2.9
5	Boys					
	$\bar{x}$	6.025	119.8	23.1	16.09	66.3
	SD	0.338	4.21	3.52	1.4	2.5
	Girls					
	$\bar{x}$	6.016	116.37	21.58	15.93	63.9
	SD	0.369	5.34	3.97	1.2	4.1

Tables 4.7a, 4.7b, 4.7c, 47d show the changes of *anthropometric variables* during the mentioned period of development. The changes in BMI were reported above. All measures increased significantly. As indicated by the results of the cross-sectional study, the increments of different bodily dimensions varied markedly. Body weight increased by 20 to 24% and height by only 9 to 10% as compared to initial values. The breadth measurements of the trunk-biacromial and bicristal breadth also increased approximately to an almost equal extent. Head circumference only increased by 1 to 2%, similar to the femoral condyles. The length of the trunk increased relatively less than the length of the lower extremities. This influenced the proportionality of the

TABLE 4.7b   Length Measures on the Extremities in Boys and Girls Followed Longitudinally Five Times (1–5; Survey E)

Measure-ment		Upper extremities (total)	Acromion -radiale	Radiale -stylion	Lower extremities (total)	Iliospinale -tibiale	Tibiale-sphyrion
1	Boys						
	$\bar{x}$	42.5	17.3	13.5	57.0	26.1	21.7
	SD	2.9	2.0	1.0	2.8	1.6	1.7
	Girls						
	$\bar{x}$	40.9	16.8	13.0	5.0	25.5	21.4
	SD	2.1	1.1	1.0	3.	1.9	2.2
2	Boys						
	$\bar{x}$	43.9	17.9	14.2	58.4	29.4	21.9
	SD	2.1	0.9	0.8	3.2	2.0	1.3
	Girls						
	$\bar{x}$	42.0	17.0	13.8	57.3	28.7	20.1
	SD	2.4	1.1	0.8	3.6	2.2	1.4
3	Boys						
	$\bar{x}$	46.0	18.8	14.7	61.7	31.1	23.1
	SD	2.2	1.0	1.0	2.7	2.0	1.1
	Girls						
	$\bar{x}$	44.0	18.2	14.3	60.2	30.4	21.7
	SD	2.5	1.0	1.3	3.4	1.9	1.5
4	Boys						
	$\bar{x}$	47.8	19.6	15.2	64.2	32.4	23.2
	SD	2.3	1.7	0.9	2.6	1.8	1.2
	Girls						
	$\bar{x}$	45.6	18.9	14.6	62.8	31.9	22.5
	SD	2.4	1.0	1.4	3.4	2.0	1.5
5	Boys						
	$\bar{x}$	50.9	21.0	16.6	67.3	35.3	25.0
	SD	4.6	2.4	1.0	11.7	2.0	1.2
	Girls						
	$\bar{x}$	48.2	20.1	15.6	67.2	34.1	24.1
	SD	2.8	1.1	0.8	3.3	1.9	1.6

body build as also shown in the cross-sectional study. The average values of BMI fluctuated slightly at the 55th to 70th percentiles.

Sex-linked differences were apparent, especially regarding height and weight. Though in this smaller group, they were not significant. The same applied to the breadth of shoulders and pelvis (biacromial and bicristal breadths). Apart from this, there were sex-linked differences in sitting height, length of the upper extremities, depth of the chest, and the circumferences of head and neck, where the values in boys were higher. Chest circumference was significantly greater in boys only during the first measurement.[236,238]

The increments of individual parameters between measurements were also evaluated; this showed the dynamics of development in boys and girls.[255]

In general, the conclusions from longitudinal measurements were in agreement with the results of cross-sectional investigations, thus confirming the developmental trends during this growth period.

TABLE 4.7c Breadth Measures on the Trunk and on the Extremities (cm) in Boys and Girls Followed Longitudinally Five Times (1–5; Survey E)

Measurement			Biacromial	Biiliocristal	Chest Depth	Hand	Wrist	Humeral Condyle	Femoral Condyle	Ankle
1	Boys	x̄	23.2	16.9	12.7	5.2	3.8	4.4	7.1	5.1
		SD	1.0	0.8	0.8	1.0	0.2	0.2	0.3	0.3
	Girls	x̄	22.9	16.5	12.0	5.2	3.5	3.8	6.8	4.8
		SD	1.2	1.0	0.8	0.4	0.7	0.7	1.2	1.2
2	Boys	x̄	23.7	17.5	12.9	5.3	4.0	4.6	7.1	5.2
		SD	1.4	1.0	0.7	0.6	0.5	0.2	0.4	0.3
	Girls	x̄	23.5	17.0	12.3	5.3	3.6	4.3	6.7	4.9
		SD	1.1	0.8	0.8	0.4	0.2	0.2	0.3	0.4
3	Boys	x̄	24.6	18.0	13.2	5.9	4.0	4.7	7.3	5.4
		SD	1.0	1.2	0.9	0.7	0.3	0.3	0.4	0.3
	Girls	x̄	24.5	17.6	12.6	5.5	3.8	4.6	6.9	5.2
		SD	1.3	1.1	1.0	0.3	0.2	0.6	0.4	0.3
4	Boys	x̄	25.2	18.5	13.1	5.9	4.1	4.8	7.5	5.6
		SD	1.0	1.0	0.7	0.4	0.2	0.3	0.3	0.3
	Girls	x̄	24.9	18.0	12.6	5.4	3.9	4.5	7.0	5.2
		SD	1.4	0.9	1.2	0.7	0.2	0.6	0.5	0.4
5	Boys	x̄	26.4	19.4	13.6	5.9	4.2	5.0	7.7	5.7
		SD	1.5	1.5	0.8	0.6	0.2	0.2	0.4	0.3
	Girls	x̄	26.0	18.5	12.9	5.5	4.0	4.7	7.0	5.3
		SD	1.2	1.1	1.2	0.6	0.3	0.2	0.7	0.4

TABLE 4.7d Circumferential Measures (cm) in Boys and Girls Followed Longitudinally Five Times (1–5; Survey E)

Measurement			Head	Neck	Chest	Waist	Arm	Forearm	Thigh	Calf
1	Boys	x̄	50.5	25.6	54.4	50.9	17.1	16.7	32.0	21.7
		SD	1.1	1.0	2.4	3.6	1.2	0.9	2.4	1.4
	Girls	x̄	49.3	24.3	52.8	49.8	16.5	16.7	32.3	21.3
		SD	1.7	1.0	2.6	3.3	1.1	1.4	2.5	1.6
2	Boys	x̄	50.9	25.4	55.7	52.8	17.2	17.0	33.1	22.7
		SD	1.1	1.2	3.2	4.7	1.5	0.9	3.1	1.4
	Girls	x̄	49.5	24.2	53.6	51.3	16.8	17.0	33.5	22.5
		SD	1.0	0.8	3.2	3.2	1.1	1.6	3.5	1.9
3	Boys	x̄	51.3	25.9	57.0	53.5	17.6	17.4	33.5	23.5
		SD	1.3	1.3	3.5	5.0	1.6	1.0	3.4	1.6
	Girls	x̄	49.8	24.8	55.6	52.3	17.3	17.0	34.7	23.4
		SD	1.2	1.1	3.6	3.5	1.3	4.1	3.6	1.9
4	Boys	x̄	51.7	25.9	58.0	54.2	17.7	17.7	34.3	23.5
		SD	1.2	1.4	3.2	4.4	1.6	1.0	2.9	1.4
	Girls	x̄	50.2	25.0	57.0	53.5	17.6	18.1	35.5	24.0
		SD	1.7	1.6	4.0	4.6	1.3	1.8	3.7	2.1
5	Boys	x̄	52.2	26.7	60.3	56.7	18.3	18.0	35.9	25.9
		SD	1.2	1.2	4.6	5.5	1.7	1.1	3.4	3.4
	Girls	x̄	50.6	25.3	58.3	53.5	17.8	18.4	36.9	24.7
		SD	1.0	1.1	4.3	3.3	1.2	1.6	3.6	1.9

TABLE 4.8   Somatic Development in Preschool Boys (n = 367) and Girls (n = 397) Followed Longitudinally. First Measurement, 4.4 Years (Boys) and 4.6 Years (Girls). Second Measurement, 1 Year Later. Third Measurement, 5.9 Years (Boys) and/or 6 Years (Girls) (Survey F)

Measurement		1 $\bar{x}$	SD	2 $\bar{x}$	SD	3 $\bar{x}$	SD
Height	Boys	107.7	4.6	115.4	3.0	118.8	2.8
(cm)	Girls	107.2	5.1	116.0	3.4	118.5	3.0
Weight	Boys	18.32	2.11	20.11	1.15	22.49	1.15
(kg)	Girls	17.78	2.41	19.10	1.32	22.31	1.17
BMI	Boys	15.8	1.4	15.02	1.5	15.93	1.3
(kg/m$_2$)	Girls	15.47	1.3	14.20	1.4	15.89	1.6
Circumferences							
Chest	Boys	55.0	2.7	59.0	2.3	59.0	3.1
(cm)	Girls	54.4	3.2	59.9	2.1	56.9	3.3
Waist	Boys	52.6	3.5	55.4	2.1	55.3	2.3
(cm)	Girls	52.0	3.3	54.9	2.2	55.0	2.2
Arm	Boys	17.2	1.4	18.1	1.0	18.3	0.8
(cm)	Girls	17.4	1.7	18.2	1.0	18.9	1.0
Thigh	Boys	32.9	2.9	—	—	34.2	3.1
(cm)	Girls	33.8	3.2	—	—	36.0	3.1

Modified from Pařízková, J. and Kábele, J., *Acta Univ. Carol. Gymnica,* 21, 55, 1985 and from Pařízková, J. and Kábele, J., *Coll. Anthrop.,* 12, 67, 1988.

A longitudinal investigation (survey F) was also made in 367 boys and 397 girls (Table 4.8) who were measured in different districts of the Czech Republic. In this case, only height, weight, BMI, and circumferential measures were evaluated. The results of the longitudinal measurements in this larger sample during about 1 ½ years revealed slightly lower BMI values than those in other groups of children, fluctuating again at approximately the 55th percentile. The average values corresponded roughly to the results of other mentioned investigations.[266–268] The results of the circumferential measurements also showed similar trends of development as in the above mentioned surveys.[242]

III. BODY COMPOSITION AND FAT PATTERN

Preschool age is characterized by a number of changes in physique. There is a trend toward linearity, which is partly reflected by BMI changes. Changes in circumferential measures also indicate variations in different body components, mainly depot fat.

At the age of 7 years, we succeeded in measuring body density using underwater weighing with simultaneous assessment of the air in the lungs and respiratory passages.[227,233] Groups of children from 7 to 16 years of age were followed up using this method.[229–231,233] The utilization of this method was reviewed more recently by Lohman.[198] Only some children who were 7 years old were able to cooperate with the underwater weighing with the simultaneous assessment of air in the lungs and respiratory passages. This procedure requires a good level of cooperation, lack of fear about submerging the head under the water, and control of breathing as instructed by the researcher. Therefore, other methods such as anthropometry, mainly skinfold thickness measurements (which correlate significantly with the percentage of body fat and enable the derivation of regression equations for the estimation of depot fat[229–231,233]), are recommended for younger school children.

More recently these relationships were again validated, and prediction of total body fat was made possible in children 7 to 10 years of age.[381] We may assume the significant correlations between skinfolds and total body fat assessed by densitometry in preschool children, as indicated by the correlations between skinfold thicknesses and body fat measured by body water measurements.[42] Other methods for body composition measurements are mentioned in Chapter 8.

As shown by previous studies, body fat varies markedly since the very beginning of life; the variation coefficients (CV) of the skinfolds, measured during the first 48 hours after birth and during the first year of life were the same as those during later growth and adulthood.[233] At birth, there already were significant sex-linked differences (e.g., a significantly larger suprailiac skinfold in newborn girls[231]) and marked differences among normal, full-term and pre-term children and/or children born from diabetic mothers.[231,233]

Subcutaneous fat changes markedly during the first year of life; first there is a significant increase and later a decrease, especially at the age of about 10 months and older. At that time, children start to walk and generally engage in more physical activity.[233]

A follow-up of the influence of breastfeeding in all our samples was difficult, as the weaning time is generally earlier in our children than in other countries, and the transition to solid food is gradual: children had mixed diets during various periods. Only in survey A did we get some information on the duration of breastfeeding.

Fuertez-Dominguez et al.[118] showed the influence of breast vs. formula feeding — children fed with adapted formula had higher sums of skinfold thicknesses and fat percentage than children who were breastfed. All other anthropometric variables, i.e., (length, weight, Rohrer's index etc.) were not affected. The influence of early weaning in our child population (about 30% of infants are still breastfed at the age of 3 months, and about 10% at the age 6 months) may also be manifested in both BMI and fatness.

The development of fat was followed up by *measurements of ten skinfold thicknesses* using two types of calipers. First, we used a modified caliper designed by Best[30] (1954), which varies from other calipers by the size of contact surfaces and the pressure exerted on the measured skinfold.[230,233] This type of caliper was selected as it makes it possible to check and to adjust the pressure exerted on the measured skinfold, and it is easy to correct; this is important when measuring very young children, especially newborns. (This caliper in our modification also has a greater range of measured values thus making it possible to measure grossly obese subjects where the range of other calipers is not sufficient). The Harpenden caliper[233,347] (which has similar characteristics and therefore gives values comparable to Lange caliper) was also used for the measurements of five skinfolds on the right and left sides.

The selection of skinfolds was meant to characterize the development of subcutaneous fat on the head, neck, trunk, and extremities. In selected surveys (A and C), the percentage of depot fat was also evaluated using Brook's formula[42] and Harpenden caliper values. Bioimpedance analysis was available for our research from the beginning of the 1990s. Without validation for children 3 to 6 years old, we preferred to continue body composition estimations using skinfold thickness measurements.

Changes in individual skinfolds (as measured by modified Best's caliper[30]) with increasing age are presented in Figures 4.2a, 4.2b, 4.2c, 4.2d. This overall trend is characterized by *a decrease of the subcutaneous fat layer in boys.* This is most apparent when we compare the values associated with the sum of skinfolds measured using both calipers in the youngest and oldest boys. *In girls there is a stagnation in the sum of all skinfolds.* At certain sites (under the chin, on the chest, in the abdomen, and in the suprailiac), there is a slight increase but at other sites the skinfolds diminish (cheek, chest, triceps, subscapular skinfolds). The deposition of subcutaneous fat is greater in the cheeks and in the extremities than in the trunk,[256] which differs from the older age categories starting with puberty.[231,233] When estimating fat ratio from skinfolds,[233] it decreased from about 14–13% to 11–10% in boys, remaining about 16% in girls.

There is always more subcutaneous fat in girls, i.e., in practically all cases the values of skinfolds are higher (Figure 4.2a, 4.2b, 4.2c, 4.2d). The differences are more apparent in the trunk. The sex-linked difference in the amount of subcutaneous fat is however manifested already immediately after the birth,[231,233] increasing later. (However, the relatively greatest differences between sexes appear at the time of puberty.[229,231,233])

Skinfold thicknesses measured by the Harpenden caliper (Table 4.9a) vary from the values ascertained by the modified Best's caliper which results from different parameters of the calipers.[233] (It is possible to convert the results assessed by one caliper to the results corresponding of measurements by an other caliper.[233]) This gives the researcher the opportunity to compare data assessed by different calipers. Measurements by the Harpenden caliper give higher values on the left side as compared to right side. In our group the number of left-sided children was low and laterality was not definitely accomplished; nevertheless the more loaded side of the body had a smaller layer of subcutaneous fat (Table 4.9b).

The fat pattern and **distribution** was evaluated with the help of indices relating the skinfolds on the trunk to those on the extremities — subscapular/triceps skinfold (i.e., "centrality index") and index, including all skinfolds on the trunk to all skinfolds on the extremities (cheek + chin + triceps + thigh

+ calf/chest 1 + 2, subscapular + abdomen + suprailac skinfolds). As evident from the average values (Figures 4.3a, 4.3b, 4.3c) the *fat pattern does not change markedly during the period of preschool age.* The centrality index decreases slightly from 3 to 5 years and then increases again at the age of 6 in boys and in girls when the skinfolds were measured using a modified Best caliper. The trend in the changes of the same index, calculated from the values of skinfolds measured with the Harpenden caliper, is the same in girls, but there is a decrease in boys. The evaluation of the second index (relating all skinfolds measured on the trunk and on the extremities), revealed a small fluctuation in boys and an increase in girls (Figures 4.3a, 4.3b, 4.3c).[254]

When we measured *five skinfolds by the Harpenden caliper* in the longitudinal study (survey E), covering a similar growth period, *a decrease in the sum of all skinfolds was again found for boys and a stagnation of values in girls* (Table 4.10). Repeated measurement of skinfolds in the same children confirmed the conclusions based on cross-sectional measurements of subcutaneous fat.[242] The centrality index changed very slightly both in boys and girls, i.e., the fat pattern remained more or less the same during preschool years. As mentioned above, genetic factors have an impact on fat distribution,[7] as shown by longitudinal studies.[172,233]

A comparison of the average values of the individual skinfold thicknesses measured in late 1950s[229–231,233] and in the present studies did not show the increase of subcutaneous fat in preschool children. An increase, however, was shown for children between the ages of 4.5 and 11.99 years in the UK measured in 1972, 1982, and 1990, respectively; these changes were associated with an increase in parental BMIs and decrease in family size.[41]

IV. SOMATOTYPES

The somatotype is a description of the morphological state of the individual at a given moment. It is expressed using a 3-digit evaluation comprised of three consecutive numbers always listed in the same order. Each number represents the evaluation of one of the three basic components of the figure and expresses individual variations in the morphology and composition of the human body. The procedure by Heath and Carter was used.[47,154]

The first component (1), **endomorphy**, relates to the relative adiposity of subjects; it relates also to thinness. This means that endomorphy expresses the amount of subcutaneous fat on a continuum from the lowest to the highest values.

The second component (2), **mesomorphy**, relates to the relative skeletal muscle development in relation to height. The second component appraises skeletal muscle development on a continuum from the lowest to the highest values. Mesomorphy may be considered lean body mass in relation to height.

The third component (3), **ectomorphy**, relates to the relative length of parts of the body. Assessment of the third component is based mainly on the index of the ratio of height to the cubic root of body weight. This index and

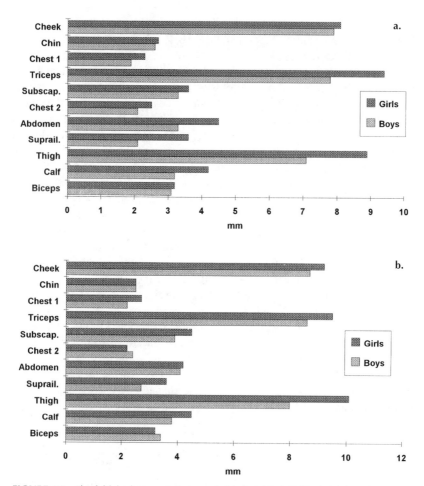

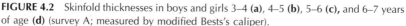

FIGURE 4.2 Skinfold thicknesses in boys and girls 3–4 (**a**), 4–5 (**b**), 5–6 (**c**), and 6–7 years of age (**d**) (survey A; measured by modified Bests's caliper).

the assessment of the ectomorphic component are closely related. The lower end of the range implies the relative shortness of various bodily dimensions and the upper end implies the relative length of various bodily dimensions.

The extreme values are at the end of each series (a continuum). This means that the low values of the endomorphic component describe an individual with a small amount of body fat, while a high value describes an individual with a large amount of fat. A low value of the mesomorphic component describes an individual with a small frame and poorly developed musculature, while a high value of this component implies marked muscular development. Low values of the ectomorphic component describe subjects with relatively short extremities and a low grade of the index height $\sqrt[3]{\mathrm{weight}}$,

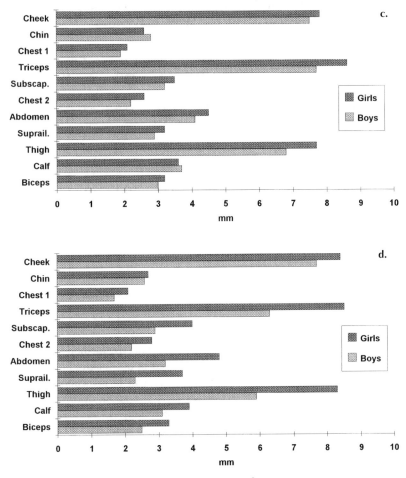

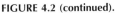

FIGURE 4.2 (continued).

while a high value of this component describes a subject with relatively long extremities and relatively long segments of the whole body with a high index.

The following data are needed for ratings: height, weight, four skinfolds (triceps, subscapular, suprailiac, calf), two bone diameters (humerus, femur), two muscle circumferences (calf, flexed arm), age and revised HWR table (height $\sqrt[3]{\text{weight}}$). The usual form for the evaluation of somatotype, as presented by Heath and Carter,[154,47] was used for preschool children, i.e., for our longitudinal study (boys n = 38, girls n = 22; survey E; see Tables 4.7a, 4.7b, 4.7c, 4.7d), and then also on the occasion of the second measurement of 367 boys and 397 girls measured in different districts of The Czech Republic (survey F; see Table 4.8).

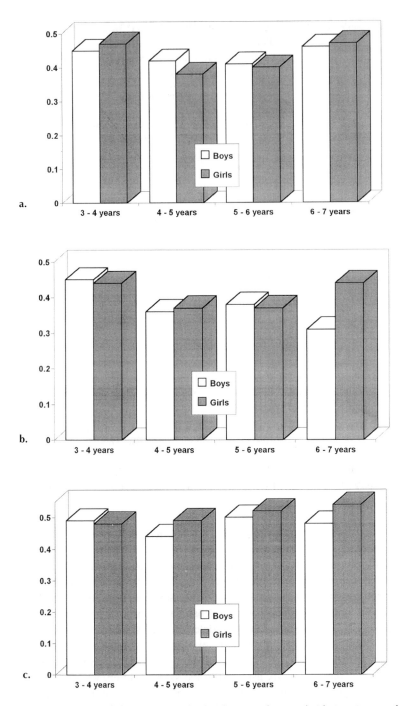

FIGURE 4.3   Indices of subcutaneous fat distribution in boys and girls 3 to 6 years of age as measured by modified Best's caliper (**a**) and Harpenden caliper (**b**), centrality index, i.e., subscapular/triceps), and by Best's caliper (**c**, index relating 5 skinfolds on the trunk/5 skinfolds on the extremities, see Figure 4.2 and Table 4.9a; survey A).

TABLE 4.10 **Skinfold Thicknesses (mm) Measured Longitudinally Five Times by Harpenden Caliper in Preschool Children (Survey E)**

Measure-ment			Triceps	Subscapular	Suprailiac	Calf
1	Boys	$\bar{x}$	9.5	5.6	4.3	5.1
		SD	2.6	2.0	1.7	1.8
	Girls	$\bar{x}$	10.0	6.1	5.2	6.0
		SD	2.4	1.9	2.5	1.8
2	Boys	$\bar{x}$	9.3	5.3	4.5	4.9
		SD	3.5	1.9	3.4	2.2
	Girls	$\bar{x}$	10.0	5.9	4.5	4.9
		SD	2.8	1.9	3.4	2.2
3	Boys	$\bar{x}$	8.9	5.5	4.6	4.8
		SD	3.2	2.7	3.4	2.3
	Girls	$\bar{x}$	9.7	6.3	4.9	5.5
		SD	2.7	3.7	3.0	2.1
4	Boys	$\bar{x}$	8.2	5.0	4.1	4.3
		SD	2.7	2.3	3.5	2.2
	Girls	$\bar{x}$	9.8	6.5	4.1	5.2
		SD	3.1	4.6	3.0	2.1
5	Boys	$\bar{x}$	8.3	5.5	4.4	4.3
		SD	3.3	3.2	3.3	2.1
	Girls	$\bar{x}$	10.0	6.4	5.0	5.3
		SD	3.3	4.6	3.8	2.3

TABLE 4.11a **Somatotypes Evaluated Longitudinally 5 Times in Preschool Children (Survey E)**

Measure-ment		Endomorphy		Mesomorphy		Ectomorphy	
		$\bar{x}$	SD	$\bar{x}$	SD	$\bar{x}$	SD
1	Boys	1.50	0.60	5.64	0.49	1.22	0.56
	Girls	2.31	0.87	5.50	0.79	1.06	0.57
2	Boys	1.37	0.86	5.45	0.66	1.37	0.53
	Girls	2.12	1.04	5.59	0.66	1.19	0.54
3	Boys	1.39	1.05	5.33	0.71	1.74	0.78
	Girls	2.20	1.03	5.43	0.79	1.47	0.79
4	Boys	1.21	1.02	5.08	0.78	2.09	0.73
	Girls	2.06	1.18	5.19	0.83	1.62	0.82
5	Boys	1.28	1.30	5.03	0.74	2.25	0.94
	Girls	2.11	1.08	4.88	0.54	2.15	0.82

Compiled from Pařízková, J., et al., *Humanbiol. Budapest,* 16, 113, 1985.

For the evaluation of body posture, a simple scale was chosen which enabled on assessment in larger population samples under field conditions. This procedure was developed by Jaros and Lomicek (see Reference 256) During the evaluation, we first ask the child, "Show how you can stand up

TABLE 4.11b Somatotypes Evaluated at the Occasion of Second Measurement of a Longitudinal Study of 367 Boys and 397 Girls, at the Age of 5.4 Years (Boys), and 5.6 Years (Girls) (See Table 4.8) (Survey F)

		Components					
Measure-ment		**Endomorphy**		**Mesomorphy**		**Ectomorphy**	
		$\bar{x}$	SD	$\bar{x}$	SD	$\bar{x}$	SD
2	Boys	1.74	0.23	5.06	0.64	2.54	0.31
	Girls	1.81	0.37	5.15	0.79	2.67	0.41

Modified from Pařízková, J. and Kábele, J., *Acta Univ. Carol. Gymnica,* 21, 55, 1985 and from Pařízková, J. and Kábele, J., *Coll. Anthrop.,* 12, 67, 1988.

before the start of exercise!" The child's posture is evaluated from the profile and from the back. If the child stands up in a stiff manner, he/she is asked to perform some simple exercises or to say something about his/her family, etc. During the evaluation, different signs were marked on the record card in three grades (1 to 3; see Appendix 1). The depth of the cervical and lumbar lordosis was given in centimeters of the deviation from a plummet dropped from the back of the child's nape. In some instances, evaluation of the abdominal wall was facilitated by dropping a plummet from the breast bone.

The lowest score (1) was the best, and the highest (3) was the poorest. Not only was the ratio of different grades in boys and girls in individual age groups used but also average values which made the statistical evaluation easier. First we evaluated body posture in the cross-sectional study of 3- to 6-year-old children in Prague (n = 238, survey A).[256]

The position of the neck (Table 4.12) was most frequently evaluated by grade 1 followed by grade 2; the worst score was only observed exceptionally. There was a trend towards somewhat poorer results in girls, but a significant difference was only recorded in 5- to 6-year-old children. The position of the back and the evaluation of the outline of the abdomen was worse; grade 2 predominated. There was a somewhat poorer trend in girls. Score 3 was again observed exceptionally.

The depth of the cervical and lumbar *lordosis* was evaluated in centimeters. Mean values are given in Table 4.12. There was a trend toward higher values in girls. ***The position of the shoulders and back*** was expressed by gradest 1 to 3, with the *average value expressing the mean grade.* No marked sex-linked differences were found. An evaluation of the ***shape of the spine*** from the back view in a standing position and when bent forward points up, however, markedly better results in girls when evaluated bent forward. These results are, in almost every age group, statistically significant. In both types of evaluations, the spine grade 1 predominates, which demonstrates the most favorable result.

TABLE 4.12   Body Posture in Preschool Children (1, Best; 3, Poorest Level; Depth of Cervical and Lumbar Lordosis in cm; Spine 1, Evaluated in Erect Position; Spine 2, When Bent Forward) (Survey A)

		Age (years)							
		3–4		4–5		5–6		6–7	
		Boys	Girls	Boys	Girls	Boys	Girls	Boys	Girls
Neck	$\bar{x}$	1.06	1.13	1.48	1.54	1.50	1.80	1.60	1.75
	SD	0.4	0.34	0.51	0.51	0.51	0.50	0.50	0.44
Back	$\bar{x}$	1.79	1.65	1.74	1.88	0.77	2.00	2.07	2.19
	SD	0.48	0.45	0.45	0.34	0.50	0.29	0.46	0.40
Abdomen	$\bar{x}$	1.56	1.74	1.96	1.67	1.77	1.8	1.80	1.94
	SD	0.61	0.45	0.36	0.48	0.43	0.50	0.41	0.44
Cervical lordosis	$\bar{x}$	2.69	2.87	2.91	3.10	3.25	3.50	3.30	3.31
	SD	0.62	0.07	0.75	0.66	0.66	0.94	0.75	0.47
Lumbar lordosis	$\bar{x}$	2.62	2.97	2.2	2.33	2.37	2.56	3.0	3.06
	SD	0.78	0.68	0.76	0.54	0.78	1.04	0.50	0.77
Shoulders	$\bar{x}$	1.53	1.35	1.91	1.71	1.73	1.88	1.60	1.88
	SD	0.56	0.48	0.59	0.62	0.52	0.72	0.50	0.62
Scapulae	$\bar{x}$	1.62	1.43	1.73	1.63	1.60	1.72	1.73	1.56
	SD	0.55	0.50	0.45	0.57	0.50	0.68	0.59	0.51
Spine 1	$\bar{x}$	1.24	1.00	1.30	1.08	1.17	1.44	1.07	1.13
	SD	0.43	0.00	0.47	0.28	0.38	0.58	0.26	0.34
Spine 2	$\bar{x}$	1.03	1.00	1.13	1.00	1.13	1.08	1.13	1.00
	SD	0.17	0.00	0.34	0.00	0.34	0.27	0.35	0.00

The worst results were recorded when evaluating the ***position of the back*** (view from profile) where grade 2 was most frequent. The same applied to ***the outline of the abdomen***. The average evaluation of the position of the shoulders (view from back) was not favorable either: grade 2 was less frequent than in the case of the back and spine. The frequency of grade 3 was a total of 7.4% of all cases, which implies a markedly impaired position of the shoulders.[256]

At this young age the impaired position of the spine was not yet associated with the impaired shape of the spine, but from the prognostic aspect, it is possible that the development of mild and later more severe scoliosis may be foreseen unless marked improvement occurs soon.

The above mentioned deviations are obviously due to an impaired and inadequate muscular tonus, as indicated also by the outline of the ***abdominal wall***, suggesting general marked flabbiness of the musculature. ***Protruding scapulae*** and ***an increased lumbar lordosis*** are other consequences of an inadequate muscular tonus.

Comparison of different age groups indicates that *posture further deteriorates with advancing age.* The depth of the cervical and lumbar lordosis increases significantly and ensues in particular, based on a comparison of the youngest age group (3 to 4 years) and the oldest one (6 to 7 years). This increase in the depth of lordosis is not only associated with the generally increasing bodily dimensions, but also with further deterioration of body posture with age. This is apparent in particular from the comparison of the youngest and oldest children as regarding the position of the neck and the outline of the back, shoulders, and abdomen. The older the child, the poorer the posture. This applies to both girls and boys.

In a large sample of 2839 boys and 2759 girls aged 6.4 years (survey B), body posture was also evaluated (Table 4.13). The results varied; in some items the results were better in boys (neck, abdomen); in others there were no differences (e.g., depth of cervical and lumbar lordosis). In some instances girls had better results (outline of the scapulae, shoulders, shape of the spine). There were also some differences related to environmental conditions (see Chapter 9).

**TABLE 4.13   Body Posture in 5598
Preschool Boys and Girls
(See Table 4.4) (Survey B)**

	Boys		Girls	
	$\bar{x}$	SD	$\bar{x}$	SD
Neck (grade)	1.28	0.47	1.34	0.49
Back (grade)	1.55	0.54	1.47	0.54
Abdomen (grade)	1.68	0.51	1.69	0.52
Cervical lordosis (cm)	2.0	1.00	2.00	1.00
Lumbar lordosis (cm)	3.0	0.90	3.00	1.00
Shoulders (grade)	1.28	0.49	1.26	0.49
Scapulae (grade)	1.40	0.45	1.31	0.49
Spine 1 (grade)	1.24	0.45	1.17	0.44
Spine 2 (grade)	1.28	0.47	1.23	0.44

A comparison of the results from our study with those assembled in the 1950s revealed, e.g., the mean value of cervical and lumbar lordosis increased and that new standards must be elaborated.[254] The changes were due to accelerated somatic development and to the increase in bodily dimensions of children equal in age, then and now; however, the generally greater weakness of skeletal muscles resulting from the lifestyle changes — especially from a reduced opportunity for spontaneous games and outdoor exercise — are considered as the main cause of poor body posture. This is more marked in larger urban agglomerations than in smaller communities (see Chapter 9).

We wanted to validate the findings on the deterioration of body posture during preschool years. Therefore, some of the children were followed up longitudinally (survey E; n = 58; see Tables 4.7a, 4.7b, 4.7c, 4.7d, 4.10, 4.11a). Body posture was evaluated using the same procedure of Jaros and Lomicek.[256]

Longitudinal observations confirmed the above mentioned results and conclusions: *with advancing age body posture deteriorated in the same children in all items* mentioned above. An unequal level of the shoulders and a protruding scapulae and abdominal wall, as compared to the thorax, were found in a greater proportion of the children during the last measurement at the age of 6 years and more frequently than during the first measurement, i.e., at the age of 3 years.[266]

Deteriorated body posture, due mainly to an inadequate muscle tone, resulting from insufficient motor stimulation and lack of exercise *during pre-school years deserves much greater attention than it has had up to now.* Adequate measures for the prevention of poor body posture, or at least a reduction of its deterioration has to start sooner than was originally assumed. For this reason, a proper system of motor stimulation and exercise should be introduced as early as possible.

V. RELATIONSHIP BETWEEN HEIGHT AND WEIGHT OF PARENTS AND ANTHROPOMETRIC VARIABLES OF PRESCHOOL AGE CHILDREN

In survey A, the height and weight of parents of children from day care centers was also assessed. In both parents, significant relationships between total height of father and mother, on the one hand, and total and sitting height and length measures of the extremities (acromion-radiale and iliospinale-tibiale) of boys and girls from 3 to 6 year, on the other hand, are most often found.

Correlations were much more frequent between the anthropometric variables of children and the height and weight of the mother than between those of the father. The father's height correlated significantly with the child's total and sitting height, weight, and waist circumference. The weight of the father correlated significantly with child's total and sitting height, waist circumference, and with the biiliocristal and femoral condyle breadth.[256]

The height of the mother correlated significantly with the child's total and sitting height, weight, circumferences of the head, neck, abdomen, forearm, thigh, calf, and with biacromial, biiliocristal, hand, femoral condyles, and ankle breadth. The mother's weight correlated significantly with total and sitting height, weight, circumferences of neck, chest, abdomen, arm, forearm, thigh, calf, and with biacromial, biiliocristal, hand, femoral condyles and ankle breadth. The relationships were weak ($r = 0.2 - 0.39$) but significant (mostly $p < 0.01$) and consistent, both in the whole sample and/or in individual age groups of boys and girls. In age and sex subgroups these relationships were similar, except for lower significance due to the smaller number of analyzed individuals.[256]

VII. OTHER SURVEYS

Numerous longitudinal studies revealed that the earlier a child develops a certain degree of fat depot ratio, the more it is possible that he/she will be fat later in life; e.g., Siervogel et al.[329] showed that weight/stature^2 at an early age correlates significantly with that at the age of 18 years. Roland-Cachera et al.[299-307] concluded the same on the basis of the evaluations in her longitudinal studies of BMI.

As reviewed by Kuczmarski et al.,[188] the *increasing prevalence of obesity* among U.S. adolescents and adults shown in the National Health and Nutrition Examination Surveys 1960–1991 indicates that the prevention of obesity early in life has become even more urgent than before.

Insulin-like growth factor-I (IGF-I) has been studied insufficiently up to now in spite of its dependence on nutrition and the possible changes that may explain a number of phenomena concerning growth. However, Wilson et al.[390] found no relationships between nutritional indicators (BMI, skinfolds, waist/hip ratio, height, weight) and dietary intake (energy, protein, fat, carbohydrates) in adolescents. However, children within normal nutritional status were followed up in this study, so there is a question as to how these relationships would manifest when malnourished and/or obese children were included. Preschool children were not followed up.

Longitudinal studies of French children led to the conclusion that the early production of IGF-1 triggering cell multiplication in all tissues precociously shows a positive association with an increased intake of protein in early childhood.[307] This is consistent with the acceleration of maturity in obese children, in which early rebound of BMI and adiposity were observed. On the other hand, when dietary intake is reduced, plasma concentration of growth hormones is increased while IGF-1 is decreased. Excess protein intake in early childhood causes obvious chronic increases of IGF-1, which reduces growth hormone levels and slows down growth in the obese.[299,307]

VIII. GENERAL CONSIDERATIONS

Growth and development during preschool age is characterized by differentiated changes of individual anthropometric variables; the greatest changes occur in length dimensions and in body weight. Breadth and circumferential measurements on the trunk and extremities change relatively less. The smallest change occurs in the head circumference, which also shows the smallest variability. Along with that, body proportionality also changes significantly. Body fat is the only variable that stagnates (in girls) or decreases (in boys); fat patterns remain nearly the same, similar to the somatotype. All of these morphological changes are related to the variations of functional development during that period. Sex-linked differences are already evident in a number of variables.

Body posture already starts to deteriorate during the preschool period. This was confirmed by both cross-sectional and longitudinal measurements. Anthropometric variables of children are significantly related to the height and weight of parents, showing genetic predispositions in preschool children similarly as fat pattern mentioned in previous Chapter 3.

When comparing the results of the measurements at the beginning of seventies and at the end of eighties, there was a trend toward slight growth acceleration and the slenderization of preschoolers. Skinfold thicknesses did not change markedly. BMI values, especially those from the beginning of the 1970s, were higher than those measured in Czech children in 1895 or as BMI values of French children.

Chapter 5

NUTRITIONAL STATUS AND DIETARY INTAKE IN EARLY LIFE

Food intake corresponding to one's needs is a prerequisite for adequate growth and development as well as for desirable nutritional status, a condition for an adequate level of functional capacity and fitness. All of this applies even more to early childhood.

"How much is enough"[377,378,380,387] (or too little or too much) is difficult to define. From the beginning of life, *"nutritional individuality"*[383] is manifested in newborns and infants. Pediatricians claim that newborns already behave in a different way during the first breastfeeding (the same applies to motor activity, crying, etc.). Some newborns accept the mother's breast quietly, drinking enough milk, while others often refuse an adequate amount. These characteristics often persist and are manifested even more markedly later in life.

During the first year of life, variability in both absolute and relative energy intake in infants was shown. Black et al.[33] showed that the variation coefficients in energy intake of infants from 2 to 18 months were between 16.9 to 23.3% (between subjects) and 10.6 to 18.1% (within subject). Bellu et al.[22] also showed a great variability of energy intake in Italian infants. Intra- and inter-individual variability ratios were found even greater than 1.

"Sensitive periods" exist in the first 2 or 3 years of life, during which humans acquire basic knowledge on what foods are safe to eat. Analyzed by Cashdan,[48] the willingness to eat a variety of foods is greatest between the ages of 1 to 2 years, declining to low levels at 4 years of age. This implies the ability *to influence the food choice early in life* in a positive or negative way, with possible delayed consequences or advantages.

The requirements for energy and protein of children are similarly specified for all other age categories; adhering to the RDAs, which correspond to the actual needs of the growing organism, is also essential in light of the future development of health. Presented information on RDAs for energy, macro-components, minerals, and vitamins were selected with respect to early age.[393–398]

I. ENERGY REQUIREMENTS

The energy requirement of an individual relates to the level of energy intake from food, which will balance energy expenditure when the individual has body size and composition and a level of physical activity consistent with long-term good health. This will allow for the maintenance of necessary and socially desirable physical activity. In children and in pregnant and lactating women, the energy requirement includes the energy needs associated with the deposition of tissues or with the secretion of milk at rates consistent with good health. This is a definition that the World Health Organization presented in the Report of a Joint FAO/WHO/UNU (Food and Agricultural Organization and United Nations University) Expert Committee, which met at FAO in Rome in 1981, which was then published by WHO in Geneva in 1985[393] and confirmed in the Report of the Scientific Committee for Food, nutrient, and energy intakes for the European Community.[398] Very few modifications have been presented since then. James and Schofield[166] elaborated further on the principles of defining the recommended energy allowances, especially with respect to physical activity, resulting energy output, and its balance with energy intake.

All requirement estimates refer to needs persisting over moderate periods of time. The corresponding intakes may be referred to as "habitual" or "usual" in order to distinguish them from intakes on a particular day. However, as a matter of convention and convenience, they are expressed on an intake basis. There is no implication, though,that these amounts must be consumed each day.[393]

Energy requirements should be defined so as to correspond to the real needs of the individual.[387] Once the level of body weight and physical activity has been fixed and the appropriate growth rate defined, there is only one level of intake at which energy balance can be achieved. As a result, this becomes that individual's requirement for energy. Even some degree of adaptation is possible, but it is assumed that such a range is fairly narrow.[393] Therefore, it is desirable to define, as exactly as possible, individual recommended energy allowances.

In case the intake is either above or below the requirement, a change in body energy stores should be expected unless energy expenditure is correspondingly altered. If such changes in expenditure do not occur, the energy store, mainly in the form of adipose tissue, will increase when the intake exceeds requirement, and decrease when it is bellow requirement.

It would be contradictory to general experience to suppose that for each individual there is one fixed set-point for body weight and adipose tissue mass compatible to adequate health. In fact, for any individual there is probably a range of acceptable body weights. However, if the imbalance is too great or continues over very long periods, the resulting changes in body weight and composition can be detrimental to function and health. In conjunction with this, risks may appear which are associated with intakes either above or below actual requirements.

Body size is the *major determinant* of the absolute requirements for energy. Variations in size are probably more significant quantitatively than metabolic adaptations. The acceptable ranges in body size were already discussed, tables of weight, height, and BMI standards as established in different parts of the world are presented (see Table 4.1, Table 5.1a and 5.1b; see Figures 4.1a, 4.1b).

TABLE 5.1a Body Weight for Children

	Boys			Girls		
Age years	−2 SD	x̄	+2 SD	−2 SD	x̄	+2 SD
3	11.4	14.6	18.3	11.2	14.1	18.0
4	12.9	16.7	20.8	12.6	16.0	20.7
5	14.4	18.7	23.5	13.8	17.7	23.2
6	16.0	20.7	26.6	15.0	19.5	26.2
7	17.6	22.9	30.2	16.3	21.8	30.2

Adapted from the World Health Organization, *Diet, Nutrition and the Prevention of Chronic Diseases,* Techn. Rep. Ser., No. 797, World Health Organization, Geneva, 1990.

TABLE 5.1b Mean Values for Height and Weight in European Children

	Height (cm)		Weight (kg)	
Age (years)	Boys	Girls	Boys	Girls
3.5	96.0	95.0	15.0	14.0
4.5	106.5	105.5	17.5	17.0
5.5	112.5	111.5	19.5	19.5
6.5	119.0	118.0	22.0	21.5
7.5	124.5	123.5	24.5	24.0

Modified from *Nutrient and Energy Intakes for the European Community,* Report of the Scientific Committee for Food, 31st Series, Directorate-General, Industry, Office for Official Publications, Luxembourg, 1993.

Although the energy and protein requirements for the process of growth are relatively small compared to those for maintenance (except in the young infant), *satisfactory growth is nevertheless a sensitive criterion for whether the energy and protein needs are being met or not.* Therefore, *the definition of satisfactory growth* is the *first and most important initial step.*[393]

As mentioned above, there is a dilemma as to whether reference standards for the growth of children in industrialized countries should be accepted universally, as relevant, or whether local standards should be used.[393] Differences were found even in the framework of an industrially developed country — children from larger urban agglomerations are usually bigger and more advanced in growth and development.[236,238,242]

Estimates of requirements based on body size are, however, an approximation, since they do not take into account body composition which may finally determine the requirements. In recent decades, the emergence of numerous methods for the estimation of body composition in living subjects (see Chapter 8) has resulted in observations on several thousand people, ranging from newborn infants to the elderly.

The neonate averages 14% of depot fat, which has gradually accumulated during the last period of pregnancy. Children of diabetic mothers are not only larger, but also have greater amount of body fat.[231,233] During the first year of life, depot fat rises to about 23% and then declines to 18% at 6 years of age.[152] This applies both to total and to subcutaneous fat, measured as skinfold thickness using a caliper.[231,233] Girls always have larger absolute amounts and relative amounts of depot fat, and this difference increases with advancing age. Individual differences in body composition may cause different energy and protein requirements in spite of the same body size. The proportion of internal organs, which have a much higher metabolic level, is considerably greater in early childhood than later on (Table 5.2).

TABLE 5.2   Metabolic Rates (MR) of Organs and Tissues in Man

	Newborn			Adult		
Organ	Weight (kg)	MR/day kcal (kJ)	% of whole body MR	Weight (kg)	MR/day kcal (kJ)	% of whole body MR
Liver	0.14	42 (176)	20	1.6	482 (2017)	27
Brain	035	84 (325)	44	1.4	338 (1414)	19
Heart	0.02	8 (33)	4	0.32	122 (510)	7
Kidney	0.024	15 (63)	7	0.29	187 (782)	10
Muscle	0.8	9 (38)	5	30.00	324 (1356)	18
Rest (by difference)	—	—	20	—	—	19
Total	3.5	197 (824)	100	70.00	1800 (7530)	100

Organ weights taken from Boyd.[41]

Metabolic rates for the neonate estimated by assuming that the metabolic rate of each organ per unit weight is the same as in the adult. The total activities of the tissues listed are expressed as fractions of the total basal energy expenditure in the adult and the neonate. The total basal metabolic rate in the neonate approximates to that measured by Benedict and Talbot;[24] no data on children 3 to 6 years of age are available.

Adapted from Boyd, E., in *Growth, Including Reproduction and Morphological Development,* Altman, P.L. and Dittmer, D.S., Eds., Washington, D.C., Federation of *American Societies for Experimental Biology,* 1962, 346; and from Benedict, F.G. and Talbot, F.B., *Metabolism and Growth from Birth to Puberty.* Washington, D.C., Carnegie Institute, Publ. No. 302, 1921.

The impact of free body mass and gender on the resting energy expenditures of children was similar to those in adult age,[133–135] i.e., the evaluation of body composition contributes substantially to the definition of energy requirement in childhood.

Assessment of energy needs[166] is based on energy expenditure. Therefore, estimates of energy requirements should be based on measurements of energy expenditure during differing periods of time and during various activities. Under conditions of dynamically changing physical activity (which are usual in small children),[133] it is very difficult to obtain exact data even when sophisticated methods (such as doubly labeled water — $^2H_2^{18}O$) are available. The the only feasible approach, then, is to estimate requirements from measurements of intake, provided that the usual growth rate of height and weight is preserved.[128] Detailed questionnaires on physical activity for parents and caretakers, e.g., teachers from day care centers, help to differentiate and categorize children when used for longer periods of time.[270]

It cannot be assumed that observed expenditure or intake levels always represent what is desirable for the maintenance of health.[52] In developing countries actual intakes may be too low to allow for what has been previously described as "leisure time" activity or "discretionary" activity. On the other hand, in the industrially developed countries the actual intake is usually excessive, and the same applies to the recommended energy allowances.[289] Moreover, in affluent societies many subjects, including young children, may be less physically active than what is considered desirable for ensuring cardiovascular health.

The basal metabolic rate (BMR) is the metabolic rate measured at optimal mental and physical rest conditions, at a comfortable temperature, 12 to 14 hours after the last meal. The metabolic rate during sleep is even lower, so the metabolic rate measured under the thesethese conditions is also defined as the resting metabolic rate.

The energy requirement per kilograms of body weight varies markedly during the lifespan. In children, the change of BMR per kilograms of body weight with age is much greater than in adults, i.e., about 5% per year between 3 and 10 years. Presently, we do not know to what extent this reflects an age-related change per se or age-related changes in body composition. The BMR per unit of weight also varies with weight and BMI: within a given age range, the BMR per kilograms is higher in short, light, and lean individuals and is lower in taller, heavier ones. For practical purposes, then, the most useful index is body weight.

Until recently, many regression equations have been used for the estimation of the resting metabolic rate, the results of which are indirect calorimetry assessments made 50 to 60 years ago. These equations were validated with new measurements of resting energy metabolism in children 5 to 16 years old and compared: the Harris-Benedict and new equations were elaborated due to the WHO/FAO/UNU expert Committee.[393] Those published by James and Schofield[166] were in best agreement with the recent measurements of many authors including Firouzbakhsh et al.[110]

Numerous mathematical analyses were tested; e.g., the conventional use of surface area or inclusion of height made no significant difference in the accuracy of prediction. Different types of equations were tested (linear, quadratic, logarithmic, etc.). The more complex functions added nothing to the accuracy of prediction. Therefore, in each age-sex group the BMR was estimated from the body weight by the simple linear equation:

Boys 3 to 10 years: kcal/day = 22.7 weight − 495 (SD = ±62)

Girls 3 to 10 years: kcal/day = 22.5 weight − 499 (SD = ±63)

These equations were also used for the estimation of BMR and for the evaluation of total energy output (adding multiples of BMR for various activities) in our studies of small children.[393]

The changes in body composition with age markedly affect energy requirements since some organs are metabolically more active than the others. Table 5.2 shows a comparison between a newborn and an adult; e.g., the neonate brain comprises about 10% of the total body weight and may account for 44% of the total energy needs of the child under basal conditions.[24] On the other hand, the energy needs for muscle metabolism at this time are very low because of the relatively small muscle mass (see Table 5.2). Data on preschool children are not available.

Some studies attempt to assess possible ethnic differences in BMR. Spurr et al.[340] measured BMR in both control and undernourished boys and girls in underprivileged areas of Cali, Colombia, but these failed to reveal any differences which could not be related to the nutritional status or to climatic conditions.

Other items in the estimation of energy requirement is *the energy cost of growth*, which includes two components: the energy value of the tissue or product formed and the energy cost of synthetizing it. The total cost will, therefore, depend on the composition of such a tissue. The energy value is the heat of combustion, without the deductions for losses in urine and feces, which are allowed for by the Atwater factors. The average values for protein, fat, and carbohydrates are 5.7, 9.3, and 4.3 kcal, respectively (24, 39, and 18 kJ) per g.[393]

In young children, a rounded-off value of energy cost *5 kcal (21 kJ) per g of tissue increment* has been widely accepted.[334] In contrast to this, a higher figure is obtained in adults for the energy cost of weight gain under different conditions. This may be because relatively more fat is laid down. However, even during growth the weight increments may have quite a different composition in children living under various conditions of dietary intake, physical activity, etc.

In the case of growth spurts, very little or no fat is laid down. This also applies to preschool age. As described in the previous chapter, skinfold thickness decreases in boys and remains stable in girls, which mainly indicates the development of lean body mass.[233]

Energy output resulting from physical activity and work vary according to age. In children, it is determined by habitual physical tasks and play. The degree of energy output depends on the *intensity and duration of such activities*. This may be estimated using *multiples of BMR*.

The calculations in children and youth are more difficult because during the same physical task, *growing subjects increase their energy output in relation to the BMR relatively less than adults.* Studies concerning age differences in the relative increase of energy output during the same work load started at the age of 12 years.[240,257] It was shown that for example during a work load of 2 w/kg body weight on a bicycle ergometer with a 11.8-year-old boy the energy output equals 5.91 BMR and in a 17.8-year-old boy is 7.18 BMR, which is 21% higher. When we compare the youngest boys with a 25.1-year-old man, where the BMR multiple during the same work load equals 7.76, the difference is 31%. These differences may be part of the reason for the lower level of spontaneous physical activity with advancing age: the strain during the same work load is relatively greater in older subjects due to a relatively greater increase of energy output in relation to BMR. This also imposes a greater demand on all systems engaged during increased work load and higher physical activity in older subjects, and vice versa for children.[240]

There are no comparable data in small children where such work loading would be possible. However, it may be assumed that especially during spontaneous dynamic activity such as running and playing, the relative increase in energy output is also correspondingly lower than in older children and/or in adults. During spontaneous play, telemetric measurements reveal to an increase in heart rate up to 220 heart beats per minute.[186,187] In the adults, the heart rate of 200 or more is considered the maximal value during a maximal work load. When we compare these maximal values with basal values at rest in children (i.e., about 100 to 115 beats/minute), we can again see that the difference between them is much smaller than in older subjects.

From these observations, it may be deduced that in small children the values of multiples of BMR which characterize the energy output during various activities will be probably different, i.e. lower than in older age categories. The validation of these multiples, however, has not yet been made in preschoolers. The example of the estimate of energy output is presented by WHO[393] for the energy requirement of a 4-year-old child (Table 5.3).

Recommendations for the energy intake established for the European Community (E.C.)[398] are based on the same principle and procedure. The E.C. document also gives direct estimates for an average energy intake of preschool children (Table 5.4).

Recently, more data on energy expenditure measured with the help of doubly labelled water are available.[75,76,288] In our studies, we used BMR multiples estimated from the increments of heart rate at rest, during moderate activity, and maximal values during spontaneous play.[186,187,233,256]

Children can manage with considerably lower energy intake compared to the actual recommended dietary allowances (RDAs) for this age category without growth deficits.[288] On the other hand, a higher energy intake does not cause most actual cases of overweight. Another question remains, however: how will such discrepancies between energy intake and output be manifested in the long run? It is also known that children with insufficient energy intake

TABLE 5.3 Example of the Estimation of the Daily Energy Expenditure of a 4.5-Year-Old Boy (Body Weight 18 kg)

Activity	hours	kcal	kJ
Sleep at 1.0 × BMR	12	456	1884
Kindergarten			
light activity at 1.2 × BMR	3.0	137	565
moderate activity at 1.9 × BMR	3.5	253	1044
high activity at 5.0 × BMR	0.5	95	392
Home			
light activity at 1.3 × BMR	2.5	123	510
moderate activity at 2.0 × BMR	2.0	152	628
high activity at 5.0 × BMR	0.5	95	395
Growth	—	80	334
Total requirement per 24 hours at 1.31 × BMR	24.0	1391	5752

Note: BMR estimated to be 913 kcal/day, 38 kcal/hod (3.82 MJ/day, i.e., 157 kJ/hod) using the regression equation of BMR of the E.C.[398] The multiples of BMR were roughly estimated from the ratio of heart rate at rest (BMR) and maximal levels achieved in preschool children, and from the comparison with similar ratios in older subjects (this ratio is much lower in children,[240] but is not yet known for preschoolers). Total energy requirement depends on the level and duration of physical activity per day, and thus varies considerably among individual children.

TABLE 5.4 Estimated Average Requirements of Energy for Children 3 to 7 Years Old

Age (years)	Average weight (kg)		Energy intake (kcal/kg)		Energy intake kJ/day	
	Boys	Girls	Boys	Girls	Boys	Girls
3.5	15.5	15.0	395	375	6100	5650
4.5	17.5	17.0	375	354	6550	6200
5.5	19.5	19.5	365	330	7100	6800
6.5	22.0	21.5	350	330	7700	7100
7.5	24.5	24.0	330	305	8100	7300

Adapted from *Nutrition and Energy Intakes for the European Community,* Report of the Scientific Committee for Food, 31st Series, Directorate-General, Industry, Office for Official Publications, Luxembourg, 1993.

decrease their physical activity, an action that is considered the "first line of defence" against malnutrition in childhood.[378]

Under the usual physiological conditions, the physical activity level in preschool children varies markedly in the same way as in older children, i.e., under the same conditions one child could be several times more active as another. This was confirmed by pedometer measurements in preschool children.[254] Therefore, it is very difficult to estimate more exactly the energy output and thus the energy requirements in individual children.

Estimation of energy output used the most common approach to be the assessment of spontaneous food intake; Birch et al.[31] showed that in children 2 to 5 years old the intake of individual children was relatively constant during 6 days in spite of a great variability of each meals during the day. There were marked differences between each child. The spontaneous intake of individual meals, though, depends significantly on food choice and preference. With very appetizing meals with a high energy density, self-control may fail. Then, the intake of protein, fat, sugar, and other components may be excessive and may not be compatible with optimal development of weight, BMI, and body composition in the present or future. Thus, parents should respect the real energy needs of the developing child, supplying an adequate and individually defined dietary allowance of energy.

II. PROTEIN REQUIREMENTS

Protein requirements are defined as *the lowest level of dietary protein intake that a person will need to balance the nitrogen losses from the body in persons maintaining energy balance at modest levels of physical activity.* In children and pregnant or lactating women, this requirement includes the needs associated with the deposition of tissues or the secretion of milk at rates consistent with good health.[103,393]

During *growth and development, more protein is necessary* to build up the body, i.e., about 2 g/kg body weight at first through third month is recommended. The period from 6 to 12 months is clearly most critical because of the rapid growth that occurs during this time and because the child increasingly relies on supplementary foods. The mean rate of nitrogen accretion during growth can be estimated using the expected daily rate of weight gain, which corresponds to the 50th percentile of usual growth standards[35,290–293,301,302] and to the nitrogen (N) concentration in the body. This is low at birth and increases to the adult value by the age of 5 years of age or sooner. The extent of the increase is important between 6 and 12 months when growth is rapid. Reported values for body N concentration at different ages were obtained using three different methods.[111,393] At some ages, the values were not in agreement.

It should not be assumed that growth always proceeds at exactly the same rate from day to day, even in normal healthy children with adequate and regular food intake. The cause, extent, and significance of these fluctuations in growth rate are difficult to assess. The variability of gain is much greater than the variability of intake. These differences may also represent day-to-day differences in the proportions of deposited fat and lean tissue, which depends both on nutritional and physical activity regimes. This applies even more to periods of recovery from malnutrition and/or from a disease, etc.

TABLE 5.5 Safe Level of Protein Intake (Milk or White of Egg Protein) of Small Children (Genders Combined)

Age years	Maintenance	Growth	Total	+2 SD	% CV	Safe level (g prot./kg BW)
	(mg N/kg per day)					
3–4	117	24	141	175	12.0	1.09
4–5	116	21	137	170	12.0	1.06
5–6	115	17	132	164	12.0	1.02
6–7	114	17	131	163	12.0	1.01

Modified from the World Health Organization.[393]

In order to maintain a satisfactory overall growth rate, any failure to take in protein one day must be compensated for on a subsequent day. The human body has a very limited capacity for storing amino acids or for drawing on the free amino acid pool for protein synthesis. Even during short periods such as 12 hours without food, the nitrogen balance becomes negative.[56] It follows that since it is impossible to foretell on which days the growth rate will be lower or higher, it is necessary to provide enough energy every day for the possible extra demand even when some sparing mechanisms under conditions of malnutrition may appear.

The estimated safe levels of N and protein calculated in this way are shown in Table 5.5.[393] These values are given for a joint group of boys and girls. This RDA refers to high quality protein (from sources such as egg white, milk, beef, fish, and the like). *Proteins should account for 12 to 13% of the energy intake.* This applies to all age categories. In *very young children,* this proportion is higher: in a 4-year-old boy with a body weight of 18 kg about *18% of energy is covered by protein,* as follows from the calculations of the intake of protein in grams per kilograms of body weight and total energy recommended dietary allowance.

Habitual home diets of some population groups may provide the same foods in different proportions, and their constituent proteins may not supply an adequate combination of essential amino acids. In such a case, when the quality is poor, a higher intake of protein is required. The safety margin is narrower for children than for adults.

Energy and protein are the two main components of foods that cannot be substituted with anything else. Energy is also derived from fat and carbohydrates and when the energy intake is not sufficient, from protein. This is especially detrimental during growth, and sufficient amounts of both energy and protein are, therefore, indispensable.

III. FATS

Another source of energy is fat, which has the highest energy content. Moreover, it contains essential fatty acids, which are indispensable to adequate growth and development.

Triglycerides are the principal lipid component of foods and the most concentrated source of energy among the macrocomponents of the diet (9.3 kcal/g, 38 kJ/g). They can enhance palatability by absorbing and retaining flavors and by influencing the texture of foods. When fats are digested, they facilitate the intestinal absorption (and perhaps also the transport) of the fat-soluble vitamins A, D, and E.

Actual RDAs specify the intake of saturated, and mono- and polyunsaturated fatty acids. The RDAs of the European Community (E.C.) specify servings for polyunsaturated fatty acids (Table 5.6a). The most important polyunsaturated fatty acids are linoleic acid, and linolenic acid (containing more than one double bond). The major polyunsaturated fatty acid (PUFA) in fish are eicosapentaenoic acid (EPA), and docosahexaenoic acid (DHA). All these fatty acids are indispensable to healthy development, while also playing a role in the prevention of cardiovascular diseases.

TABLE 5.6a   Population Reference Intakes for all Healthy Preschool Children, European Community

	Age group (years) 4–6
Protein (g/kg BW)	1.0
n-6 PUFA (% dietary energy)	2
n-3 PUFA (% dietary energy)	0.5

Adapted from *Nutrient and Energy Intakes for the European Community,* Report of the Scientific Committee for Food, 31st Series, Directorate-General, Industry, Office for Official Publications, Luxembourg, 1993.

Fatty acids can be utilized directly as a source of energy by most body cells, with the exception of erythrocytes and cells of the central nervous system, cells which normally use glucose as the major energy source. Excess energy is stored principally as triglycerides in adipose tissue, the percentage of which varies markedly in the organism with age, sex, nutritional status, and physical activity regime.

The recommended dietary allowance for fat is defined as 30% of the total energy intake or less. Usual consumption of fats is mostly higher, which was found for different population groups in most industrially developed countries. However, children who had different ratios of their dietary energy covered by fats did not show differences in growth.[326]

Linoleic acid should account for 1 to 2% of total dietary calories, for infants consuming 100 kcal/kg body weight per day, only 0.2 g/kg body weight. For adults, a minimal adequate intake of linoleic acid is 3 to 6 g/day; RDAs for young children are intrapolated.[396–398]

The strongest dietary determinant of the blood cholesterol is the level of saturated fatty acid intake. The cholesterol concentration of the diet has an appreciable, but usually smaller, influence. In the past decade, considerable attention was also given to the potential role of dietary factors in the etiology and prevention of cancer. Increased consumption of fats is considered a risk factor.

Regarding the influence of diet and its composition on the development of the thesethese diseases, there has been already evidence that these factors influence the human organism from the very beginning of life.[396–398] Therefore, not only during childhood, but also during pregnancy, an adequate diet can play an important role in health development and in the prevention of these diseases later in life.

IV. CARBOHYDRATES

Carbohydrates, an important source of energy, should account for more than a half of the energy intake. This follows from the recommendations for protein and fat. However, in small children, where the percentage of energy covered by protein is higher due to higher amounts of protein per kilograms of body weight, at least 52 to 54% of energy should be covered by carbohydrates.

The intake of sugar should not exceed 10% (larger amounts involve the risk of dental cavities and a risk of elevated blood cholesterol and triglyceride level), and the percentage of fiber ought to amount to 20% of the total energy intake. The latter is hygroscopic, promoting normal elimination. A fiber-rich diet may also promote satiety. Some fiber components, including oat bran and pectin, lower plasma cholesterol levels, either by binding bile acids or by other mechanisms. Diets rich in plant foods with an increased amount of fiber are inversely related to the incidence of cardiovascular diseases, colon cancer, and diabetes. In the U.S.,[397] the percentage of energy covered by various macro-components of diet did not generally correspond to the thesethese standards, i.e., carbohydrates covered 45.3% of energy in adult men, 46.4% in adult women, and 52% in children 1 to 5 years of age.[397] Similar conclusions also apply to the dietary intake in the Czech Republic.

V. MINERALS AND TRACE ELEMENTS

A positive *calcium* balance is required for bone formation until peak bone mass is achieved. The mineralization of bone continues for some years after longitudinal bone growth has ceased. Most of the accumulation of bone minerals occurs in humans by the age of about 20 years, but some mineral is added during the third decade.

A high-calcium food consumption pattern established in childhood may be related to bone density in postmenopausal women.[123] The most promising nutritional approach to reducing the risk of osteoporosis in later life is to ensure a calcium intake that allows the development of each individual's genetically programmed peak bone mass during the formative years, especially during childhood.[320,397,398]

Regarding the growth period, Calcium accretion averages 140 to 165 mg/day and may be as high as 400 to 500 mg/day during puberty.[123] An intake of 800 mg/day is recommended for both sexes from ages 4 to 10 years and later on 1200 mg/day.[397] The RDAs of the European Community[398] (E.C.) are lower. These amounts can easily be obtained if dairy products are included in the diet (see Table 5.6b).

Another essential component of bone is ***phosphorus***, where it is present at a mass ratio of 1 phosphorus to 2 calcium. Children and adults absorb 50 to 70% of the phosphorus in normal diets and as much as 90% when the intake is low.[197] Phosphorus is present in nearly all foods. Major contributors of phosphorus are protein-rich foods and cereal grains, milk, meat, poultry, and fish. Cow's milk contains more calcium and phosphorus than does human milk, and the ratios of the elements differ widely. The RDAs for the E.C. are lower than those for the U.S. (Table 5.6b).

The requirement for phosphorus is usually set equal to calcium RDAs for all age groups except the young infant. It was accepted that a 1:1 ratio of calcium to phosphorus will provide sufficient phosphorus for most age groups, but if the calcium intake is adequate, the precise ratio of these minerals is unimportant. The RDA for phosphorus is 800 mg for children 1 to 10 years[397,398] (Table 5.6b).

Magnesium modulates many biochemical and physiological processes and is indispensable to them as the Mg-ATP complex. The highest concentrations of magnesium are found in whole seeds such as nuts, legumes, and unmilled grains. More than 80% of the magnesium is lost by removal of the germ and outer layers of cereal grains. No data exist on the magnesium requirements of young children, however, 80 to 170 mg/day is recommended for children from 1 to 10 years of age (Table 5.6b), i.e., about 6 mg/kg body weight. The RDA of the E.C. (1993) is 7- 4.2 mg/kg weight from 6 months up to 15–17 years i.e., from 4 to 6 years the RDA is 120 mg/day (Table 5.6b,[397,398]).

Iron, a constituent of hemoglobin, myoglobin, and a number of enzymes, plays an important role in ensuring an optimal level of overall functional capacity and an adequate aerobic power during all periods of life, starting with early childhood. When the iron supply in the food is sufficient, its absorption is regulated to keep the body iron content constant. Iron absorption increases under conditions of its deficiency. However, this response may not be sufficient to prevent anemia in subjects whose intake of available iron is marginal.

TABLE 5.6b   Comparison of Recommended Dietary Allowances of Minerals for Preschool Children (4 to 6 Years), of National Research Council[397] and European Community[398]

Minerals	NRC	E.C.
Calcium (mg)	800	450
Phosphorus (mg)	800	350
Magnesium (mg)	120	—
Iron (mg)	10	4
Zinc (mg)	10	6
Iodine (μg)	90	90
Selenium (μg)	20	15
Copper (mg)	1.0–1.5	0.6
Manganese (mg)	1.5–2.0	—
Fluoride (mg)	1.0–2.5	—
Chromium (μg)	30–120	—
Molybdenum (μg)	30–75	—
Potassium (mg)	—	1100

Adapted from *Nutrient and Energy Intakes for the European Community,* Report of the Scientific Committee for Food, 31st Series, Directorate-General, Industry, Office for Official Publications, Luxembourg, 1993; also compiled from *Recommended Dietary Allowances,* 10th Ed., National Research Council, National Academy Press, Washington, D.C., 1989.

Impaired iron status is manifested in three stages:

1. Diminished stores manifested by a fall of plasma ferritin, and no functional deterioration evident
2. Iron-deficient erythropoiesis in which the hemoglobin level is within 95% of the reference range for age and sex, and the working performance may be impaired
3. Iron deficiency anemia in which total blood hemoglobin levels are reduced below normal values and severe iron deficiency anemia is characterized by microcytosis and hypochromia

For males and females over 4 years of age, anemia is defined as a hemoglobin level below 13 g/dl and 12 g/dl, respectively. In children, iron deficiency is associated with apathy, reduced attention, irritability, and the reduced ability to learn. Milder forms of anemia may be connected with poor school performance. From about 6 months to 4 years, iron deficiency may be due to a low iron content of milk while the body is growing rapidly, and iron reserves are low. Iron availability may be enhanced by simultaneously consuming foodstuffs containing vitamin C. Increased consumption of bran can limit absorption of iron.

From birth to the age 3 years, infants not breastfed should have an iron intake of approximately 1 mg/kg body weight per day. Children and adolescents need iron, not only to maintain hemoglobin concentrations, but also to increase their total iron mass during the growth period. The iron requirements of children and adolescents are considered to be slightly higher than those of adults. A dose of 10 mg/day is recommended for children. RDAs of E.C. are lower[397,398] (see Table 5.6b).

Zinc is an essential element for humans as a component of some enzymes. Its deficiency is manifested by loss of appetite, growth retardation, skin changes, and immunological abnormalities. Experiments in laboratory and domestic animals have shown that zinc deficiency during pregnancy may lead to developmental disorders in the offspring.[397] Pronounced zinc deficiency in men, resulting in hypogonadism and dwarfism, has been found in the Middle East. Marginal zinc deficiency was also observed in a survey of apparently healthy children who exhibited suboptimal growth, poor appetite, and impaired taste acuity, along with a low hair zinc level.[148] Increasing zinc intake by 0.4 to 0.8 mg/kg brought about marked improvement. Supplementation of infant formulas to increase zinc levels resulted in increased growth rates in males, but not in females.[374]

Animal products provide about 70% of the zinc intake, followed by zinc from cereals. The bioavailability varies in different foodstuffs. The recommended U.S. allowance for children is 10 mg/day and 6 mg/day in the E.C. allowances (see Table 5.6b). Lower intake in preadolescent children resulted in lower hair and plasma zinc levels, along with retarded growth (tenth percentile). The rate of linear growth improved as a result of supplementation with zinc to the level of the RDA.[374] Excessive intake of zinc can cause the impairment of various immune responses, decrease of HDL-cholesterol, etc.[397]

Iodine is an integral part of the thyroid hormones thyroxine and triiodothyronine. Its deficiency can lead to a wide spectrum of diseases, ranging from severe cretinism with mental retardation to barely visible enlargement of the thyroid. Endemic goiter continues to be a worldwide problem. Iodine deficiency disorders can be prevented, but not cured, by providing an adequate iodine intake. The prevalence of goiter decreased considerably in all countries where iodized salt was introduced. Natural goitrogen sources are cabbage or cassava.[397]

In the coastal areas, seafoods, water, and iodine containing mist from the ocean are important sources of iodine, whereas further inland, the iodine content of plants and animal products is variable, depending on the geochemical environment, fertilizing, feeding practices, and food processing. In these areas, iodized table salt is a reliable source, providing 76 μg of iodine per gram of salt.[397]

The RDAs for children are 70 to 90 μg/day both in the U.S. and the E.C. (see Table 5.6b). Excess intake of iodine, i.e., 1 mg/day, did not produce indications of physiological abnormalities in children.[397–398]

The role of ***selenium*** in human nutrition was demonstrated by the association of low selenium status and Keshan disease, a cardiomyopathy which primarily affects young children and women of childbearing age in China. A large-scale intervention trial involving several thousand Chinese children showed the value of selenium in preventing this disease. The most important sources of selenium are liver, kidneys, and seafood. The content of selenium in grains and seeds depends on the content of this trace element in the soil. Small amounts are also in vegetables and fruit.[397]

RDA for selenium were extrapolated from the values of adults, i.e., 10 to 15 µg/day as little is known about the selenium requirements for children (Table 5.6b).

Other indispensable trace elements are **copper, manganese, fluoride, chromium,** and **molybdenum.** Their function, bioavailability, RDA, etc.,[397] have been described in Table 5.6b.

VI. VITAMINS

A. FAT SOLUBLE

Vitamin A comprises a group of compounds essential for vision, growth, cellular differentiation and proliferation, reproduction, and the integrity of the immune system.[397] Vitamin A deficiency is found most commonly in children under 5 years of age, mainly in the Third World countries, and is usually due to an insufficient dietary intake. Deficiency also occurs as a result of chronic fat malabsorption. The RDAs for children (400 to 500 µg/day) were extrapolated from infant values to the adult level on the basis of body weight. No differentiation between genders is necessary.

The RDAs for the U.S. and the E.C. are give in Table 5.6c. A single dose of 60 milligrams of retinol in oil (60,000 RE or 200,000 IU) has been successfully used prophylactically in Asian preschool children.[397] About 1 to 3% of children have transient toxic symptoms without lasting effects.

Vitamin D (calciferol) is essential for proper skeletal formation and for mineral homeostasis. Vitamin D deficiency in children causes deformation of the skeleton, resulting from the inadequate mineralization of bones. In industrially developed countries, milk and other foods are fortified with vitamin D, and rickets are very rare in these countries. When skin is sufficiently exposed to sunlight, the amount of vitamin D synthetized can meet the requirements. Its amount depends on the area of skin exposed, the time of exposure, and the wavelength of the ultraviolet light.

The allowance for children older than 6 months has been set at 10 µg (400 IU)/day (Table 5.6c). Because the complete maturation of the skeleton is not achieved until the third decade, this allowance is recommended through 24 years. There is a problem as to whether usual sources of vitamin D are sufficient (milk, eggs, butter, etc.) without enough sun exposure. However, in many industrialized countries, such as the U.S., these foodstuffs are fortified by sufficient amounts of vitamin D.[397,398]

Vitamin E, or tocopherols, are known biochemically as antioxidants, i.e., they prevent propagation of the oxidation of unsaturated fatty acids by trapping peroxyl free radicals. In vitamin E deficiency, the oxidation of PUFA (polyunsaturated fatty acids) is more readily propagated along the cellular mem-

TABLE 5.6c **Comparison of Recommended Dietary Allowances (RDAs) of Vitamins for Preschool Children (4 to 6 Years), National Research Council (NRC) and of European Community (E.C. Population Reference Intakes)**

Vitamin	NRC	E.C.
A (μg RE)	500	400
D (μg)	10	10
E (mg alfa TE)	7	0.4 (/g PUFA)
K (μg)	20	—
C (mg)	45	25
Thiamin (mg)	0.9	100 (μg/MJ)
Riboflavin (mg)	1.1	1.0
Niacin (mg NE)	12	—
B$_6$ (mg)	1.1	15 (μg/g protein)
Folate (μg)	75	130
B$_{12}$ (μg)	1.0	0.9
Biotin (μg)	25	—
Pantothenic acid (mg)	3–4	—

Modified from *Recommended Dietary Allowances,* 10th Ed., National Research Council, National Academy Press, Washington, D.C., 1989; and from *Nutrient Energy Intakes for the European Community,* Report of the Scientific Committee for Food, 31st Series, Directorate-General, Industry, Office for Official Publications, Luxembourg, 1993.

brane, leading to cell damage and eventual symptoms, mainly neurological. During steady growth in early childhood, an intake increasing from 6 mg for the reference child of 13 kg body weight at 1 to 3 years of age to 7 mg to 10 years should be satisfactory for the average diet (Table 5.6c). The RDAs for the E.C. give the value of 0.4 mg α-tocopherol equivalents per 1 g of PUFA.[398] In children, vitamin E deficiency occurs mostly in those with congenital disorders.

The *vitamin* K content of commonly consumed foods is not known exactly and therefore is not given in food composition tables. Green leafy vegetables are the best source. Small but significant amounts of vitamin K are also in the milk and dairy products, meats, eggs, cereals, fruits, and vegetables. Another potentially important source of vitamin K is the bacterial flora in the jejunum and ileum. In the absence of specific information about the vitamin K requirement of children, RDA values for them are set at about 1 μg/kg body weight for both the U.S. and the E.C. (see Table 5.6c). Toxic effects of excessive amounts ingested are not known.[397,398]

B. WATER SOLUBLE

Vitamin C (L-ascorbic acid) cannot be synthetized by humans; it affects functions of leukocytes and macrophages, immune responses, wound healing, and allergic reactions. It also increases the absorption of inorganic iron.[397]

The major source are vegetables and fruits. Vitamin C status is usually evaluated from clinical deficiency, plasma (or blood) levels (less than 0.2

mg/dl), or leukocyte concentrations. Vitamin C must be continuously supplied in the food. The RDAs for children are 25 to 45 mg/day[397,398] (see Table 5.6c).

Thiamin (B₁) deficiency is associated with abnormalities of carbohydrate metabolism related to the decrease in oxidative decarboxylation. Dietary sources of thiamin include unrefined cereal grains, brewer's yeast, organ meats, lean cuts of pork, legumes, seeds, and nuts. Daily RDAs for children were approximated at 0.5 mg/1000 kcal (or 100 µg/MJ), which provides for variability in requirements (see Table 5.6c).

Riboflavin (B₂) functions primarily as a component of two flavin coenzymes — flavin mononucleotide (FMN) and flavin adenine dinucleotide (FAD) catalyze many oxidation-reduction reactions. Clinical signs of ariboflavinosis are rare; nevertheless, children's diets must contain adequate amounts of riboflavin: 0.8 to 1.2 mg/day of riboflavin is recommended (see Table 5.6c). No cases of toxicity are known.

Niacin is used here in a generic sense for both nicotinic acid and nicotinamide and the PP-factor. Nicotinamide functions in the body as a component of two coenzymes — nicotinamide adenine dinucleotide (NAD) and nicotinamide adenine dinucleotide phosphate (NADP). The best source of niacin is meat. Tryptophan in the diet can contribute to the niacin supply due to possible conversion. No data exist on the niacin requirements of children. The RDAs are set at 6.6 NE/1000 cal (NE — niacin equivalent) or at 9 to 13 mg NE/day (1.6 mg/MJ, see Table 5.6c).[397,398]

Vitamin B₆ comprises three chemically, metabolically, and functionally related forms — pyridoxine (pyridoxol PN), pyridoxal (PL), and pyridoxamine (PM). The richest sources are chicken, fish, kidney, liver, pork and eggs, unmilled rice, soy beans, oats, whole-wheat products, peanuts, and walnuts. Information on requirements of children are scarce. The RDA is 1.0 to 1.4 mg/day[397] or 15 µg/g protein[398] (see Table 5.6c).

Folate and folacin include compounds that have nutritional properties and a chemical structure similar to those of folic acid (pteroylglutamic acid, or PGA). Folates function metabolically as coenzymes which transport single carbon fragments from one compound to another in amino acid metabolism and nucleic acid synthesis. Deficiency of this vitamin leads to impaired cell division and to alterations of protein synthesis, which manifests most markedly in aidly growing tissues.[397,398]

Folate is widely distributed in foods. Evidence of defective DNA synthesis is seen as the hypersegmentation of cells and abnormality in the sensitive deoxyuridine suppression test. Megaloblastic bone marrow and macrocytic anemia are late consequences of deficiency.[397] The folate RDAs for healthy children between 1 and 10 years are interpolated from allowances for infants and adolescents, i.e., 50 to 130 µg/day (see Table 5.6c). There is no evidence about the benefit of excess folate intake, but some potential for toxicity may exist.[397]

Vitamin B₁₂ (cobalamin) stimulates erythropoiesis and acts as a coenzyme in amino acid metabolism. Cyanocobalamin is commercially available as vitamin

B_{12} in pills. This form is water soluble and heat stable. Animal and dairy products (where they accumulate from bacterial synthesis) are the primary dietary source of vitamin B_{12} in different forms. The RDAs for children 1 to 5 years of age are about 0.05 μg/kg body weight/day, i.e., 1 μg/day (see Table 5.6c). The real intake of the child population is usually higher. An additional non-dietary source of small amounts of absorbable vitamin B_{12} may be bacteria in the small intestine of humans. An insufficient supply of vitamin B_{12} results in macrocytic, megaloblastic anemia, and neurological symptoms, due to demyelination of the spinal cord and brain and the optic and peripheral nerves. In other less specific symptoms also occur (e.g., sore tongue, weakness). The cause of this deficiency in the industrially developed countries may mostly be malabsorption.

Biotin contains sulfur, and is essential for humans and other species. It is contained in different foods and is synthetized in the lower gastrointestinal tract by microorganisms and some fungi. Biotin is an integral part of enzymes, transporting carboxyl units and fixing carbon dioxide in animal tissue. The conversion of biotin to the active enzyme is dependent on magnesium and adenosine triphosphate (ATP). The RDAs for children and adolescents gradually increase from infant values (10 to 15 μg/day) to adult values (see Table 5.6c). No toxicity was reported in conjunction with intakes as high as 10 mg daily.[397]

Pantothenic acid, a vitamin of the B-complex, is a component of the coenzyme A molecule. It is important in the release of energy from carbohydrates, in the degradation and synthesis of fatty acids, in gluconeogenesis, in the synthesis of such vital compounds as sterols, steroid hormones, porphyrins, and acetylcholine, and finally in acylation reactions in general. In children of younger school age (7 to 9 years), diets that met the recommended allowances for all other nutrients provided 4 to 5 mg of pantothenic acid daily.[397] The RDAs for children are extrapolated from infant values (2 to 3 mg/day) to adult ones (see Table 5.6c).

VII. METHODS FOR THE EVALUATION OF DIETARY INTAKE

The goal of nutrition surveys is to define a population and/or an individual in terms of a specific factor, i.e., dietary intake and resulting nutritional status, related to a number of characteristics of the human organism. These comprise morphological, functional, biochemical, and psychological variables. Most often, it is designed to identify malnutrition, which can vary in character.

Quite often a diet that seems to correspond to the rules of rational nutrition may be unsatisfactory because it does not meet the real needs of the subject in question. This happens most frequently in hypokinetic individuals who have a very low energy output and who need to not only reduce the amount of food ingested but also to pay increased attention to their diet in order to ensure a well balanced and satisfactory diet without any deficiencies. On the other hand, *active individuals with a high level of energy output* do not need to care so much about the composition of their diets because they can eat abundantly; *in a larger amount of food, a deficient intake of some essential nutritional items is less likely to occur.*

The classic approach for the determination of nutritional status can provide dietary, biochemical, and clinical data. It is generally agreed that dietary surveys evaluate current food intake, biochemical data, recent nutritional status, and clinical evaluations of long-term nutritional history. The results of these three approaches do not necessarily correlate with each other.[161,283]

Generally, the information on the nutrition of a population can be supplemented by agricultural data, vital and health statistics, anthropometric studies, and others, such as various dietary surveys. Most commonly used methods are household food consumption, food list, food record, weighed household consumption, individual food consumption assessment. Estimation by recall is generally used for a 24-hour period only.

Food records must be kept by the individual of food eaten during varying lengths of time, usually 3 to 7 days. *Weighed intake* may be obtained by having a subject or a trained person weigh all food consumed during a given period of time. In spite of accuracy of the actual data, there are some limitations: subjects are prone to try to find shortcuts and thus to change from their usual eating patterns. It is used mostly in laboratory and metabolic ward studies.[283] *Diet history* is designed to uncover the usual food intake and dietary habits over a longer period of time. Most often, it is obtained with an *interview*.

Biochemical evaluation is mostly limited to blood and excreta in human metabolic studies in nutrition surveys. *Clinical evaluations* include physical examination of the subjects, which was the earliest means of evaluating nutritional status since the knowledge of nutrients evolved from the observation of deficiency syndromes. Signs used in nutrition surveys are found on hair, face, eyes, lips, tongue, teeth, gums, glands, skin, nails, subcutaneous tissue, muscular and skeletal system, and internal systems (gastrointestinal, nervous, cardiovascular).[283]

All of the mentioned methods were repeatedly analyzed by numerous expert committees of the World Health Organization.[393–396] Regarding mutual relationships, dietary and biochemical data correlate more closely than either criterion correlates with clinical examination.[161,283]

VIII. DIETARY INTAKE AND ENERGY OUTPUT IN CZECH PRESCHOOLERS: RESULTS OF CROSS-SECTIONAL AND LONGITUDINAL SURVEYS

Food intake studies in the preschool period have been relatively rare. Most studies of this sort were performed in infants, mostly during their stay in some institution. Recently, 1675 of U.K. children from 1.5 to 4.5 years of age were followed up.[141,143] Previous measurements of this sort in U.K. children were executed in 1967 (Department of Health, 1975). Otherwise, mainly school children were followed up.

Our initial measurements were made in a day care center in Prague, where it was possible to cooperate with the director and all staff members, i.e., teachers, cooks, and other employees. In the first survey (G; n = 84), we recorded food ingested by individual children, entered daily for 1 week on food record forms by teachers and cooks in the kindergarten for all individual children followed up. In the second study (H; n = 52), the overall dietary intake in individual children during the whole day and week was recorded, including both food ingested in the center, as in survey G. This was supplemented by data from the parents, who entered all foods ingested by the child during the rest of the day and during the weekend. Also, measurements of anthropometric variables, skinfolds, step test, and motor and sensomotor development were evaluated with the help of the thesethese procedures and tests.

The dietary intake of individual children was assessed with an analysis of the composition of meals and foods ingested. The amount of composition of the food was evaluated using a computer program based on the composition of local foods, which is used widely for other population groups in The Czech Republic (National Institute of Public Health, Prague, Ing. Z Roth). The results were compared with national and other (WHO, E.C.) recommended dietary allowances.

The recommended allowance (RDAs) for energy intake in children 4 to 6 years old in our country[171] was 1550 kcal, i.e., 7120 kJ. The diet should contain 60 g of protein, 50 g of fat, and 234 g of carbohydrates. These RDAs (which were previously even higher) differ markedly from RDAs of WHO,[393] the European Community,[398] and the U.S.[397] (i.e., energy is either adjusted according to energy output assessed individually, or taken from tables[398]). There is also a differentiation according to individual years (i.e., energy recommendation for 4-year-old children is lower and for 6 year olds is higher than those in our country) and gender (i.e., RDAs for energy is lower for girls). The RDAs for protein in the European Community[398] is 1 g/kg body weight/day, which is much lower than in Czech RDAs; the same approach is applied in the U.S.[397] The recommended value for U.S. children 4 to 6 years old is 24 g/day, contrasting with 60 g/day for Czech children.

At the time of our measurements, the daily menus for the children in kindergarten were prepared centrally.[256]

The results of a 5 day follow up (survey G) in 84 day care centers children showed that 85% of our daily recommended allowance for energy was already met during the day in the day care centers (where children spent, on the average, 7.3 hours/day). The children eat, as a rule, three meals (unless they go home earlier, which was not the case during our observations).

Carbohydrates accounted for 49.3% of the energy intake, fats for 39.3%, and proteins for 14.4%. When we evaluated the nutrient intake in relation to dietary allowances at that time, the fat intake corresponded to 98.5% of the allowance, and the protein and carbohydrate intake corresponded to roughly 80%.[171] Where the diet of the children at home was investigated, it was found that they had breakfast, an afternoon snack (in case they left earlier and did not have it in the kindergarten), and a complete, balancedsupper.

These data indicate that, on average, *the energy intake of the investigated children was excessive.* Although there was always a ***considerable variability*** in the energy intake of different children, the teachers tried to ensure that the children ate all their helpings of meat, fruit, etc. and thus the variability of the energy intake was due to carbohydrates or possibly fats.[239,256]

The assessments of food intake were repeated in several studies, cross-sectional and longitudinal, again along with other measurements (morphological, functional, biochemical, motor performance, etc.). In the following group of preschool children (survey H, boys n = 31, girls n = 21), it was possible to measure food intake, not only in the day care centers where the teachers and cooks recorded the intake of meals of individual children, but also at home, with the help of the parents who were involved in the study and cooperated by entering the data on food consumption at home during the whole week. The results are shown in Tables 5.7a and 5.7b, which confirm the the the observations on the excessive food intake of preschool children. The results of this comparison concerns Czech RDAs; if we compare these data with other RDAs, the relative intake would be even higher.

TABLE 5.7a   Dietary Intake/Day of Czech Preschool Children, Aged 4–5 Years (Boys, n = 31; Girls, n = 15, Survey H)

		Energy (kJ)	Protein (g)			Fat (g)			Carbohydrate (g)
			Total	Animal	Plant	Total	Animal	Plant	
Boys	x̄	9190	74.0	50.8	23.3	84.3	67.5	16.9	294.8
	SD	2380	20.7	17.9	6.9	26.5	21.9	16.1	82.7
Girls	x̄	9140	71.2	46.9	24.3	80.4	64.7	15.8	301.7
	SD	2450	19.6	18.2	6.5	36.3	35.0	13.8	87.6
RDA*		7120	60.0	40.0	20.0	55.0	—	—	234.0

Note: * RDA used in The Czech Republic.[171]

Adapted from Pařízková, J., et al., *Growth, Fitness and Nutrition in Preschool Children,* Charles University, Prague, 1984 and from Kajaba, I., et al., *Čas. Lek. Čes.,* 131, 198, 1992 (in Czech).

Energy intake was higher by about 31% in boys and by about 30% in girls. The intake of the absolute amount of proteins (g) was higher by 23 to 24% in boys and by 18 to 19% in girls. *If we compare the intake of protein with the E.C. or the U.S. RDAs, the intake would be about three times higher than those recommended in these countries for preschool children.*

When we compare the average intake of *fat* with actual Czech RDAs,[171] it was 53% higher in boys and about 46% higher in girls. The intake of

TABLE 5.7b **The Intake of Minerals and Vitamins/Day in Preschool Children, Aged 4–5 Years (Survey H)**

		Minerals		Vitamins			
		Ca	Fe	B₁	B₂	PP	C
Boys	x̄	1122	10.7	1.1	1.4	12.8	63.5
	SD	568	5.7	0.4	0.9	5.6	30.6
Girls	x̄	1076	9.9	1.1	1.2	12.0	63.3
	SD	678	4.1	0.4	0.4	4.3	34.1
RDA*		900	12.0	0.7	1.0	11.0	55.0

* RDA used in The Czech Republic.

Modified from Pařízková , J., et al., *Growth, Fitness and Nutrition in Preschool Children,* Charles University, Prague, 1984 and from Kajaba, I., et al., *Cas. Lek. Ces.,* 131, 198, 1992 (in Czech).

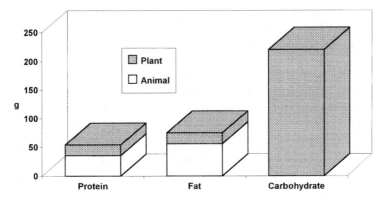

FIGURE 5.1 Intake of protein, fat, and carbohydrates in preschool boys and girls (survey I).

carbohydrates was higher by about 25% in boys and by about 28 to 29% in girls. Neither the E.C. nor the U.S. RDAs give special values for fat and carbohydrate intake, so Czech data can not be compared. Again, though, an excess could be assumed.

In survey H the intake of ***calcium*** was higher by 24 to 25% in boys and by 19 to 20% in girls, in the comparison to Czech RDAs.[171] When compared with the RDAs for Ca, it would be nearly 2.5 times as high for the E.C.[398] and 1.4 times as high for the U.S.[397] This applies to boys although the difference would be slightly lower for girls.

The **iron** intake in boys was lower by about 11% and by about 16 to 17% in girls compared to Czech RDAs.[171] The intake of iron would correspond to the U.S. RDAs and would be more than double compared to those of the E.C.[397,398]

The intake of **vitamin B₁** was higher than recommended by 15 to 16% in both boys and girls. (RDAs for thiamin for U.S.[397] preschool children are slightly lower compared to the E.C.;[398] it is expressed in relation to energy intake in MJ; see Table 5.6c). The intake of **vitamin B₂** was about 40% higher in boys and 20% higher in girls. Because the RDAs of the E.C. and the U.S. are higher, the consumption of this vitamin by our group of children would have corresponded better to these RDAs than to Czech ones.

The intake of **niacin** was about 16% higher in boys and about 9% higher in girls, and the intake of vitamin C was higher than recommended by about 15%, both in boys and girls. The E.C. and U.S. RDAs for **vitamin C** are lower[397,398] (see Table 5.6c), so the excess intake of this vitamin would be even more marked when compared with these RDAs.

Regarding the **sex-linked differences,** the intake of energy and all other items was almost always slightly higher in boys compared to girls (with the exception of vegetable protein and carbohydrates), but the differences were not significant because of a great interindividual variability, i.e., high values of CV (see Tables 5.7a and 5.7b).

The trend toward higher energy intake in preschool boys can be explained by a slightly higher weight and leanness; in addition, practical experience and evaluation by the teachers in day care centers showed almost regularly slightly higher levels of spontaneous physical activity in boys, which could be responsible for the trend of increased energy intake. This was also proved by DuRant et al.[89,90] when using Children's Activity Rating Scale (CARS). These measurements showed, moreover, a higher level of activity in summer and in spring than during the winter and ethnic differences in activity levels in Anglo-, African- and Mexican-American children aged 3 or 4 years.

When we evaluated the **ratio of macrocomponents,** i.e., the percentage of energy provided by protein, fat, and carbohydrates, the results were not satisfactory. In boys the energy ratio of protein was about 13%, of fats was about 34%, and of carbohydrates was 53%. In girls the energy ratio of individual nutrients was about 13:32:55. This indicates once more that the amount and percentage of fat was too high; the recommendations of the World Health Organization[396] emphasize that less than 30% of energy should be provided by fat and more than 50% by carbohydrates.

The **practical outcomes** of these assessments are *the individual recommendations to the parents* on how to improve the diet of their children, mainly by decreasing the amount of fat and protein and by increasing the consumption of carbohydrates (especially of complex carbohydrates). Girls had slightly better composition of diet, but the differences in our groups were not significant. General instructions also included increased consumption of vegetables and fruits and reduced sugar consumption.

Increased intake of total and saturated fats was also shown in U.S. children: in 80% of children, this intake was higher than the recommended levels.[168,352] The level of urbanization affected the most of nutrient intake variables, followed by race. Living in a rural area and being black were significant predictors for higher intakes of total and saturated fat, cholesterol, and sodium. By introducing meals containing a smaller amount of fat, a significant reduction of fat intake was achieved.[352]

Until recently, the computer program used in The Czech Republic did not permit the evaluation of saturated and polyunsaturated fats, cholesterol, sugar, fiber, etc.; the use of foreign programs cannot give exact results (International Union of Nutritional Sciences, IUNS; Federation of European Nutritional Sciences, FENS; European Academy of Nutritional Sciences, EANS, etc., do not permit the use of programs with different databases). The analysis of the intake of individual foodstuffs showed that *children consumed more sugar* (especially as sweets) and *less fruit and vegetables than generally recommended*. Although there was no vitamin C deficiency in the whole group, in a number of children the intake of this vitamin was quite low (but not as low as the RDAs of the E.C.[398]), as indicated by the values of CV. The same also applied to some other dietary components, e.g., especially to the calcium and iron intake.

The values of somatic development — height, weight, and BMI — did not reveal markedly elevated values and/or obesity. However, the delayed effects of such a diet with too much proteins and fats may appear later in school age and/or during adolescence.[299,306] This was shown by higher BMI values in the upper percentiles, starting with 7 years of age in Czech children.[294] All this may be related to increased health risks later in life as mentioned above.[360]

Large interindividual variability of food intake was also shown, i.e., an excessive intake was not recorded in all children. For example, the values of CV of the intake of energy was 24 to 26; of proteins, 27 to 28; of fats 31 to 32 in boys and about 45 in girls; and of carbohydrates, about 28 to 29. Variability was even greater regarding the intake of minerals and vitamins (see Table 5.7b), i.e., the values of CV were 41 to 63 for calcium and iron intake, about 36 for vitamin B_1, 64 to 65 for vitamin B_2, 35 to 43 for niacin, and around 50 for vitamin C. These values indicate that in some cases the intakes were not only excessive, but were also occasionally deficient. This was found when evaluating children individually and day-by-day. However, on a long-term basis and even within 1 week, the variations were usually compensated for and on the average, no real deficiencies were found. However, some intakes were lower than desirable.[254]

Correlation analysis showed the closest relationship between the intake of energy and that of carbohydrates (r = 0.92), then of fat (r = 0.85), and finally of protein (r = 0.82). Correlation coefficients r were always higher for animal rather than for plant fat and protein.[254]

Food intake was also assessed in our ***longitudinal measurements*** of children mentioned in Chapter 4 (study E). At the time of the first measurement of 36 boys and 22 girls, the dietary intake was examined using the same procedure as mentioned above. However, due to a greater need for cooperation, at the time of the second and third measurement we were only able to assess the dietary intake in a smaller number of children. Therefore, they were not always the same children in all measurements. On the whole, though, the conclusions based on the sort of diets ingested by preschool children revealed that their composition, the mutual relationships of various components, the inter- and intra-individual variability, etc. were nearly identical, as described above.

The results of both cross-sectional and longitudinal measurements of dietary intake made during the same growth period of growth, i.e., 4 to 6 years (G, H, E) revealed that

1. There was approximately the same dietary intake in both genders, with a trend toward higher intake in boys; this applied both to cross-sectional and longitudinal surveys (see Table 5.7a and Table 5.7b). The differences between boys and girls were not significant, and the interindividual variability was great.
2. During repeated measurements, dietary intake showed a slightly increasing trend which was not significant during the period from 4 to 6 years, mainly due to a great variability.[254,256]

All these studies were made in Prague, where the economic level has always been the highest of The Czech Republic. When we compared the results with the data assessed in other parts of our country, we found different results: Prague children had a higher dietary intake than, e.g., children from a small town (16,000 inhabitants) about 60 km from Prague (survey I). These children also had a smaller body size and different motor abilities (Chapter 9; Figure 5.1).

When evaluating the dietary intake of children followed up on different occasions, we can find the reason for *an elevated BMI* and for some other variables concerning body fat: *the dietary intake, especially that of fat, but also that of protein, was too high.* The intake of energy obviously did not correspond to the needs of the organism.[179]

This was also confirmed by the estimation of energy output, using the above described approach for the analysis of energy requirements recommended by WHO (see Table 5.3). These evaluations could not be made in all children, but only in a subsample, using questionnaires where the activities of children (specified activities, duration) were entered by kindergarten teachers and by parents. The results showed that the estimated energy output was lower than the energy intake, by about 20% (see example). We had no opportunity to use the doubly labeled water method.

IX. FOOD INTAKE AND ENERGY OUTPUT
IN OTHER CHILD POPULATIONS

A great variability in food and nutrient intake was also observed in other studies of children, e.g., in Asian children by Sheffield.[150] The between-person variation, as measured over a period by weight intake data, was high and comparatively larger than the within-subject variability. For energy the between-subject variability was 26% at 4 to 12 months and 36% at 12 to 24 months. A variability of a similar sort already appears, however, at the beginning of life, similar to the variability in infants.[22]

Johnson et al.[168] showed that in U.S. children aged 1 to 10 years the nutrient intake was mostly affected by the level of urbanization; this was followed by the impact of race. Living in a rural area was a significant predictor for a higher intake of total fat, saturated fatty acids, cholesterol, and sodium. Mean annual household income had no significant effect on any of the diet quality measures. In an average diet, vitamin E, vitamin C, iron, and zinc intakes were below recommended levels. The percentage of calories from total and saturated fats and mean sodium intakes were above recommended levels.

In the U.K., the intake of fats increased up to 40% of the levels of energy in the late 1950s, with little change until the late 1970s.[341] Trends were similar in all age groups. These results differ from the pattern in the U.S., where a decline in mortality from coronary heart disease can be seen. In preschoolers in the U.K., the fat intake is 35.9% of energy.[141]

Low intake of vitamin C was shown even in a country where fruit is cheap; in Latino children in the U.S., it was lower than recommended levels.[19]

There is a problem with alternative diets for young children (macrobiotic, vegetarian, etc.). The long-term consequences of all of the diets mentioned above concerning nutritional, metabolic, and functional status of children were not yet reported, which would be a decisive factor to the evaluation of their longitudinal impact during growth period. Because it is very difficult to ensure an adequate composition of alternative diets in line with the RDAs for young children, it is necessary to be very careful; perfect nutritional knowledge on the required composition and/or supplementation of such diets is limited, so it is better to choose normal diets (however, even such diets can have inadequate composition and deficient amounts of certain items!).

Measurements of dietary intake (during 4 days) in 1657 U.K. children[141] from 1.5 to 4.5 years of age showed in the oldest subgroup (3.5 to 4.5 years) markedly lower energy, nutrient, vitamin and mineral content compared to those in Czech children, which cannot be explained by the slightly different age of groups compared. Although the dietary intake of U.K. preschool children was also higher than local RDAs, a considerable difference in dietary intake of Czech and U.K. children is obvious. Actual values of BMI in Czech and U.K. children, however, do not differ significantly.

Data on energy expenditure in young children have been sparse up until now, especially in the industrially developed countries; however, using the method of doubly labeled water revealed a number of important measurements under field conditions.[196,288] In young children, especially infants, data on energy intake correspond much better to the data on energy output than in older subjects. However, in *children 3.5 to 4.5 years old, the weighed dietary record gave an energy intake greater than the expenditure measured by doubly labeled water,*[75,141] which confirmed the conclusions from our observations. Similar results have been reported in slightly older children.[196] This may be a significant bias which could ultimately lead to obesity (provided the measurements are exact), the elevated prevalence of which was reported recently in the U.S.[188] and elsewhere during adolescence.

Goran et al.[135] examined the components of daily energy expenditure in children 4 to 6 years old, characterized for body weight, height, heart rate, and body composition from bioelectrical resistance. Total energy expenditure (TEE) was measured over 14 days under free living conditions using doubly labeled water. Resting energy expenditure (REE) was estimated using indirect calorimetry, and activity energy expenditure was calculated from the difference between the TEE and the REE. The mean value of the assessed TEE was markedly lower than the RDA for energy for this age group. Activity related energy expenditure was estimated to be 267 kcal, i.e., 1117 kJ/day. The TEE was most closely related to fat-free mass (FFM), body weight, and REE. When the TEE was adjusted for the FFM, a significant correlation with the heart rate was observed. When evaluated collectively, 86% of interindividual variations in the TEE were accounted for by the FFM, heart rate, and REE. *The results of this study also indicate that the present RDAs for energy are unnecessarily high,*[288] which could be one of the reasons for an increasing prevalence of obesity later on. This applies even more to Czech children.

In another study, Dauncey[72] showed that the evidence from direct and indirect calorimetry suggests the possibility of the alteration of 24-hour energy expenditure by 20% by altering the differences in minor spontaneous activity. This compares with values in the order of 10% from moderate overfeeding and somewhat less than this during mild cold exposure. Individual variability in 24-hour energy expenditure can, therefore, be accounted for not only by the differences in resting metabolism and the thermic responses to energy intake and temperature, but also by differences in minor activity. *Even fidgeting can contribute significantly to energy expenditure in restless children.*[72]

Davies et al.[76] measured total energy expenditure using the doubly labeled water technique and compared it with 1991 U.K. recommendations for energy intake. These results add to the growing literature[91,92,196,289] which indicates that *energy expenditure in young children is significantly below previous estimates, i.e., by 10 to 12%. Secular changes in habitual levels of physical activity might be responsible for reduced energy output* as shown previously by Durnin et al.[91] and recently by Schlicker et al.[318] Davies et al.[75,76] assessed the ratio of total energy expenditure/basal metabolic rate (TEE/BMR) and TEE minus BMR in 77 preschool children. The TEE was measured using the doubly labeled water technique, and BMR was predicted from body weight. Body fat was assessed by measuring the total body water via stable isotope dilution. Correlation analysis of the results showed that low physical activity level was associated with high level of body fat. This was also demonstrated in previous surveys of Czech children.[270,271]

The estimates of energy expenditure for children published by FAO/WHO in 1973 gave much higher values than those compared to the actually measured values. Since some dramatic fall in the BMR of children during the last decade could hardly be assumed, *only changes in behavioral patterns, i.e., overall lowering of physical activity*[92] *level, may explain the discrepancies between assessed energy expenditure of children*[142] *and previous RDAs for energy.*[393] The differences found between these RDAs for energy and the level of energy expenditure measured by Griffiths and Payne[142] was of the same range as the differences in energy expenditure of children from obese and normal weight children.[142,143]

Physical activity and motor development level, which display such a large variability, can be influenced by a number of factors.[391] The results of Wolanski and Siniarska[392] showed that parallel to genetic and maternal factors cultural factors in a particular society (traditional customs, social practices, etc.) determine motor traits in children.

Genetic factors obviously play an important role in the development of physical activity and energy expenditure.[298] The level of spontaneous physical activity in 24-hour cycles during 1 week was assessed in monozygotic and dizygotic twins.[121,194] Under physiological conditions, the level of physical activity was quite stable over a certain period of time, as observed for energy intake.[31,233] Days with a higher level of spontaneous physical activity were alternated with days in which the activity level was lower. The resulting value for 1 week was a relatively stable characteristic for a particular child.

There was more resemblance in the level of spontaneous activity during the same period in monozygotic than in dizygotic twins.[194] Another study using a film recording method showed that monozygotic twins resembled each other more regarding **biomechanical stereotype** when performing the same physical task (e.g., running, jumping, etc.), than normal siblings or non-related children of the same age.[332]

Griffiths and Payne[142] assessed energy expenditure in 4- to 5-year-old children born to either normal or obese parents, in whom a different level of physical activity may be assumed. The values of integrated pulse rate for the day were measured and were individually calibrated for the oxygen consumption (measured with a continuous flow diaferometer). *Energy expenditure was significantly lower in children of obese parents.*

Birch et al.[31] recorded a lower energy intake in 2- to 5-year-old U.S. children comparable in weight (and obviously also age) than in Czech children. The composition of the diet in U.S. children was quite different (see Tables

5.7a and 5.7b). U.S. diets were lighter, with more fruit and less fat. A great variability in the food intake of children was also found; in this study, though, the age and weight range was much wider than in our study, so it is difficult to compare the results. These authors also found a great variability in individual meals and a negative correlation between the energy intake of one meal to the next one. Negative correlations predominated. This indicates the existence of some orderly control mechanism, which is regulated over a longer period of time, under conditions when a child is free to consume meals according to spontaneous choice.

Genetic similarities in response to negative energy balance caused by *exercise* in adult identical twins with constant energy intake were observed. Intrapaire resemblance in the changes of body weight, fat mass, skinfolds, abdominal visceral fat, fasting plasma triglycerides and cholesterol, maximal oxygen uptake, and respiratory exchange ratio was found.[40]

Regarding the relationships between dietary intake and energy output, the measurements using doubly labeled water during a 7-day period again showed in 5-year-old children that the total free-living energy expenditure (TEE), including physical activity, (assessed by questionnaires) was considerably lower than the recommended dietary allowances (1370 ± 222 vs. 1807 ± 310 kcal/day, $p < 0.001$). The resting metabolic rate (RMR) was slightly higher than the predicted RMR. Physical activity accounted for only 7% of the TEE. The index of activity, assessed as the difference between the measured TEE and the predicted TEE, correlated positively with sports leisure activity assessed in the questionnaire. It was concluded that the TEE in 5-year-old children yields lower values of energy expenditure by about 400 kcal/day compared to current estimates. This might be due to lower than expected levels of physical activity.[112] However, it is necessary to be cautious regarding the interpretation of data using various methods — e.g., the use of the food-frequency questionnaires significantly overestimates energy intake measured in children.[174]

The imbalance between energy intake and output,[92] the impact of which might not be manifested immediately, is obviously a serious risk for later obesity and other health risk factors. This was also indicated by some experiments on laboratory animals.[158]

One of the reasons *for supressed fat deposition is a high level of spontaneous physical activity, a common characteristics of preschool age.* Later on, when the level of activity is diminished (as it occurs at the beginning of primary school both at school and during leisure time[263]), the excess intake may already manifest itself in apparent overweight or even obesity. This starts to show itself in younger school children and worsens later — especially if the overall dietary regime and physical activity does not improve. The influence of parental practices on children's food intake is important[184] and the same applies to general lifestyle.

X. RECOMMENDED DIETARY ALLOWANCES FOR PRESCHOOL CHILDREN: IS THERE A NEED FOR REVISION?

With increasing frequency, we encounter the opinion that not only the actual food intake but primarily the recommended energy allowances for children are too high. The effort to feed the child abundantly is certainly well motivated and is the result of experiences from previous centuries when a bigger and fatter child survived more often or was in better shape than a smaller, leaner child. Old painting masters presented as an ideal the "little angels" who are nowadays considered as obese. Energy reserves were good for coping with gastrointestinal, respiratory, and other illnesses, especially in early childhood. This may still apply to Third World countries.

However, under present conditions in industrially developed countries such a situation is not necessary due to the development of medical care. The delayed consequences of an imbalance between energy intake and output since the beginning of life have been considered. As shown by our previous studies, the percentage of depot fat correlated significantly positively with total serum cholesterol and triglycerides, i.e., the fatter the preschool child, the higher the serum level of cholesterol and triglycerides.[243] Donker et al.[86] also found a significant positive correlation between the Quetelet index (which expresses basically the same as a BMI) and cholesterol in children and youth aged 4 to 19 years. However, such a relationship was not proven in child populations in Spain which may be due to the Mediteranian diet.[93] Dietary intake was also followed in preschool children in Yugoslavia, and intervention was made according to the level of their serum lipids.[278]

These relationships indicate that excess dietary intake resulting in actual or delayed fatness are risk factors which enhance the development of atherosclerosis and/or ischemic heart disease later in life. Atherosclerosis is now defined as a "pediatric problem."[395] Obese children generally become obese subjects.[81]

Nutritional data from the second National Health and Nutrition Examination Survey (NHANES II) were analyzed in order to assess dietary patterns of a representative sample of children, starting with the first year of life. The results showed that the average U.S. child's diet is relatively high in total and saturated fat and low in the ratio of polyunsaturated and saturated fat. These dietary patterns[178] deviate from current dietary recommendations of World Health Organization, among other organizations.[397,398]

The percentage contributions of specific macronutrients to total energy intake in the U.S. study were as follows: total fat, 35 to 36%; total carbohydrates, 49 to 51%; and protein, 15 to 16%. This is in contrast to current expert recommendations for the period of growth, i.e., up to 30% of energy covered by fat, 15% by protein, and 55% by carbohydrates. The observed intake of saturated fats in U.S. children was 13% of energy in contrast to a recommended level of 10%. There were also some racial differences — white children ingested more carbohydrates and less fat than black children, who had more cholesterol in their diet. The amount of protein did not differ. More wholesome dietary intake patterns were suggested for U.S. children.[178]

Another comparative analysis by Albertson et al.[8] showed trends after a 10-year interval, i.e., 1978 and 1988 in U.S. 2- to 10-year-old children: 14-day food consumption diaries showed that the intake of most dietary macro-components of food remained constant. However, daily vitamin and mineral intakes were lower in 1988 than 10 years before. The intake of most nutrients remained higher than U.S. RDAs. For more than half of the children the intakes of calcium, zinc, and vitamin B_6 were below RDAs. These results also indicate the necessity for permanent monitoring of food consumption patterns in children.

As shown by Shea et al.,[325] higher amounts of fat are not indispensable for normal growth; the status children with different fat intake, i.e., 27.1% vs. 38.4% of energy (i.e., lowest and highest quintile), were compared. Children who consumed a lower percentage of energy provided by fat also consumed significantly less total calories, saturated fat, cholesterol, calcium and phosphorus, carbohydrates, thiamin, niacin, vitamin A, and vitamin C. No differences were evident in growth stature across quintiles, in spite of all differences in dietary intake mentioned. However, possible later changes in growth were not followed up more.

Recent surveys by Gregory et al.[141] showed higher than necessary energy and macrocomponent intake in preschool children in the U.K. confirming previous conclusions *on necessary revision of RDAs.*[289] The measurements in children of the Czech Republic revealed, as mentioned above, much higher dietary intakes, especially fat and protein, which may be one of the causes of the numerous health problems in the Czech population later in life.[360]

However, the *RDAs for fat must be adhered to,* especially foe the *essential, long-chain fatty acids.* Their deficiency may effect *the maturation of central nervous system, including visual development and intelligence.* The intake of fat *should not be restricted to under 30% of energy intake* until the age of 2 years.[151] The same applies to many other essential items of children's diet.

Individuals with higher energy output can eat more without the risk of enhanced fatness or possible marginal deficiencies due to reduced food intake. It is therefore, *more plausible to return to former behavioral patterns with increased physical activity than to adapt the dietary intake to reduced energy output with lowered food intake.*

It is also highly desirable to introduce a healthy composition, i.e., ratio of macrocomponents of diet early in life when nutritional habits are established,[48] and an adequate and/or inadequate food choice may be taught and practically introduced. This includes an adequate amount and mutual ratio of foods ingested, with a satisfactory amount of fiber, a limited amount of sugar and saturated fats, and adequate amounts of other food items. According to recent changes of lifestyle, though, it would be recommendable to correct the energy output and the overall energy balance with increased physical activity and exercise — this may be a more natural way to improve fitness and health.

Chapter 6

FUNCTIONAL DEVELOPMENT DURING EARLY CHILDHOOD

"The weaker the body, the more it gives orders; the stronger it is, the more it obeys."

Jean Jacques Rousseau

Physical fitness is a complex of prerequisites that allows an organism to react in an optimal way to various environmental stimuli. This is an essential component of health. Therefore, *its examination is also essential for the evaluation of the health status of any human being, not only in relation to eventual sport activity.* The human being was born as an active subject, so he/she should be examined as such — during activity. This applies to all age categories, including preschool age children.

Impaired physical activity and fitness often appears as a result of either a markedly reduced or an over abundant food supply. Inadequate diet has a significant impact on functional development as well as on the level of spontaneous physical activity of the human organism. All this can cause deviations from normal growth and development. In addition, lack of physical activity, which contributes to an inadequate energy balance and has an undesirable impact on lipid metabolism,[233] plays a role in the pathogenesis of some diseases manifested in later life.

I. COMPLEXITY OF PHYSICAL FITNESS

Physical fitness can be evaluated by assessing the functional capacity of various body systems involved during physical work loads of different degree and character. Fitness implies optimal reactions to demanding situations — both heavy work loads and accompanying environmental stress.

However, the assessment of physical fitness has been frequently restricted to the evaluation of one system only — mostly *cardiorespiratory* and/or *motor fitness* or to the determination of *total work output*, which under special situations may depend primarily upon *muscular strength, endurance,* or *skill*. Thus, the interpretation of nutritional and other environmental stimuli varies considerably, depending on the approach used. Comprehensive and well-integrated evaluation of physical fitness still needs substantial methodological development.

When correlations are sought between diet and fitness, the individual aspects of physical fitness must be differentiated. Along with the morphological prerequisites, physical performance is determined by the summation of aerobic and anaerobic processes, depending largely on the cardiorespiratory system, with a contribution from neuromuscular function and psychological factors. All of this varies during different periods of life, especially during childhood.

Even a small child may develop a strain during different physical tasks and work loads, which can be quite intense. As mentioned above, telemetric measurements during a game, running round, fighting, etc. showed the heart rate reaching a frequency of 200 to 220 heart beats per minute.[186] This of course never lasts very long, and a child spontaneously interrupts demanding activity. We may assume that all systems necessary for performing such tasks are mobilized and are functioning on a high level. All of this may be markedly *influenced by diet* and by *adaptative processes to different regimes* of *physical activity early in life*.

As compared to morphological and nutritional data, there have been much less data available up to now on functional capacity, cardiorespiratory fitness, and gross and fine motorics in preschool children.

II. CARDIORESPIRATORY FITNESS

The ability to carry oxygen to the working tissues — particularly to the active muscles (aerobic power) — depends on the efficiency of the cardiorespiratory system. It can be evaluated by measuring the oxygen consumption at a given power output, along with the necessary factors such as heart and ventilation rate, the respiratory volume, the carbon dioxide output, or the respiratory gas exchange ratio (R).

A. METHODS OF TESTING

The maximal oxygen uptake is usually measured during a work load on a treadmill, on a bicycle ergometer, or in mounting steps (single, double, triple, etc.).[211,242,331] The maximal oxygen uptake during a load may be expressed in either absolute or relative terms (e.g., per kg body weight and/or lean body mass or per heart beat). The selection of the test depends on the aim of the study and on the kinds of subjects tested (age, sex, degree of adaptation to a work load, environmental conditions, financial resources, etc.).

With preschool age children, testing on a *veloergometer* would be difficult, since adhering to a regular rhythm and number of rounds per certain period of time (as an indispensable condition for testing and comparing individuals) is practically impossible for very young children. Methodical experiments with a specially constructed veloergometer for our laboratory proved that 4- to 6-year-old children were able to tread on the veloergometer, although irregularly, with intervals of different duration, and so on. Adherence to the conditions of veloergometer testing was only possible in 6-year-old children. With younger children, cooperation was even more difficult, in spite of their enthusiasm to use the bicycle ergometer. (Veloergometers exist with a special device that shows an attractive picture only when a certain frequency of pedaling is achieved and kept; we had no opportunity for such equipment).

Using a ***treadmill*** was also only possible for children older than 5 years.[254] At that age they were able to run on it with a safety belt inserted through a pulley. *A maximal work load, though, was not used for both ethical and physiological reasons,* even in children of this age. As shown by our methodical experiments, 3- and 4-year-old children were, on the whole, unable to accept the running carpet below their feet, so this work load could not be generally used for our studies of cardiorespiratory fitness when we wanted to compare age changes during the preschool period, i.e., from 3 to 6 years.[49,50,256]

Using a mask for measuring oxygen intake and carbon dioxide output was also not feasible. The only exception were children at least 5- to 6-year-olds who were able to tolerate the mask and were able to breathe normally with it, not only at rest, but also during a work load. The same applied to cooperation with the experimental worker, so as to gain reliable and comparable data. Hoods can hardly be used during different work loads for reliable measurements.

Therefore, it was necessary to choose from a test which would be natural for children, guaranteed to assure as much as possible *homogeneous conditions for all subjects from 3 to 6 years of age,* with the ability to get reliable results comparable in all age categories mentioned. From all of the possibilities regarding the peculiarities of preschool age, as well as the accessibility of equipment, we finally chose, after longer testing, a ***modified step test*** as a submaximal work load of an aerobic character.

This test was executed in agreement with the modification of Čermák et al.[49,50] (Appendix 2). The rate was 30 steps per minute; the height of the step was 25 cm, which was adequate, on the average, for all children tested (it was, of course, not possible to adjust the height of the step to everybody's body height, or better yet, to everybody's distance from the center of gravity and/or length of lower extremities from the ground) and 30 cm for the oldest children. In kindergartens, small benches were used, and the height was adjusted with the help of mats.

As a preschool child is unable to mount a step with a regular rhythm and rate, the experimental worker always mounted alongwith two children, whom she held lightly by the hand, thus regulating the rhythm throughout the test, but without assisting the child with mounting the step. The heart rate was recorded using leads from the chest. The initial experiments were executed with the help of a multichannel recorder of Alvar and Co., and the heart rate was then obtained from the records. Later on, a specially-constructed calculator which gave alternatively the values after 30 seconds for one child and after another 30 seconds for the other child (who were tested simultaneously) was used.[256] As shown by methodical measurements, heart beat totalizers, Sporttesters, and other apparatuses constructed for the registration of heart rate in older subjects and/or adults were not usable for preschool children.[254]

Before the examination, the child rested for about 15 minutes. Then, the heart rate was assessed during *3 minutes of rest*, then, in the course of *5 minutes while mounting the step*, and finally, in the course of *5 minutes of recovery*. In total, the heart rate was recorded during 13 minutes. We also evaluated whether a **steady state** (i.e., the stabilization of heart rate during the work load, without permanently increasing until the end of the mounting) was established or not, and, if so, during which minute of the work load.

In addition to the shape of the curves of the heart rate during the above mentioned intervals, other indicators were investigated to characterize the general response to a load and to indicate the economy of this reaction. **Indices** (see Appendix 2) described previously by Čermák[49,50] were used for this purpose. These indices render general characterization of the capacity of the cardiovascular system possible (e.g., *how much work is performed per one heart beat*), thus also rendering the comparison of different age groups of boys and girls possible, where marked morphological and functional changes during the preschool period of their development occur.

B. RESULTS OF CROSS-SECTIONAL AND LONGITUDINAL SURVEYS

Average values at rest, as measured in survey A, corresponded to standards given in pediatric textbooks in all age categories examined. Mean rest values declined significantly with increasing age and did not differ (except in two cases) in boys and girls (Figures 6.1a and 6.1b).

The heart rate during *mounting of the step increased* on the average by *about 30 to 45%*. In the younger children (i.e., 3 to 4 years), in light of the higher rest values, the relative increase during a work load was somewhat smaller than in older children (6 to 7 years). Similar to heart rates during rest, the mean values of the heart rate also declined during mounting the step with advancing age. Sex-linked differences were only recorded in exceptional instances (Figures 6.1a and 6.1b).

Evaluation of the steady state revealed that it was established in all children, approximately during the second minute of the step test. *The establishment of the steady state was more rapid in older children* (Figures 6.1a and 6.1b).

During the *recovery period, the values of the heart rate returned relatively rapidly to the values at rest*. The values of the heart rate during the fifth minute of recovery did not differ significantly from the values recorded during the first 3 minutes of rest. In older children the values of the heart rate during recovery were again lower than those in younger ones (Figures 6.1a and 6.1b).

An evaluation of total values of the heart rate at rest, during a work load and during recovery, respectively, supplemented the evaluation from previous experiments (Figures 6.1a and 6.1b). A marked *decline in the values of all indicators was observed with advancing age,* i.e., of the mean heart rate after 3 minutes of the initial rest period, the sum of heart beats during 5 minutes of

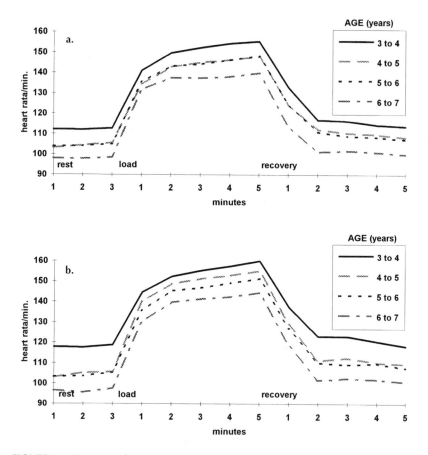

FIGURE 6.1 Heart rate during step test, i.e., 3 minutes rest, 5 minutes work load (mounting a step), and during 5 minutes of recovery in boys **(a)** and girls **(b)** of different age (survey A).[233,254,256]

work load (A) and 5 minutes of recovery. In spite of slightly higher average values of heart rate in girls, no significant sex-linked differences were observed.

In line with the calculation of the indices (see Appendix 2), i.e., net heart rate increase during work load, cardiac efficiency index 1 and 2 (Figures 6.2a and 6.2b), net heart rate during recovery and Brouha's step test index (Table 6.1) indicate *an improving economy of cardiac work during a work load in older children.*[256] An increasing effectiveness of cardiac work in relation to performed physical work is also evident. This is manifested in particular by the cardiac efficiency index (which relates the total number of heart beats during the work load and recovery to the amount of performed work; Appendix 2 for formula; Figures 6.2a and 6.2b) and in other indicators. *Brouha's index also increased markedly* (Table 6.1), indicating an improvement of cardiac efficiency during a load and a better economy of cardiac activity during the

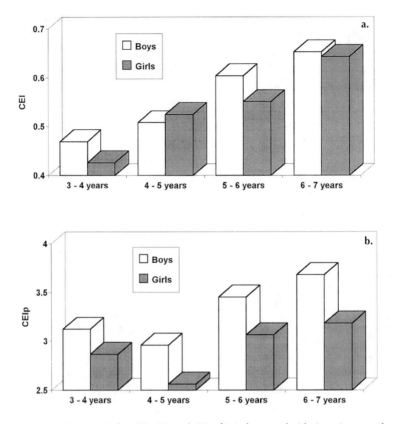

FIGURE 6.2 Step test index CEI$_1$ **(a)** and CEI$_2$ **(b)** in boys and girls 3 to 6 years of age (survey A).[254,256]

step test. In older children the increased amount of circulating blood and thus a more ample oxygen supply to the tissues during a load was obviously due to the increase of the stroke volume. This is a functional advantage for the organism during physical activity. It coincides with the increasing level of spontaneous physical activity during the preschool period and with improving motor performance.[254,256]

As mentioned above, *sex-linked differences were sporadic.* Girls tended to have somewhat higher values of heart rate during the load and during recovery. These differences were significant, however, in rare instances only. In the economy of cardiac activity, marked sexual differences were not observed. It could be expected that such differences might have appeared during a maximal work load, which were not used in our studies.

With regard to the *relationships of anthropometric variables and response of the circulation* during step test, the absolute values of heart rate during the step test and recovery correlated significantly negative, i.e., *the older and*

TABLE 6.1 Results of Brouha's Step Test Index (STI) in Children from 3- to 4- and 6- to 7-years of Age (Survey A)

Age (years)	Boys		Girls	
	$\bar{x}$	SD	$\bar{x}$	SD
3–4	87.1	8.0	82.8	6.5
4–5	91.4	9.2	90.6	7.4
5–6	92.2	10.2	92.7	10.4
6–7	99.9	9.9	98.3	10.9

Note: SD, standard deviation.

Modified from Pařízková, J., et al., *Growth, Fitness, and Nutrition in Preschool Children,* Charles University, Prague, 1984.

TABLE 6.2 Correlation Coefficients of the Relationship Between Anthropometric Variables and Indices of Cardiorespiratory Efficiency (index CEI_1, CEI_2, and Brouha's Step Test Index) in Preschool Children (Survey A)

	CEI_1	CEI_2	Brouha's index
Height	0.752**	0.254*	0.399**
Weight	0.884**	0.353**	0.334**
Length of lower extremities	0.718**	0.222*	0.376**
Breadths			
Biacromial	0.773**	0.287**	0.357**
Biiliocristal	0.631**	0.238*	0.274**
Circumferences			
Chest	0.793**	0.322**	—
Abdomen	0.637**	0.254*	—
Arm	0.704**	0.259*	—
Forearm	0.737**	0.236*	0.241*
Thigh	0.732**	—	—
Calf	0.7526**	0.228*	0.252*
Skinfolds			
Sum of 10 (modified Best)	0.239*	—	—
Sum of 5 (modified Best right)	0.238*	—	—
Sum of 5 (Harpenden right)	0.223*	0.276**	0.262**
Sum of 5 (Harpenden left)	0.578**	0.257**	0.202*
Bone age	0.462**	—	—

Note: CEI_1, CEI_2, Brouha's step test index (STI) — see Appendix 2; ** $p < 0.01$; * $p < 0.05$.

Modified from Pařízková , J., et al., *Growth, Fitness, and Nutrition in Preschool Children,* Charles University, Prague, 1984.

bigger the child, the lower the heart rate during work load and recovery. In relation to the indices of cardiorespiratory efficiency, i.e., index CEI_1, CEI_2, and Brouhas's step test index, the situation is reverse (Table 6.2). The same applies to bone age, which characterizes the level of maturation of the child.[256]

All indicators concerning the development of the child from 3 to 6 years, including the increasing circumferential and breadth measurements, correlated positively with the characteristics of the economy of work of the cardiorespiratory system. In our sample, which did not include malnourished and/or overweight children, this also concerned skinfold thicknesses that decreased during this age period — slightly in girls and more markedly in boys. Therefore, the correlation coefficients for CEI_1, CEI_2 (Figures 6.2a and 6.2b) and Brouha's step test index with skinfolds are much lower than for the other anthropometric variables and/or bone age (Table 6.2).[254,256] Only skinfolds measured on the left side correlated more closely with the indices of the cardiorespiratory efficiency.

This correlation analysis was also made in individual age groups where these relationships were rarely apparent; however, even within the framework of one age subgroup, the age was not exactly the same. As marked changes occur in preschool children even within trimesters, the impact of age was always significant. When the group was really homogeneous with age, the relationships between body size and cardiorespiratory efficiency (and also some motor tests) were not obvious; this was mostly marked in older children.[233,256]

Measurements of heart rate during the step test were also made repeatedly in the ***longitudinal studies*** of the same children followed up five times from 3.3 to 6.0 years along with morphological, motor etc., characteristics (survey E; Table 6.3) using the same protocol as in cross-sectional investigations. Although the total work performed (expressed in kpm) increased significantly during the step test, the heart rate during all stages of step test decreased. However, the heart rate also declined in older children at rest, similar to those in our cross-sectional measurements of study A (see Figures 6.1a and 6.1b). In the course of work load during each subsequent examination the heart rate was also lower; the same applied to the heart rate during recovery.

With advancing age the work load was performed more economically and efficiently. This was proved also when comparing the average values of cardiac efficiency index (CEI_1, step test index; see Table 6.3) during the first and fifth measurements.[254,256]

In this respect, the results of longitudinal survey E confirmed the trends of development in the response of cardiovascular system to a work load as assessed in the cross-sectional survey A. During the period from 3 to 6 years, important functional changes in the cardiovascular system obviously occur, meaning less strain for the child because of improved cardiorespiratory efficiency (Table 6.3).

The above mentioned changes render a gradual increase of the work load possible and, in particular, its prolongation which is impossible at a younger age. Children 5 to 6 years old were able to tolerate a defined work load without

TABLE 6.3 Changes in Cardiac Efficiency Index (CEI₁) and Brouha's Step Test Index in Preschool Children Followed Up Repeatedly (Five Measurements 1–5; Survey E)

Measurement	1	2	3	4	5
CEI_1					
Boys					
$\bar{x}$	0.47	0.53	0.57	0.64	0.85
SD	0.07	0.09	0.08	0.08	0.08
Girls					
$\bar{x}$	0.43	0.47	0.51	0.59	0.80
SD	0.07	0.07	0.10	0.10	0.10
Step test index					
Boys					
$\bar{x}$	87.2	92.5	91.1	99.1	103.3
SD	8.0	8.7	6.0	9.0	8.9
Girls					
$\bar{x}$	82.9	88.2	90.5	92.8	98.0
SD	6.3	10.5	9.7	10.56	10.1

major fatigue. This applies to an aerobic work load of medium intensity which partly has an endurance character.

C. SURVEYS IN OTHER CHILD POPULATIONS

Cardiovascular functions (heart rate and blood pressure at rest, heart rate response) were also tested by Baranowski et al.[15] in 3- to 4-year-old children with different infant nutrition, along with different heights, BMIs, and seven skinfolds. Infant feeding practices were not related to cardiovascular functioning. DuRant et al.[89,90] also followed up on cardiovascular fitness along with somatic characteristics and blood lipids.

In the available literature we did not find results of a comparable study; more recently, Italian,[104] Turkish,[359] and Senegalese[25,26] preschool children were examined.

III. MOTOR AND SENSOMOTOR DEVELOPMENT: GROSS AND FINE MOTORICS

Several tests were selected to characterize, in a more comprehensive way, different aspects of motor development. The tests should be representative of a certain motor faculty, adequate and natural regarding the stage of development, easy to perform under laboratory and/or field conditions, reproducible, and reproductible. Numerous methical measurements were performed; there was also an attempt to use tests that are part of children's usual play.[233,235,236,238,242,247,251,255,256]

A. METHODS OF TESTING
1. Speed
A 20 m dash was evaluated mostly outdoors on a playground or path in a park, not on a pavement or concrete. The child stands ready at the starting line, dressed in suitable light clothing and gym shoes. At the starting line is one person giving the order: "Ready, set, go!" The second person is at the finish line recording the time in seconds and tenths of seconds with a stop watch. After a 10 minute rest, the run is repeated, and both times are recorded for every child. Two children run simultaneously, but the time is only recorded for one child (Appendix 3).

2. Endurance
Endurance was tested in 4-year-old (and older) children (survey E) using a *500 m run-and-walk*. This test was performed in a suitable stadium or on a road. Ahead of the children, an instructor ran to make sure to set a suitable speed of both running and/or alternative walking, according to the possibilities of the children tested. This arrangement was indispensable as in the case of the step test. These kinds of activities are monotonous and uninteresting for this age period, so it was necessary to guide the children and to adjust the running speed so they will be able to finish this test. Endurance time was also tested in young children using the Bruce walking treadmill protocol to voluntary exhaustion. This method, however, is too demanding for some young children. In addition, such a method requires certain laboratory equipment, and requires the children to visit a particular institution.

3. Muscle Strength and Skill
Muscle strength in Czech preschoolers had already been measured by Matiegka[209] at the end of the last century. *Hand grip strength* was included in our surveys, assessed by a special dynamometer designed for the hands of the small children in our laboratory[233,256] based on a tensometric principle. Instruction and a demonstration made by an experimental worker preceded the experimental measurements. Two attempts were always made, and the better result was finally evaluated, as those in other performance tests.

Standing broad jump is for both testing the *explosive strength of lower extremities* and also partly a *test of skill*. The experimental worker demonstrates the jump and instructs the child "to swing your arms and then to jump as far as possible!" The child makes two attempts; both performances are recorded in centimeters, from the toes to the last foot mark of the child as in tests for older subjects. Care must be taken that the child does not start the jump while standing on the mat, but when standing on the floor. He/she then jumps onto a low mat.

Throwing a tennis ball characterizes both *the explosive strength of the upper extremities* as well as the *skill* of the child. The child stands at the line and throws the ball with an upper arch. Two attempts with each arm are made.

This is preceded by a demonstration by the experimental worker. The result of this performance is measured by a tape measure with an accuracy of a tenth of a meter.

4. Balance

Walking on a beam (at the height of about 25 to 30 cm) unassisted (but supervised) should be a *test of audacity as well as of skill and balance*. The task is considered fulfilled (grade 1) when the child has walked over the whole beam without touching the floor. When he/she touches the floor, even with just the tip of the foot, the task is not considered fulfilled (grade 2). This test is carefully followed as with all others, and the experimental worker is ready to assist in the case of marked imbalance of the child.

Standing on one leg is also a test for the ability to balance one's own body. It is demonstrated once by the experimental worker, then one attempt (the first attempt of the child) is evaluated. The task is fulfilled when the child does not touch the floor for a period of 10 seconds (recorded using a stop watch). The other leg may be bent.

The forward roll (one attempt) is evaluated according to a detailed scale from one to five (see Appendix 3). The best performance is the highest score, of five. Instructions are as follows: "Stand on the mat (not on the floor), make a 'window' with your legs wide apart, and do a forward roll as best as you can!" After doing the forward roll the child should sit on a mat.

5. Rhythm, Response, and Coordination

Walking at a given rate (one attempt), the experimental worker beats a drum at a rate suitable for a preschool child's gait. The child adheres to the rate given by the drum and marches about 20 steps in a desired direction. The standard of walking is also evaluated under the heading "body posture". The rate is given by the drum (fulfilled, 1; not fulfilled, 2). This test shows the child's ability to adhere to a given rhythm.

The task of **catching a ball (8 cm diameter)** is a test of prompt response, anticipation, and skill as detailed in Appendix 3. Each task is only performed after a demonstration by the experimental worker. The thrusting requires throwing the ball two to three times above the child so that he/she can catch it. Only one attempt is evaluated (unless the experimental worker throws the ball badly, then the procedure must be repeated; see Appendix 3).

The open and close the hands test[256] is an important indicator of senso-motor development and psychomotor coordination, as well as of the observing ability of the child (Appendix 4). The experimental worker demonstrates each procedure five times. Before doing so, he/she says "Watch what I am doing carefully and then you will do it yourself!" The demonstration is not commented on verbally so the child can watch attentively. When the child performs, we again abstain from any comments, verbal or otherwise. The first attempt (1) is evaluated (see Appendix 4). This test includes six items, each which

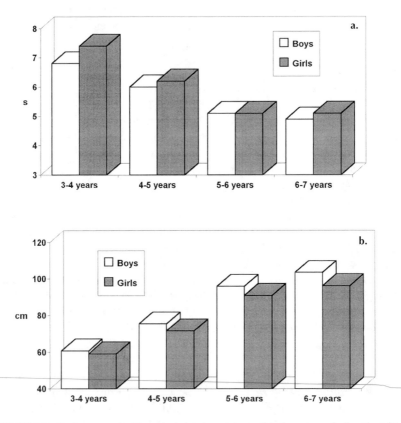

FIGURE 6.3 Performance in 20 m dash **(a)**, broad jump **(b)**, throwing a ball with right **(c)** and left hand **(d)** in boys and girls 3 to 6 years of age (survey A).[254,256,258]

gradually become more difficult. We evaluate whether the child fulfills the task (score 1) or does not fulfill the task (score 2). *Orientation in the space* and in one's body scheme is also evaluated after the first trial (see Appendix 4; fulfilled 1; not fulfilled, 2) In addition, *testing of laterality* renders the evaluation of the dominant hand, leg, and eye possible(Appendix 4).[256]

B. RESULTS OF MOTOR AND SENSOMOTOR TESTING

Speed, i.e., performance in the *20 m dash* (survey A), increased with advancing age, i.e., the time for covering this distance was lower in older children compared to younger ones. The performance level was also *better in boys than in girls in all age categories* (Figure 6.3a). This was shown also in survey B (Table 6.4). The same applied to the results of broad jump: longer jump in older children, and better results in boys (study A, Figure 6.3b; survey B; Table 6.4).

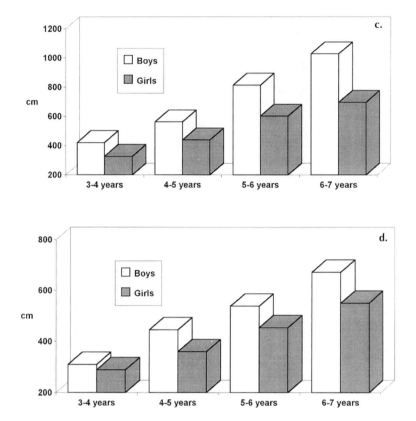

FIGURE 6.3 (continued)

**TABLE 6.4   Motor Performance in Boys and Girls 6.4
            Years Old (Survey B)**

Test	Boys		Girls	
	$\bar{x}$	SD	$\bar{x}$	SD
20 m dash (s)	5.43	1.13	5.69	1.27
Broad jump (cm)	108.5	20.8	101.7	20.4
Throwing ball/right hand (cm)	1068.6	386.8	688.8	218.8
Throwing ball/left hand (cm)	681.8	237.5	528.3	159.8

Adapted from Pařízková , J., et al., *Growth, Fitness and Nutrition in Preschool Children,* Charles University, Prague, 1984.

***Throwing a ball** with both hands was also better in older children, and
in boys compared to girls.* In this case, the sex-linked differences were usually
significant (Figures 6.3c and 6.3d).

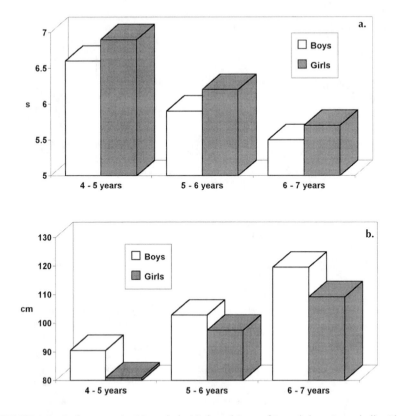

FIGURE 6.4 Performance in 20 m dash **(a)**, broad jump **(b)**, and throwing a ball with right **(c)** and left hand **(d)** in boys and girls 4 to 6 years of age (survey C).[236,238]

During the preschool years there are remarkable improvements in performance each year. This is most apparent when we compare children 3 to 4 and 6 to 7 years old: average values for the time in the 20 m dash are significantly shorter, the jump and throwing a ball significantly longer (Figures 6.3a, 6.3b, 6.3c, 6.3d). The results of survey B (children 6.4 years old; Table 6.4) showed very similar results compared with the oldest age category of survey A (Figures 6.3a, 6.3b, 6.3c, 6.3d). Sex-linked differences in this larger sample were always statistically significant.[256]

Physical performance in age groups from 4 to 5 up to 6 to 7 years was tested several years later in another cross-sectional study of 1848 boys and 1864 girls (survey C) and in 506 boys and 499 girls (survey D). The conclusions of these measurements were similar, i.e., the improvement of motor performance with increasing age, with significantly better results in boys (Figures 6.4a, 6.4b, 6.4c).[238] Performance in the 20 m dash tended to be worse than that in survey A and in boys as compared to survey C. The results of the broad jump and the ball throw were about the same.

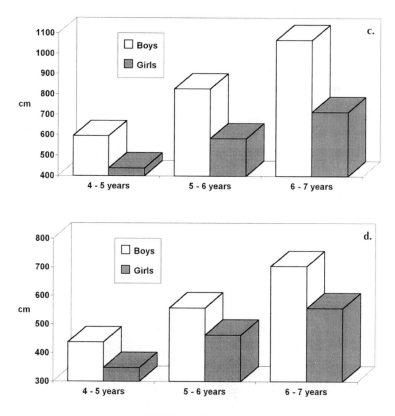

FIGURE 6.4 (continued)

Tests of motor performance correlated significantly positive with the results of step test, i.e., the reaction of the cardiorespiratory system to this work load was closely related to the performance in the above mentioned tests (Table 6.5). Cardiac efficiency index I (CEI I) correlated most closely with the performance in the 20 m dash, broad jump, and throwing a ball.

The results in **hand grip strength** *(right and left) were significantly better in boys.* Average values were also significantly higher for the right hand, both for boys and for girls (survey A, Figure 6.5). In this case the results also improved significantly with age.[238] Data of Matiegka[209] from 1929 showed maximal strength of the right hand of 5-year-old children to be 2.5 kp, i.e., 24.5 N, and in 6-year-old children to be 9.0 kp, i.e., 88.3 N, i.e., much lower values than measured in our recent studies. *These secular changes in hand grip strength appeared along with the increase in body size and BMI.*

In tests of *skill* (survey A), *girls tended to perform better*, which was manifested in particular, in standing on one leg (i.e., lower average values mean a better result; see methods) or in the forward roll (higher value means better result). There were no marked differences in walking at a given rate and catching a ball in different modifications (study A; Table 6.6).[254,256]

TABLE 6.5 Relationships (Correlations Coefficients r) Between the Results of Step Test and Motor Performance in Preschool Children (Survey A)

Tests	20 m dash	Broad jump	Throwing ball	
			right	left
CEI_1	−0.568**	0.566**	0.502**	0.463**
CEI_2	−0.215*	—	0.258**	0.231*
Step test (Brouha)	−0.330**	0.362**	0.273**	0.298**

Note: ** $p < 0.01$; * $p < 0$.

Adapted from Pařízková , J., et al., *Growth, Fitness and Nutrition in Preschool Children,* Charles University, Prague, 1984.

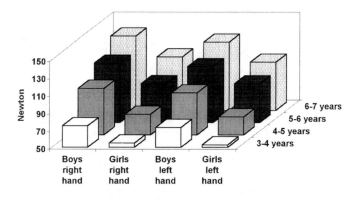

FIGURE 6.5   Hand grip strength of right and left hands in boys and girls 3 to 6 years of age (survey A).

In survey B with a greater number of children, *girls had better results in tests characterizing skill,* i.e., walking on the beam, standing on one leg, forward roll, walking at a certain rate. Only in the last variety of catching a ball (i.e., throwing it vertically above the child who catches the ball from the air; Table 6.7) were the results slightly better in boys. All sex-linked differences, although not very great, were statistically significant in this large sample (Table 6.7).[254,256] The results of the evaluation of **sensomotor development,** i.e., the "open and close hands test", in Prague children (survey A) did not show any significant sex-linked differences in any of the six items of this test. The same applied to the testing of spatial orientation and laterality (Table 6.8a).

The level of sensomotor development improved with advancing age, similar to the results of other motor tests. In more simple parts of the test requiring the opening and closing of the hands these age differences were not apparent. All of the children were able to perform them successfully from the beginning

TABLE 6.6   Results of Skill Tests in Preschool Children (Survey A)[256]

Skill		Age (years)							
		3–4		4–5		5–6		6–7	
		Boys	Girls	Boys	Girls	Boys	Girls	Boys	Girls
*Crossing	x̄	1.38	1.43	1.17	1.17	1.03	1.08	1.13	1.00
horizontal beam	SD	0.49	0.50	0.38	0.38	0.18	0.27	0.35	0.00
*Standing on one	x̄	1.56	1.26	1.25	1.04	1.13	1.04	1.07	1.13
leg	SD	0.50	0.45	0.44	0.20	0.34	0.20	0.26	0.34
**Forward roll	x̄	2.50	2.70	3.54	3.38	3.97	4.52	3.67	4.13
	SD	1.33	1.71	1.25	1.47	0.76	0.92	1.34	1.15
*Walking in rhythm	x̄	1.68	1.52	1.17	1.25	1.10	1.08	1.27	1.25
	SD	0.47	0.51	0.38	0.44	0.30	0.27	0.46	0.44
*Catching									
ball 1	x̄	1.85	1.65	1.25	1.29	1.07	1.08	1.07	1.06
	SD	0.36	0.48	0.44	0.46	0.25	0.27	0.26	0.25
ball 2	x̄	1.65	1.61	1.17	1.17	1.03	1.08	1.00	1.06
	SD	0.49	0.50	0.38	0.38	0.18	0.27	0.00	0.25
ball 3	x̄	1.97	1.91	1.79	1.88	1.53	1.48	1.53	1.50
	SD	0.17	0.29	0.41	0.34	0.50	0.51	0.51	0.51
ball 4	x̄	1.71	1.78	1.46	1.29	1.23	1.24	1.33	1.25
	SD	0.46	0.42	0.51	0.46	0.43	0.43	0.49	0.44

Note: * grade 1 (fulfilled); ** grade 5 (best score); * grade 2 (not fulfilled); ** grade 1 (worst score). Values above 1.0 indicate the percentage of children with grade 2.

Compiled from Pařízková , J., et al., *Growth, Fitness and Nutrition in Preschool Children,* Charles University, Prague, 1984.

TABLE 6.7   Skill Development in Preschool Children 6.4 Years Old (Survey B)

Skill	Boys		Girls	
	x̄	SD	x̄	SD
*Crossing horizontal beam (grade 1–2)	1.08	0.27	1.06	0.23
*Standing on one leg (grade 1–2)	1.15	0.36	1.12	0.33
**Forward roll (grade 5–1)	4.15	1.10	4.36	1.01
*Walking in rhythm (grade 1–2)	1.21	0.40	1.15	0.36
*Catching a ball 1 (grade 1–2)	1.17	0.38	1.13	0.34
ball 2*	1.13	0.33	1.11	0.31
ball 3*	1.34	0.48	1.34	0.47
ball 4*	1.28	0.49	1.29	0.45

Note: * grade 1 (fulfilled); ** grade 5 (best score); * grade 2 (failed); ** grade 1 (worst score).

Compiled from Pařízková , J., et al., *Growth, Fitness and Nutrition in Preschool Children,* Charles University, Prague, 1984.

of our measurements. Even 3-year-old children were able to imitate without making mistakes on the more simple actions.

More marked differences with advancing age were found as in the separate opening and closing of either the right or left hand (item 6), where

TABLE 6.8a   **Sensomotor Development of Preschool Children of Survey A (Results of "Opening and Closing Hands"; See Appendix 4.; Grade 1, Fulfilled; Grade 2, Failed). Lower Average Values Mean Better Results**

Age (years)			1	2	3	4	5	6
3–4	Boys	x̄	1.06	1.44	1.47	1.76	1.88	1.97
		SD	0.23	0.50	0.50	0.43	0.32	0.1
	Girls	x̄	1.04	1.43	1.39	1.87	1.87	1.91
		SD	0.20	0.50	0.49	0.34	0.34	0.28
4–5	Boys	x̄	1.00	1.08	1.04	1.25	1.38	1.54
		SD	0.00	0.28	0.20	0.44	0.49	0.50
	Girls	x̄	1.00	1.08	1.03	1.21	1.33	1.67
		SD	0.00	0.28	0.18	0.41	0.48	0.48
5–6	Boys	x̄	1.00	1.00	1.03	1.10	1.17	1.50
		SD	0.00	0.00	0.18	0.30	0.37	0.50
	Girls	x̄	1.00	1.08	1.08	1.20	1.28	1.60
		SD	0.00	0.27	0.27	0.40	0.45	0.50
6–7	Boys	x̄	1.00	1.00	1.00	1.07	1.20	1.47
		SD	0.00	0.00	0.00	0.25	0.41	0.51
	Girls	x̄	1.00	1.00	1.00	1.13	1.38	1.44
		SD	0.00	0.00	0.00	0.34	0.50	0.51

Modified from Pařízková , J., et al., *Growth, Fitness and Nutrition in Preschool Children,* Charles University, Prague, 1984.

the differences between the youngest and oldest children were greater. The more complicated the test, the poorer the result in the youngest age group. The relatively greatest improvement with age was observed in items 4 and 5 of the test (Table 6.8a).

The *last item* (the most difficult) improved the least with age, i.e., the *level of sensomotor development still remained at a relatively low level*; e.g., approximately like the results from items 2 and 3 of this test at the age of 3 to 4 years. Evidently, the sensomotor development before entering primary school still remains at a low level and is only finished during school years.

High levels of performance in spatial orientation were attained in the youngest children. There were no errors in the 6- to 7-year-old children (Table 6.8b).

The results of the laterality test were poorer, although they improved significantly with advancing age (Table 6.8b). Similar to the test of "opening and closing hands", this test still found a fairly low level of performances, even in the oldest category of preschool children.

As indicated by the observations of Keogh,(see Reference 256) even at the age of 7 years, California school children did not completely master the open and close the hands test. Sensomotor development evaluated by means of this test improves during younger school age and only reaches real maturity later. Data in older children were not obtained so far, and there are no available data on the same test in the literature. These trends do not differ significantly according to sex with increasing age.

TABLE 6.8b   Results of Testing of Spatial Orientation and Laterality in Preschool Children of Survey A (see Appendix 4; Grade 1, Fulfilled; Grade 2, Failed)

Age (years)			Spatial orientation		Laterality	
			1	2	1	2
3–4	Boys	$\bar{x}$	1.06	1.03	1.59	1.88
		SD	0.23	0.17	0.50	0.32
	Girls	$\bar{x}$	1.09	1.09	1.74	1.96
		SD	0.28	0.28	0.44	0.20
4–5	Boys	$\bar{x}$	1.13	1.04	1.38	1.58
		SD	0.33	0.20	0.49	0.50
	Girls	$\bar{x}$	1.04	1.04	1.54	1.67
		SD	0.20	0.20	0.50	0.48
5–6	Boys	$\bar{x}$	1.03	1.00	1.23	1.40
		SD	0.18	0.00	0.43	0.49
	Girls	$\bar{x}$	1.00	1.00	1.40	1.56
		SD	0.00	0.00	0.50	0.50
6–7	Boys	$\bar{x}$	1.00	1.00	1.20	1.20
		SD	0.00	0.00	0.41	0.41
	Girls	$\bar{x}$	1.00	1.00	1.31	1.63
		SD	0.00	0.00	0.47	0.50

Modified from Pařízková , J., et al., *Growth, Fitness and Nutrition in Preschool Children,* Charles University, Prague, 1984.

The test of "*opening and closing the hands*" in children 6.4 years old (survey B; Table 6.9) shows *higher levels* of concentration, attention, and imitating capacity, as well as the possibilities of a well-coordinated, more refined activity of the upper extremities *in girls*. This was apparent in particular in the more complicated parts of this test (see items 3 through 6 in Appendix 4). The percentage of girls who completed these tests was well above the percentage of boys. The same applied to spatial orientation (Table 6.9; see item 2 in the Appendix 4) and laterality test 1. The remaining tests characterizing sensomotor development in survey B did not differ in 6.4-year-old boys and girls.

The relationship between the results of individual motor and sensomotor tests was also analyzed. Figure 6.6 shows the results of the tests of independence in 3712 boys and girls aged 4 to 6 years (survey C). *There were mostly very close relationships between the results of the individual performance and skill tests.* Therefore, for practical purposes it is possible to use only fewer selected motor and sensomotor tests to get more general information on the development of motor abilities.[266]

As in the testing of cardiorespiratory efficiency by the modified step test, children were followed in longitudinal studies from 3.5 to 6.0 years regarding their motor development (study E). Repeated measurements of the same children again confirmed the results of cross-sectional examinations: the level of performance in running, jumping, and throwing improved significantly with

TABLE 6.9   Sensomotor Development in Preschool Children 6.4 Years Old (Survey B; grade 1 and 2)

Sensomotor test	Item	Boys $\bar{x}$	Boys SD	Girls $\bar{x}$	Girls SD
Opening and closing hands	1	1.03	0.16	1.02	0.15
Opening and closing hands	2	1.09	0.28	1.09	0.29
Opening and closing hands	3	1.10	0.30	1.09	0.28
Opening and closing hands	4	1.34	0.47	1.30	0.46
Opening and closing hands	5	1.33	0.47	1.30	0.46
Opening and closing hands	6	1.72	0.45	1.67	0.47
Spatial orientation	1	1.02	0.10	1.02	0.14
Spatial orientation	2	1.02	0.10	1.01	0.10
Laterality	1	1.29	0.45	1.28	0.45
Laterality	2	1.33	0.48	1.36	0.48

Adapted from Pařízková , J., et al., *Growth, Fitness and Nutrition in Preschool Children*, Charles University, Prague, 1984.

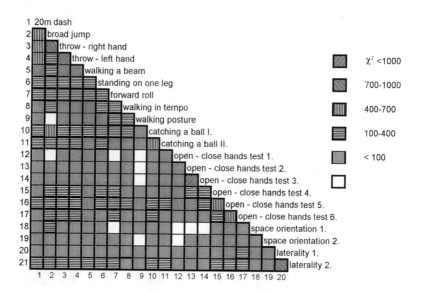

FIGURE 6.6   Relationships among the results of motor performance and skill tests in preschool children tested by χ^2 (survey C).

advancing age, and the results were always better in boys. The hand grip strength increased with age and was also greater in boys.[255] This was in contrast to the results of step test; apparently, the *sex-linked differentiation is only manifested in tests motivated toward maximum performance* and not in that of medium intensity.

All above mentioned sensomotor tests were also repeatedly performed. As mentioned in conjunction with cross-sectional comparisons, marked improvement with increasing age was found.[255]

TABLE 6.10 **Correlation Coefficients Between the Results of Performance Tests Measured Three Times at Different Ages in Preschool Children (Survey E)**

Discipline	Measurement		
	1st–2nd	1st–3rd	2nd–3rd
Boys			
20 m dash	0.677**	0.714**	0.857**
Broad jump	0.709**	0.422*	0.661**
Throwing a ball (right)	0.321	0.516**	0.374
Throwing a ball (left)	0.356	0.634**	0.450*
Hand grip strength (right)	0.533**	0.477*	0.424*
Hand grip strength (left)	0.488**	0.532**	0.336
Girls			
20 m dash	0.647**	0.633**	0.598**
Broad jump	0.554*	0.750**	0.204
Throwing a ball (right)	0.655**	0.714**	0.678**
Throwing a ball (left)	0.390	0.495*	0.461*
Hand grip strength (right)	0.515*	0.462*	0.479*
Hand grip strength (left)	0.587**	0.379	0.365

Note: Statistical significance, $p < 0.01$**; $p < 0.05$*.

Compiled from Pařízková , J., *Wld. Rev. Nutr. Diet.,* 51, 1, 1987 and from Pařízková , J., et al., *Humanbiol. Budapest,* 16, 113, 1985.

Individual stability of motor development was shown by intercorrelations of the results measured in individual children at the occasion of the first and second, the first and third, and the second and third measurements in survey E (Table 6.10), i.e., from about 3.5 to 6.0 years. The closest relationships were found for speed (20 m dash) and in the broad jump at the beginning and end of our measurements.[266]

Further analyses of the results in motor tests in the individual years *did not always show more favorable results in larger children in the same age category.* In some cases, performance was better in larger peers, but quite often, smaller children of comparable age were more fit, especially in running and in skill tests.[254]

Another longitudinal study, made several years later along with morphological measurements (survey F) from about 4.5 years up to 5.9 through 6.0 years, also confirmed, in three consecutive measurements, a significant improvement in motor performance with age and better results in boys (Figures 6.7a, 6.7b, 6.7c, 6.7d). Mutual comparison of the results of the same tests in study E and F were complicated because of the slightly different average age of the individual groups of children followed in these particular surveys; it was not possible to keep our measurements completely identical to homogeneous samples in relation to age.

In study F, the evaluation of performance in the ***500 m run-and-walk*** (Figure 6.7d) was also evaluated, but only starting at the age of 5 years and 4 months in boys and 5 years and 6 months in girls. In this endurance test,

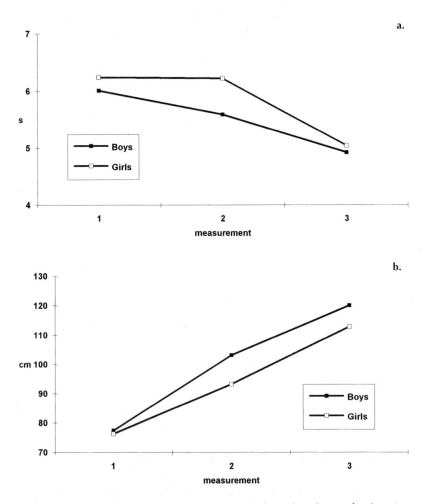

FIGURE 6.7 Changes of the performance in 20 m dash **(a)**, broad jump **(b)**, throwing a ball with right hand **(c)**, and 500 m run-and-walk **(d)** in boys and girls followed up longitudinally from 4.4 years (boys) and 4.6 years (girls; survey F), then 1 year later, and finally at the age of 5.9 years (boys), and 6 years (girls).[239,267]

there were significant *improvements* again with *advancing age and significantly better results in boys.* Girls in survey F performed better in skill tests as in the other groups mentioned above.[242]

Performance in *tests of fine motorics and coordination of the hands* (open and close the hands test) improved significantly between the first and second measurement of survey F in both girls and boys. On the other hand, the results of the third and last measurement were significantly worse, in both boys and girls. However, girls always had better results compared to the boys, especially during the second and third measurement.

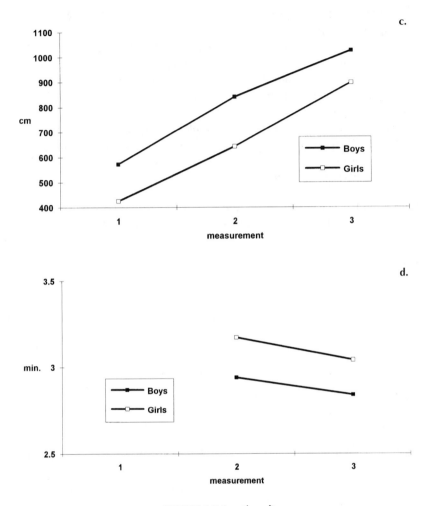

FIGURE 6.7 (continued)

Performance in the test of copying pictures improved in boys and girls during all measurements. Girls had significantly better results than the boys, during the first and third measurement.[207,208]

Orientation in space and in relation to one's own body was tested during the first and third measurement of study F. The results were significantly better in the last measurement. In both cases, girls had markedly poorer results than boys.

Laterality was tested only during the first and third measurements. The results were worse during the third measurement compared to the results of the first one. This shows a shift toward ambivalence in the development of preschool children.[242] In this case, sex-linked differences were not observed.

C. MOTOR DEVELOPMENT IN ESTONIAN CHILDREN OF PRESCHOOL AGE

Oja and Jurimae[222] measured preschool children in Tartu, Estonia. The goal of their investigation was to develop a battery of tests for measuring motor abilities in preschool children and to validate the tests used elsewhere for Estonian children of preschool age which have never been followed up in this respect before.

Somatic development is shown in Table 6.11, i.e., the values of height, weight, and BMI of children measured in various kindergartens in Tartu. The average values do not differ significantly from international standards and/or from the values measured in Prague children.

TABLE 6.11 Anthropometric and Motor Performance Variables of Preschool Children in Tartu, Estonia (n = 932)

		Boys	Girls	Boys	Girls
Age (months)	$\bar{x}$	54.2	53.5	65.9	65.7
	SD	3.8	3.7	3.6	3.4
Height (cm)	$\bar{x}$	107.0	106.4	114.2	112.8
	SD	4.4	5.3	5.0	5.1
Weight (kg)	$\bar{x}$	18.0	17.5	20.1	19.5
	SD	2.0	2.2	2.4	2.6
BMI (kg/m²)	$\bar{x}$	15.7	15.4	15.4	15.2
	SD	1.2	1.4	1.2	1.3
3 minute run (m)	$\bar{x}$	333.9	324.5	366.7	349.3
	SD	37.4	36.0	38.1	34.8
Broad jump (cm)	$\bar{x}$	88.2	84.7	105.4	100.1
	SD	17.3	16.1	17.5	14.6
Bag throw — right (cm)	$\bar{x}$	472.8	359.6	609.1	439.7
	SD	144.1	93.4	172.7	110.3
Bag throw — left (cm)	$\bar{x}$	337.0	300.9	433.8	363.6
	SD	90.6	74.8	114.3	83.4

Modified from Oja, L. and Jürimae, T., Assessment of motor ability in 4- to 5-year-old children, in press, 1995.

Regarding **motor abilities**, the standing long jump, the two-handed sand bag throw (150 g), the 4 by 10 m shuttle-run, the 3-minute run, sit-ups, and the sit-and-reach were used to test children 4- to 5- and 5- to 6-years old. As shown in previous studies, the performance of children improved significantly with age. *Motor performance was better in boys* (Table 6.11) *while girls had better results in flexibility tests.* Correlation analyses showed that the results of motor ability testing were often dependent on body height and weight, but not on BMI. Tests of fine motorics were not made.

The results of Tartu children were somewhat better than the results of surveys A, B, and E[255,256] made in the 1970s, but they were lower when comparing newer data from surveys D and F.[242,256] In this case, Czech children were also more advanced in somatic development. In other tests used in the Estonian survey,[222] only the previous data of Cratty[62,63] were available for comparison.

Generally, the results of the same tests applied in both Tartu and Prague children did not differ markedly, because the conditions of life and daily regime of children also were quite similar.

IV. METABOLIC AND BIOCHEMICAL CHARACTERISTICS

Most often, it is ofinterest to gather data on blood lipids for the early screening of possible at risk subjects. The document of the World Health Organization on "Prevention in childhood and youth of adult cardiovascular diseases"[395] focuses on the earliest periods of life, including preschool age, regarding the necessary measures for the prevention of the development of risk factors.[2,127,141] Therefore, in additional surveys H, I, J serum lipid levels were also measured. In conjunction to the evaluation of body composition the creatine kinase activity was also assessed as an indicator of muscle mass in children.

A. METHODS AND SUBJECTS

Serum lipids were estimated in the morning after an overnight (12 to 14 hours) fast. Only a light breakfast was permitted, i.e., cup of herbal tea, half a roll, and no fats. Total cholesterol, high density lipoproteins (HDL-C), and low density lipoproteins (LDL-C) were estimated using Boehringer tests. Triglycerides were assessed using Lachema tests in the World Health Organization Regional Lipid Reference Center in the Institute of Clinical and Experimental Medicine (IKEM) in Prague.[270,271]

The *creatine kinase activity* in the blood was assessed in our laboratory using the Boehringer tests.[343] The average measurement error of all biochemical methods used was 2 to 4%.

The mentioned assessments were performed in a smaller group of Prague children in day care centers (n = 22; subgroup of survey H, i.e., group 1, age 3 to 5 years). Preliminary analyses did not show any significant sex-linked difference in the biochemical variables in this sample. Further measurements were repeated in groups of children from other localities and will be discussed later.

Along with the assessment of serum lipids, cardiorespiratory efficiency was tested, using the modified step test as described above (see p. 113). Simultaneously, the dietary intake and skinfold thicknesses were measured, and the body composition was evaluated using formulas of Brook.[42] Mutual relationships of all variables followed were also analyzed.

B. RESULTS: BLOOD LIPIDS AS RELATED TO SOMATIC DEVELOPMENT, DIETARY INTAKE, AND CARDIORESPIRATORY EFFICIENCY

Mean values of height and weight did not differ significantly from standard values for this particular age category with an average age of 4.9 ± 0.52 years.[291,292] The average value of body mass index (***BMI***) was 16.2 ± 0.3, which was close to the 70th percentile of Czech standards,[35] i.e., similar to other samples of Prague children it was slightly higher than the corresponding 50th percentile.

The *percentage of **body fat*** was 16.0 ± 4.0%, *the absolute amount of lean* body mass was 16.1 ± 1.8 kg. Regarding somatic development, the children in this particular group did not differ significantly from the average child population of The Czech Republic.

A special index expressing the robusticity of lean body mass (LBM) development was also evaluated, i.e., *LBM kg/10 cm body height*. The value of this index was 1.46 ± 0.10 kg.[271]

With sex-linked differences, only body weight was significantly higher in boys compared to girls, who were slightly, but insignificantly, older than girls. There was a higher absolute amount of LBM as well as a higher index LBM kg/10 cm height in boys. These sex-linked differences, however, were not statistically significant in this group of preschool children. Therefore, mean values for all children together are given. There were no significant sex-linked differences in the serum level of serum lipids as in U.K. children.[141]

Average values of ***serum lipids*** are given in Figure 6.8. These values did not differ significantly from those given by other authors.[2,3,127] However, the comparison with recent data on serum lipids in children in the U.K.U.K. showed significantly lower values of ***total cholesterol***, significantly higher values of ***triglycerides***, and the same values of ***HDL*** in slightly younger U.K. children (3.5 to 4.5 years old[141]).

As in other variables, there was a marked interindividual variability apparent, which was greatest for triglycerides (0.34 to 0.89 mmol/l, CV = 30.8%) and smallest for total cholesterol (3.6 to 6.2 mmol/l, CV 15.6%). HDL values varied from 0.6 to 1.6 mmol/l (CV = 20.1%) and LDL from 2.1 to 5.0 mmol/l (CV = 23.3%).[271]

Values also did not differ markedly from those ascertained from older Czech children.[284] No significant relationship of blood lipids, above all HDL, to the level of physical fitness was found. Our data indicate that the cardiac efficiency index in preschool children varied more on a constitutional basis and was not significantly related to HDL.

In Czech school children (11 to 12 years old) extreme values of total cholesterol ranging from 2.6 to 7.4 mmol/l in boys, with an average value of 4.32 mmol/l, were found.[284] For girls the values ranged from 2.6 to 8.2 mmol/l, with a mean value of 4.4 mmol/l. Energy intake in these children was also higher than the RDAs of The Czech Republic[171] and of the European Community (E.C.),[398] mostly due to a high ratio of energy derived from fat.[284]

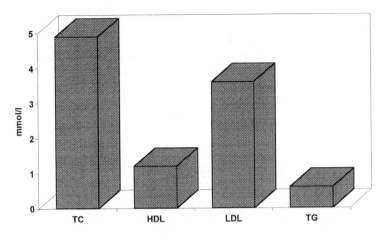

FIGURE 6.8 Blood lipid level (total, HDL, LDL cholesterol, triglycerides) in a group of preschool boys and girls (survey I)

Resting values for ***creatine kinase*** were 42.2 ± 14.4 U/l, which varied from 26.6 to 85.6 U/l (CV = 34.1%). The creatine kinase activity was approximately half the value normally assessed in the adults.[271] We did not find any values for children of this age in the literature.

In other variables assessed, the ***intake of energy and other dietary components*** (see Figure 5.1) corresponded roughly to the recommended dietary allowances (RDAs) for Czech preschool children[171] and was slightly, but not significantly, higher in boys. The fat intake was approximately 35% higher than the RDAs for Czech children. The difference from the U.S. and the E.C. RDAs (Tables 5.6a and 5.6b) is much greater, i.e., the intake of energy and macrocomponents was again much higher in Czech children.[271]

The variability of food intake was marked as usual. The values of CV for total energy was about 28%, about 34% of proteins, 34% of fat, and 35% of carbohydrates. The average value for one week's energy intake for individual children varied from 5.9 to 9.32 MJ/day.

The results of the ***step test*** again showed that the work load used was not excessive. The steady state was established during the second and third minutes of mounting, and the heart rate returned to rest values during the second to fourth minute of recovery. The curves of heart rate during step test were comparable to previous results (survey A, Figures 6.1a and 6.1b).

The calculation of the step test and cardiac efficiency indices showed a marked variability (CV about 10%). With sex-linked differences, boys tended to have better results (i.e., a smaller increase in the pulse rate during the work load, higher values of both indices), but these differences were not statistically significant. Generally, the reactions of the heart rate to this work load did not differ from those found previously in larger groups of children.

There were *no significant mutual* **relationships** *between somatic variables, percentage of depot fat, dietary intake, and blood lipid values in this group of 22 children.* (Significant positive relationships were found, however, in a larger sample of 54 preschool children for the percentage of body fat on the one hand, and both total cholesterol and triglycerides, on the other hand.[243]) However, the *index LBM kg/10 cm height* correlated significantly in this group with the cardiac efficiency index (CEI, r = 0.696, *p* < 0.001), *the creatine kinase activity* (r = 0.436, *p* < 0.05), *and fat intake* (r = 0.489, *p* < 0.05), thus revealing the importance of the development of lean body mass in cardiorespiratory efficiency.[271] At this age, the consumption of fat seems to have an influence on the development of lean body mass.

Creatine kinase activity as an indicator of muscle mass was also significantly related to the development of lean body mass, as already characterized by the above mentioned index at this growth period. The influence of fat intake — which was increased as compared to RDA — did not yet cause obesity, but rather it caused an accelerated development of lean body mass.

We had no opportunity to assess similar characteristics in parents, so the relationships between parent and child could not be analyzed.

V. STUDIES OF BIOCHEMICAL VARIABLES, BLOOD PRESSURE, AND FATNESS IN OTHER POPULATIONS

DuRant et al.[89] examined somatic variables, blood lipids, and activity in 4- to 5-year-old children followed up during 2 years. The waist/hip ratio assessed during the first year was inversely correlated with total body cholesterol (TCh) and low density lipoprotein (LDL) levels. On the basis of multiple correlation analysis, the sum of seven skinfolds, height, and gender explained the 15.4% variation of the triglyceride (TG) levels. *The sum of seven skinfold measurements was inversely correlated with the high-density lipoprotein (HDL) level.* The sum of seven skinfolds measured during the second year correlated positively with LDL/HDL and TCH/HDL ratios. These results indicate, as in our previous study,[271] a significant relationship between the accumulation of body fat and blood lipids at a young age.

Higginbotham et al.[157] considered the association between Type A behavior patterns (TABP) and serum cholesterol levels. The effects of TABP may be related to the usual coronary heart risk factors (CHRF) already early in life. However, no significant differences in serum cholesterol were found among young children (5 to 6 years old) differing in ethnicity, in gender, and/or in TABP. LDLC and triglycerides differed significantly according to gender and ethnicity.

Blood pressure was also investigated by Gutin et al.,[146] along with fat distribution and fitness (submaximal treadmill test), in children 5 to 6 years old. *Diastolic blood pressure was inversely related to the level of fitness* in boys and girls and positively related to fatness in boys. *Systolic blood pressure was positively related to fatness* in boys and girls. When using multiple regression including parental blood pressure, fatness pointed up the significant variance in systolic blood pressure for both boys and girls. This variance in diastolic blood pressure only applied to boys. *Central deposition of fat had the greatest influence*, i.e., large values of skinfold thicknesses on the trunk and less on the extremities, again only applying to *boys*. Fitness and fatness were inversely related in both sexes. Even in small children, then, it is possible to find the same risk factors for increased blood pressure as in much older individuals.

VI. GENERAL CONSIDERATIONS

As shown by all formerly mentioned cross-sectional and longitudinal measurements, there are many general considerations in the functional development of preschool children:

- A significant improvement of performance occurs in all age categories during preschool age, i.e., from 3 to 6 years[250,252,259]
- *In testing cardiorespiratory fitness by modified step test only exceptionally* significant sex-linked differences appeared in spite of a slight trend for higher values of heart rate during work load in girls when a medium aerobic work load is induced
- *Boys have significantly better results in performance tests* such as the 20 m run, the 500 m run-and-walk, jumping and throwing a ball, i.e., in the tests where a *competitive aspect for maximal effort* is involved. Boys also tended to have better results in orientation tests in space and in relation to one's own body
- *Girls normally had better results in skill tests* such as walking on a beam, walking at a given pace, forward roll, standing on one leg, as well as in relation to indicators for sensomotor development, i.e., the "open and close hands test". The same applies to the "draw-a-man-test" and other tests for fine motorics
- In all parameters measured, there appeared a marked *variability*, i.e., children showed characteristic individual features in the level of performance in various tests, as well as in the attitude to performing different types of exercise and physical activity. This indicates that some of the children demonstrated quite an enthusiasm to participate in our testing (and also in exercise and physical education in day care centers in general), while others had to be more stimulated to take part in all these activities. The combination of various favorable predispositions and/or handicaps for physical activity and performance characterized the above mentioned "motor individuality"
- *"Motor individuality"* had a *stable trend of development* as shown by significant correlations between the results in various disciplines measured in individual years of longitudinal survey E[266]

- Significant *relationships* were found between the results of individual motor and sensomotor tests as shown by χ^2 analysis: when a child showed a good level of performance in one physical task, it can be assumed that he/she will have a similarly good result in another task and *vice versa*. For practical purposes, a battery of selected tests would be sufficient (see Chapter 12)
- As shown by the better performance of children from survey A in, for example, the 20 m dash, compared to other Prague children measured during the same period (B), the role of optimal pedagogical guidance in the physical education of children is essential to achieving adequate motor development at preschool age (see Chapter 10).

The conclusions of these measurements reveal the remarkable dynamics of functional development during preschool age, i.e., motor stimulation and physical education of children should be differentiated by age. The same applies to sex-linked differences,[62,63,256] which require a different approach to the physical education of boys and girls at preschool age.[250]

No relationships between BMI and body fat to dietary intake appeared. Fat intake only correlated positively with the index LBM kg/height cm, i.e., only with more robust development of LBM. This also seems to confirm the conclusion that the development of obvious obesity does not yet appear at preschool age, in spite of more supporting factors. BMI also did not correlate with the level of performance in preschool children of the same age and the level of serum lipids.

Chapter 7

THE INFLUENCE OF DIFFERENT DEGREES OF DIETARY INTAKE ON SOMATIC DEVELOPMENT AND PHYSICAL FITNESS

"Everyone has the right to a standard of living adequate for health and well-being of himself and his family, including food …"

Universal Declaration of Human Rights, 1948

There is a long-standing ideal that adequate food should be a fundamental human right. After 1948, when the *Universal Declaration of Human Rights* was proclaimed, other such declarations followed. The *International Covenant of Economic, Social and Cultural Rights* (1976) states "The State Parties to the present Covenant recognize the right of everyone to an adequate standard of living for himself and his family, including adequate food, clothing and housing and also recognize the fundamental right of everyone to be free from hunger."

In the *Convention on the Right of the Child,*[400] two articles address the issue of nutrition. Article 24 proclaims "State Parties recognize the right of the child to their enjoyment of the highest attainable standard of health," and thus they "shall take appropriate measures to combat disease and malnutrition" through the provision of adequate nutritious foods, clean drinking water, and health care. Article 27 indicates that the State Parties "shall in case of need provide material assistance and support programmes, particularly with regards to nutrition, clothing and housing."[175]

There might have been some progress with these ideals,[321] but the situation of those who are most vulnerable and defenseless in the society — children and youth — has still been unsatisfactory in many parts of the world. As a result, a call to action was also given by the Commission on Global Governance[399] in 1995 because in some parts of the world, the situation is not improving.[401]

I. GROWTH AND DEVELOPMENT

Stunting and *wasting* have been recognized in many populations suffering from malnutrition. Stunting, i.e., small body size due to deficits in linear growth, is extremely common in the countries of the Third World, where energy and protein requirements cannot be met. In some countries, almost 50% of children have been classified as stunted,[376–378] so its significance cannot be ignored in relation to public health care. Signs of severe malnutrition, including stunting, may be observed even in the industrially developed countries. The most common causes of such a phenomenon are poverty and accompanying ignorance,[44,286] unfortunately quite common even in places where it is avoidable.

The Expert Committee of a Joint FAO/WHO/UNU Consultation[393] accepted the view that *children of different ethnic groups basically have the same growth potential,* and that *the cause of widespread growth retardation is principally environmental.*

Satisfactory growth is a sensitive criterion, whether energy and protein needs of the child are met.[319,379] The *definition of satisfactory growth is also the first step in estimating the requirements of infants, and children.*[51,52] For that reason, the evaluation of the growth level holds an important place in many scientific disciplines.

Early onset of stunting has adifferent etiology among populations of varying biological, environmental, and cultural circumstances. Powerful determinants of an infant's size at birth and during the first 6 months of life are maternal size at the beginning of pregnancy and weight and fat gain during pregnancy and lactation.[218]

As mentioned above, a *dilemma* has materialized as to *whether reference standards for the growth of children in industrialized countries should be accepted as universally relevant* or *whether local standards should be used.* Children in many developing countries are already smaller at birth compared to those born in industrialized countries, and they then grow at a slower rate during infancy and early childhood.

In some discussions, stunting has been classified as a sort of adaptation to adverse environmental conditions and lack of food. A small child needs less food, and thus survival is promoted in such a case when food is in short supply.[322] This is the concept of costless adaptation (FAO 1988), which has aroused a great deal of emotional discussion.[20,131,132,206,377,378]

"Small but healthy" was postulated by Seckler,[322] when body size was above a certain limit. This concerns more cases of marginal malnutrition than truly severe malnutrition. Many authors, e.g., Satyaranayana et al.,[315–317] claim that this justifies a certain degree of malnutrition and poverty and does not correspond to the human rights that should be the same for all human beings, including sufficient food and the development of one own's genetic potential. We may only comment that "small but healthy" is better than "small, sick, and unfit". This general hypothesis may be rephrased in the following way:

stunting is a compromise with environmental stress, perhaps the best that can be achieved under the circumstances.[378]

With preschool children, in the places where nutrition problems are coming under control, such as in Latin America, the 1990s have brought about continued improvement. In the two worst affected regions in numbers and prevalence, though, the situation is worrisome. Sub-Saharan Africa is deteriorating, and South Asia is only improving slowly, if at all.[401] Coming years will be decisive for the resolution of this problem.

II. THE INFLUENCE OF DIFFERENT DEGREES OF NUTRITION

Wasting is associated with a *low weight for height* which, especially in young children, is associated with an increased risk of morbidity and mortality.[393] This type of severe weight deficit is generally found only in a small proportion of children. A higher incidence of this type of malnutrition is only found during famines. The extra amount of energy and protein needed for catch-up growth has been calculated in some detail in studies on the rehabilitation of malnourished children. The role of urea salvage in the adaptation to low intake of protein and energy was described.[164] Representative values for the energy cost are about 5 kcal, i.e., 21 kJ/1 g of tissue laid down. Protein cost is 0.23 g/1 g of deposited tissue (0.16 g deposited at 70% efficiency of metabolic processes).

Waterlow[378] summarized the data on the influence of malnutrition on somatic growth, especially on height and weight. Data on other anthropometric variables have still been very rare. Some data for circumferential measurements and skinfolds are available. Arm circumference was selected, along with height, as a representative measure of wasting, using the "Quack stick" (i.e., a stick for measuring total body height and a mark for critical values of arm circumference) used by Quakers under field conditions in developing countries.[45]

A formula for the evaluation of arm muscle circumference (AMC) is another variable that makes the evaluation of the degree of malnutrition possible.[163] Similar formulas were also derived by other authors.[10]

Body composition in relation to body water was simultaneously followed up by Field et al.[107] in malnourished children using $^{18}H_2O$ and bioimpedance analysis. Regression equations for the assessment of body composition were derived from BIA measurements. Vettorazzi et al.[363] also used BIA for the estimation of total body water in malnourished children.

Some observations indicate that the effort to achieve larger body size does not always coincide with fulfilling the potential for factors such as high levels of cardiorespiratory fitness, positive health, and long life expectancy.[155,308,309]

Experience with *long surviving individuals* (up to the ninth decade) indicate that they mostly had *very modest and austere diet in childhood.* They also did not grow too fast and *did not achieve large body size in adulthood*[155,214] as a result of marginal malnutrition.

In his experimental model with laboratory animals, Ross[308,309] showed that *restriction of dietary intake had a significant impact on the duration of life.* The restriction of the protein component had only a small but significant effect in two dietary groups allotted rations on an isocaloric basis. A restricted carbohydrate intake with resultant restriction of energy intake enhanced life expectancy. Restricting the intake of both protein and carbohydrates with restriction of energy intake, though showing no pronounced effect early in life, enhanced life expectancy to the greatest degree because of the beneficial effects later in life.[308,309]

Under *ad libitum* conditions of feeding, the mortality patterns were considerably different than those under restricted conditions. When the identical diets used earlier were employed in all groups except the one fed a relatively low protein ratio (8%) and high in carbohydrates, the lifespan was one half to one third that of the groups of rats fed a restricted diet.[308] Rats ingesting *ad libitum* a diet with 30% protein (casein) also started to die much earlier than rats on a diet of normal composition.

Data concerning life tables and national food balance sheets[341] for populations from 96 countries[119] indicate that life expectancy at birth increases with total calories, with the overall quality and quantity of the diet, and with the ratio of fat to proteins. The ratio of carbohydrates to fats is negatively associated with level of mortality. However, evidence indicates that the main effect of the ratio of fats to proteins is reversed when diets are high in quality, and that all of the effects tend to saturate at high nutrient availability. Variation in nutrition is also strongly associated with the international variation in age patterns of mortality. *When life expectancy is held constant, populations with higher quality diets tend to have lower childhood mortality but higher adult mortality.*[119]

The definition of the limit of dietary intake for acceptable and/or satisfactory functional development, along with a desirable body size, also considering the genetic potential, is surely a very difficult task. Even in a healthy privileged population, a wide range of variation exists in the size of children. The reasons for this are mostly of genetic character, and the size of the mother seems to be of great importance. In developing countries, a body weight of 40 kilograms is considered a risk factor for reduced birth weight;[120] children born with very low birth weight are usually unable to catch up completely, remaining smaller until adulthood. In the U.S. only 1% of women have a lower body weight than 40 kilograms;[132] therefore, the risk of babies with reduced birth weight is very small in this country.

In the industrially developed countries, the wide range of variation in body size is not related to health, well-being, or physiological function per se. However, in communities where children's growth is limited by environmental factors — especially inadequate food — there is an evidence of an association between functional impairment and deficiencies in linear growth. In such situations, it is very difficult to differentiate the effects of malnutrition from those of other aspects of social deprivation.[64] Further research is, therefore, necessary for the elucidation of the main mechanism resulting in small body size — whether it is only a handicap or a result of meaningful adaptation — because minor limitations of genetic potential might not be harmful. Eventually, non-maximal realization of one potential may render possible more marked realization of another potential — especially of a functional one — such as skill, speed, endurance, etc.

Full realization of all human potentials would be the optimal goal of health and nutritional care. However, environmental conditions do not always permit this. Then, it is necessary to decide what is primary and preferable: *functional potential of an organism might be, especially under special conditions, more important than the maximal body size*; satisfactory function may exist even in a small organism.

As mentioned above, children in the developing countries of the Third World also start with a lower birth weight, which is an additional risk. In epidemiological studies of childhood undernutrition it is conventional to accept −2 SD from the median of weight as the cut-off point between "normal" and "malnourished". This corresponds approximately to the third percentile (or 80% of the median for weight,[376] and 90% for height. However, inadequate dietary intake resulting in low body weight is a risk also for low income children elsewhere.[43,287]

There is very little precise information on the age up until which the capacity for catch-up is retained. It seems probable that this is possible until the end of the adolescent growth spurt.[393]

III. SURVEYS IN POPULATIONS VARYING IN DIETARY INTAKE

The follow up of Czech children only provided a limited opportunity to analyze the influence of dietary intake, since the situation was relatively uniform, and cases of markedly reduced food intake were exceptional. Surveys on functional capacity and motor development of children with severe and/or marginal malnutrition are still very rare up to now. The influence of nutrition in preschoolers can be mainly analyzed in some surveys of subjects with different levels of food intake.

A. SOMATIC DEVELOPMENT
1. Italian Survey
Preschool children with reduced rather than ample energy and protein intake were followed by Ferro-Luzzi et al.[104] This study not only included data on growth, but also dietary intake along with functional capacity and performance using the modified step test (see Chapter 6).

A sample of 2241 children was obtained by selecting representative numbers of children from two areas — Central and Southern Italy — characterized by contrasting conditions of life. This concerns, *inter alia,* dietary intake and the level of physical activity.

Dietary intake was followed in a subsample of 550 children. Analysis of the composition of the diet showed *marginal malnutrition in preschool children from Southern Italy,* characterized by lower socioeconomic status, compared to children of the same age from Central Italy and Rome who had a higher intake of energy and macrocomponents and a better diet. Growth retardation, i.e., *smaller body size,* was obvious in a greater proportion of children from Southern Italy. The values of BMI were generally slightly higher in children from Central Italy.

Skinfold thicknesses and the calculated amount of total fat were significantly higher in children from Central Italy than those from the poorer sections of the population in the South, suggesting that at least part of the extra energy available for children was deposited as fat.[104] The values of individual skinfold thicknesses and fat pattern could not be compared with those of Czech or of other children because only values from the sum of four skinfolds were given.

2. Turkish Survey

Turnagol et al.[359] measured children younger and older than 4.5 years in Ankara. These children could not be classified as malnourished; nevertheless, their food intake was somewhat different as compared to Czech and Italian children, making a comparison of morphological and functional variables related to dietary intake possible.

The energy and macrocomponent intake in children from Ankara was lower than, for example in Prague children of similar age and/or children from central Italy (Tables 7.1a and 7.1b). The intake of protein was similar to that of children in Southern Italy and lower than that in Rome or Prague children. (The highest intake of protein was found in Rome children from the highest social strata i.e., about 63 to 67 g/day who also had the highest values of height and weight. On the other hand, Prague children had the highest fat intake. The intake of total energy did not differ in Rome and Prague children, similar to the values of height and weight.) The vitamin and mineral intake of Turkish children (see Table 7.1b) varied; e.g., the intake of Ca and Fe was lower than the U.S. RDAs,[397] and higher than EC population reference intakes;[398] the intake of vitamin C is higher than the U.S. RDAs or the EC population reference intake.

Height and weight did not seem to be different in children from an Ankara day care center. However, when we compare e.g., *breadth measurements*, the values were significantly lower in Ankara children compared to Prague ones, except for biacromial and femoral breadths. *Circumferential measurements* did not seem to differ significantly. The comparison was rendered difficult

TABLE 7.1a **Dietary Intake of Preschool Children in Ankara, Turkey, Aged <54 or >54 Months at the Occasion of the First and the Second Measurement (M) 4 Months Later**

	Age (months)	M		Energy (kJ)	Protein (g)	Fat (g)	Carbohydrates (g)
Boys	<54	1	$\bar{x}$	6397	49.2	66.0	189.7
			SD	1074	6.6	15.0	31.5
		2	$\bar{x}$	6422	49.2	58.7	201.1
			SD	940	7.0	11.6	46.8
	>54	1	$\bar{x}$	7134	56.4	71.2	213.6
			SD	955	12.1	14.2	39.7
		2	$\bar{x}$	7142	55.0	68.9	221.7
			SD	841	10.1	10.6	42.8
Girls	<54	1	$\bar{x}$	6177	47.2	60.7	189.7
			SD	1079	8.4	13.5	47.2
		2	$\bar{x}$	6417	51.3	60.1	201.7
			SD	852	8.4	10.1	44.3
	>54	1	$\bar{x}$	6814	52.7	66.5	209.7
			SD	938	10.2	10.7	32.7
		2	$\bar{x}$	6885	59.0	58.7	209.5
			SD	825	11.3	11.6	36.3

Note: SD, standard deviation.

Compiled from Türnagöl, H.H., et al., Proceedings of the Symposium *Human Growth, Dietary Intake and Other Environmental Influences,* 13th ICAES, Mexico City, 1993, Pǎrízková, J. and Douglas, P.J., eds., Danone, Paris, 1995, 8.

because the exact age of children before and after 4.5 years was not given, and the measured group from Ankara included a small number of children. According to the values of CV, though, there important differences do not seem to exist.

With *skinfolds*, it was possible to compare Prague and Ankara children. Turkish children had slightly higher values of individual skinfolds measured by a Harpenden caliper, compared to Prague children, which was only the case when a morphological variable had a higher value in Ankara children.

Age differences and developmental changes proceeded like those in Prague children. Sex-linked differences in Ankara children had the same characteristics as those in Czech children, i.e., girls were slightly smaller, their skeleton was less robust, and the deposition of subcutaneous fat was greater.[359]

Somatotype was also evaluated in Ankara children. Mesomorphy was a dominant component in Ankara children as in Prague children of corresponding age. The endomorphic component was slightly higher in Turkish girls, and the mesomorphic and ectomorphic components were higher in boys. Somatotypes changed much less with advancing age during the preschool growth period than any other morphological characteristics given in absolute values (kg, cm).[359]

TABLE 7.1b   The Intake of Minerals and Vitamins in Preschool Children (<54 and >54 Months Old) on the First and Second Measurements (M) in Ankara, Turkey

	Age (months)	M		Minerals Ca (mg)	Fe (mg)	Vitamins A (IU)	B$_1$ (mg)	B$_2$ (mg)	PP (mg)	C (mg)
Boys	<54	1	x̄	691	8.7	4970	0.83	1.12	8.1	95.0
			SD	267	1.5	2492	0.13	0.33	1.5	40.6
		2	x̄	575	9.1	5443	0.85	1.00	10.0	100.0
			SD	259	2.5	4581	0.17	0.31	3.7	47.9
	>54	1	x̄	651	10.1	6209	0.95	1.15	10.0	94.0
			SD	342	1.9	3935	0.13	0.44	3.0	47.1
		2	x̄	709	10.1	5491	0.92	1.21	9.8	100.4
			SD	306	1.5	4797	0.18	0.46	2.1	51.8
Girls	<54	1	x̄	650	8.1	4746	0.80	1.05	8.5	105.4
			SD	209	1.9	2627	0.05	0.30	2.6	52.7
		2	x̄	671	8.7	4323	0.79	1.12	9.4	83.2
			SD	306	2.6	3086	0.13	0.36	2.6	40.4
	>54	1	x̄	678	10.2	6492	0.96	1.20	9.7	97.7
			SD	347	1.7	3650	0.13	0.49	1.6	42.6
		2	x̄	828	8.8	4582	0.97	1.28	10.8	102.6
			SD	257	1.9	2197	0.11	0.31	27	51.8

Adapted from Türnagöl, H.H., et al., Proceedings of the Symposium *Human Growth, Dietary Intake and Other Environmental Influences,* 13th ICAES, Mexico City, 1993, Pařízková , J. and Douglas, P.J., eds., Danone, Paris, 1995, 8.

3. Senegalese Survey

Bénéfice[25,26] followed mild-malnourished children in Senegal and compared them to their normally nourished peers. The children came from two villages in west-central Senegal (Diokhane and Ndandol in Bambey county) and from a small coastal town, Mbour. The inhabitants of this region are Muslims, ethnic Wolofs, or in the case of Mbour, Lebous fishermen, a related tribe. Their basic *diet* is the same: rice and fish at midday and millet or sorghum gruel in the evening. A study of food consumption showed more than half these families to be short of food caloriesduring the rainy season. Protein energy malnutrition in this region ranks highest in Senegal.

Forty-four boys and forty-four girls were divided into three cohorts according their year of birth (1983–1985), i.e., the children were 3.4, 4.5, and 5.5 years old at the beginning of the follow up. These children were then examined longitudinally, i.e., three times between October 1988 and November 1989. The interval between the first and second examination (5 ± 1.5 months) was shorter than the one between the second and third examination (6.4 ± 0.5 months). Only healthy children were recruited for the study. The height of these children at the beginning of the study was close to the National Center for Health Statistics (NCHS) median, but they were *delayed in weight growth.* A total of 18% of the children had a height-for-age deficit between –1 and –2 from the NCHS distribution and 36% had a weight-for-height deficit of the same order. Only 19 children attained the median for height and for weight-for-height. There were no significant sex-linked differences, and the proportion of wasted or stunted children did not change during the study.

Repeated measurements showed regular growth, but they were still deficient compared to NCHS. On the average, Senegalese children were 1.5 years behind in weight development and 3 to 6 months behind in height compared to the mentioned standards.[25,26]

4. Zapotec Survey

Malina et al.[202–204] followed somatic development in children 6 to 14 years old with different degrees of malnutrition in Mexico. Smaller body size was mostly apparent in malnourished children; the deficit in growth was relatively greater in older children.

B. FUNCTIONAL DEVELOPMENT: CARDIORESPIRATORY FITNESS
1. Italian Survey

Ferro-Luzzi et al.[104] followed a subsample of 326 Italian preschool children from the above mentioned study with different degree of dietary intake, examining the response of the respiratory system to a constant medium intensity work load, i.e., modified *step test*, as described in Chapter 6.

In this study, sex-linked differences were observed, i.e., boys had better results than girls in this functional test (in smaller samples of Czech children, a trend for better results in boys did not reach the level of statistical significance). The work efficiency of the cardiovascular system also improved with advancing age, obviously due to the increase of stroke volume in older children.

The results of the step test, especially of the cardiac efficiency index (CEI), correlated significantly with a number of characteristics of body composition, i.e., with arm and thigh muscle area (cm^2) and with fat free body mass (kg) (r values were from 0.568 to 0.872, all highly significant). The closest relationship was found for the absolute amount of fat free body mass and CEI. No relationship was found for dietary intake and CEI.

When the groups were compared on the basis of belonging to high and low income families or to rural vs. urban environment, and on the basis of their level of spontaneous physical activity, as described by parents and teachers in the questionnaire (specially designed for this purpose), no significant differences were found.[104]

However, grouping the children by the usual geographic criteria, South andcentral, and on the basis of their dietary intake and nutritional status, the *cardiorespiratory efficiency was much better in the marginally undernourished children from the south*. In these children the energy intake was significantly lower, and the values of skinfold thicknesses were also lower in relation to the calculated total amount of body fat. However, *fat free body mass and arm*

and thigh muscle areas were the same or only very slightly smaller in boys
and girls from the south compared to children from the central part of Italy.[104]

Evidently, marginal malnutrition did not markedly reduce fat free, lean
body mass and also did not interfere with a good level of performance during
a step test in preschool children. The response to work load was better than
in bigger and fatter children with higher food intakes from Central Italy.
Because burdening of the organism by a greater amount of fat may be a
disadvantage during a dynamic work load (includes weightbearing), it seems
understandable that smaller and leaner children performed on a higher level
during a work load of this sort. The situation would be, no doubt, different
during a work load requiring muscle strength (static work load) or even during
the same work load in children with a more serious degree of malnutrition.
Similar results were found previously in prepubertal children, differentiated
in a similar way, examined in Tunisia.[233]

2. Turkish Survey

The step test was also used for the follow-up of preschool children in
Ankara. The average values of the heart rate at rest, during work load and
during recovery did not differ significantly from the values assessed in Prague
children (see Figure 6.1). Türnagöl et al.[359] only gave average values of heart
rate during rest, then during a 5-minute work load and finally during recovery
(Table 7.1c), i.e., it was not possible to compare the course of a steady state,
and/or the speed of recovery by minutes during work load and recovery. In
addition, the average age of the individual groups of Ankara children did not
correspond exactly to the average age of the group of Prague children.

Therefore, only the values of the cardiac efficiency index (CEI) were
compared in several cases when the age of the children was comparable. This
concerned the CEI evaluated for the second time in Ankara girls less than 54
months old and Czech girls 4 to 5 years old or the CEI in boys less than 54
months old measured for the second time compared to Prague boys 4 to 5
years old. The average values of CEI were significantly higher in Prague
children (see Table 7.1c; Table 6.1; Table 6.3; Figures 6.2a and 6.2b). As
mentioned above, the values of height, weight, BMI were not different, but
there were variations in breadth measures, skinfolds, and dietary intake. In
these cases, the average values were higher in Prague children.[359] This may
indicate more accelerated development in Prague children which was, in some
cases, accompanied by slightly better results in cardiorespiratory fitness.

This comparison concerned children from larger cities. The comparison
of preschool children with different dietary intake and different physical
regimes in Italy (i.e., those from the central and from the south), concerned
children from large and small communities.[104] All of these data seem to indicate
that, as in older age categories,[233] *the higher level of cardiorespiratory fitness*
at an early age is related to more modest nutrition to prevent the deposition
of excess body fat and on the *opportunity for exercise* which is usually better
in smaller communities than in larger urban agglomerations.

TABLE 7.1c   Results of Step Test in Preschool Children from Ankara,
Turkey on the First and Second Measurements,
4 Months Later

Age (months)		Boys				Girls			
		<54	<54	>54	>54	<54	<54	>54	>54
Measurement		1st	2nd	1st	2nd	1st	2nd	1st	2nd
	n	14	14	15	15	16	16	10	10
Rest	x̄	110.5	111.4	104.2	107.7	109.6	113.7	108.0	112.3
	SD	5.9	9.3	9.3	10.2	12.4	10.2	11.3	10.7
Work load	x̄	149.3	152.3	150.2	152.6	156.8	164.2	156.7	162.3
	SD	14.5	15.6	13.0	16.2	9.0	10.6	12.2	16.9
Recovery	x̄	115.9	118.0	115.2	115.0	117.1	123.2	121.3	121.6
	SD	6.7	10.1	10.8	9.4	9.5	11.9	12.0	12.4
CEI 1	x̄	0.44	0.45	0.57	0.58	0.45	0.45	0.51	0.52
	SD	0.04	0.06	0.06	0.06	0.9	0.8	0.09	0.08
Brouha's index	x̄	87.4	86.0	88.6	88.1	88.0	83.0	88.3	84.1
	SD	5.3	8.3	10.10	7.5	7.3	8.4	7.7	8.2

Note: Average values of heart rate at rest, during 5 minutes work load and during 5 minutes recovery.

Modified from Türnagöl, H.H., et al., Proceedings of the Symposium *Human Growth, Dietary Intake and Other Environmental Influences,* 13th ICAES, Mexico City, 1993, Pařízková , J. and Douglas, P.J., eds., Danone, Paris, 1995, 8.

3. Senegalese Survey

Bénéfice[25,26] followed the reaction of the heart rate in the modified step test carried out as described before (Appendix 2). The results (Figure 7.1) indicate that the heart rate at rest, during exercise and during the recovery period was higher in Senegalese children than in Czech children. The reaction of the cardiorespiratory system to this type of work load was less efficient than the one in Czech boys. The reaction to work load, i.e., the change of heart rate during mounting the step was similar to that of Czech girls, who increased their heart rate more slightly than boys. However, heart rate during the recovery decreased more slowly in Senegalese children, as compared to both Czech boys and girls (Figure 7.1), which indicates also a lower level of cardiorespiratory efficiency in this particular test.

This difference might be partly due to the influence of varying habits resulting from different conditions of life.[25,26] Children in a Senegalese village are obviously less adapted to mounting steps for 5 minutes than children in the industrially developed countries. Differences in cardiorespiratory fitness between children in different countries, i.e., different ethnic, cultural, etc. settings, many require other types of tests.

C. MOTOR DEVELOPMENT

Some differences may appear when more marked chronic nutritional deficiencies are manifested. Although in this case, it is also necessary to

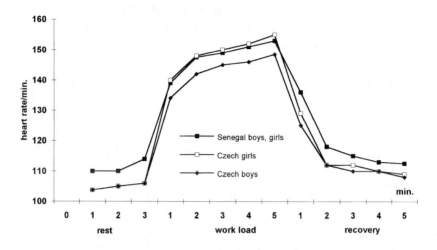

FIGURE 7.1 Comparison of heart rate during the step test, i.e., 3 min rest, the 5 min mounting the step, and during 5 min recovery in Senegalese and Czech children.

differentiate between the degrees of malnutrition and various aspects of physical fitness characterized by various motor tests: it seems obvious that, for example, speed running and skill tests (and not only those which were used in our studies) do not depend on body size, and the status of marginal malnutrition does not interfere. This may also manifest itself in adulthood e.g., Ethiopian long distance runners, who are shorter and skinnier than most runners, do not seem to have an abundant or even a satisfactory diet from the beginning of life and sometimes even later. Even so, they were still able to get gold medals just like the bigger and better fed American, Scandinavian, and many athletes from other countries.

Another example are gymnasts who are mainly within the 25th to 23rd percentile for height, weight, and BMI and who are still capable of a physical performance uncomparable to their peers with better nutrition and larger body size.[241] Of course, adaptation processes and training started early in life (even in preschool age; this is also specific for this sport discipline) are indispensable to such a performance level. On the whole, though, this example shows that ample nutrition and body size are not decisive factors for the intense training and achievement of top performance of this sort, i.e., gymnastics,[241] which requires mainly perfect neuromuscular coordination and skill. According to growth standards, gymnasts display a sort of marginal malnutrition, sometimes accompanied by deficiencies of some vitamins and minerals,[241] which must be supplemented.

1. Turkish Survey

There are very few data on skill and physical performance testing of small children with different degrees of nutrition. Türnagöl et al.[359] assessed some of the mentioned faculties, e.g., performance in *20 m dash* and *broad jump* (Table 7.1d). Again, the exact comparison with Prague children is difficult according to age, although the average values indicate markedly better results in Prague children in comparison to Ankara children. This includes both boys and girls.

TABLE 7.1d   Motor Performance in Preschool Children (<54 and >54 Months Old) on the First and Second Measurements (M) in Ankara, Turkey

	Age (months)	M		20 m run (s)	Broad jump (cm)	Hand right (kp)	Grip left (kp)
Boys	<54	1	x̄	7.15	59.1	5.1	4.7
			SD	0.89	13.7	2.3	1.9
	<54	2	x̄	6.37	66.2	6.4	5.9
			SD	0.84	13.45	2.3	2.5
	>54	1	x̄	5.65	66.4	8.6	8.6
			SD	0.71	14.6	2.9	2.9
	>54	2	x̄	5.36	81.3	8.8	8.3
			SD	0.61	17.1	2.9	2.9
Girls	<54	1	x̄	7.54	60.3	4.1	4.0
			SD	1.0	14.0	1.2	1.1
	<54	2	x̄	6.79	63.5	5.4	5.0
			SD	0.78	15.7	1.5	1.6
	>54	1	x̄	6.04	64.2	6.9	6.4
			SD	0.83	15.5	1.9	2.0
	>54	2	x̄	5.69	76.8	7.7	6.3
			SD	0.06	11.45	1.9	1.5

Adapted from Türnagöl, H., et al., Proceedings of the Symposium *Human Growth, Dietary Intake and Other Environmental Influences*, 13th ICAES, Mexico City, 1993, Pařízková , J. and Douglas, P.J., eds., Danone, Paris, 1995, 8.

Türnagöl[359] followed longitudinally other parameters of motor development, e.g., *squat jump*, *counteractive jump* and *sit-and-reach* . There was an improvement in motor performance with increasing age, with better results in boys, similar to other groups of preschool children measured before.[236,238,242,247,254,256]

In the results of the comparison between Ankara and Prague children, it seems that besides slight differences in dietary intake and some parameters of body size, the reason for some of the differences in motor skill may be conditioned by cultural characteristics and by kindergarten teaching programs. Prague children were obviously more adapted to running this distance and/or jumping than Ankara children. Therefore, the difference does not seem to be due to some functional handicaps; this is also indicated by the very few differences in the results of the step test.

However, it would be interesting to find out whether these discrete differences would increase further and become significant later in life. This would obviously depend, though, not only on dietary intake and way of life, but also on the ability to adapt to physical work loads of this type, which may follow during later growth periods. Further measurements in the same subjects would be necessary to define the role of genetic and constitutional factors in these ethnic differences already manifested during preschool age.

2. Senegalese Survey

Bénéfice[25,26] followed the results in *20 m dash*, *broad jump*, *ball throw* and *muscle strength* in Senegalese children (Table 7.2), by repeating them three times. These children suffered from mild malnutrition and somatic deficiencies in growth and development as mentioned above.

After dividing the children into four nutritional groups according to their height-for-age and weight-for-height deficiencies, it was found that normal and thin children scored higher in the various tests than children who were underweight or who were both underheight and underweight. In this study, the contrasts in nutritional status were more marked than in the other above mentioned studies.

TABLE 7.2   Motor Performance and Abilities in Preschool Children in Senegal

Age group (years)	3–4		4–5		5–6	
	18		34		36	
n	$\bar{x}$	SD	$\bar{x}$	SD	$\bar{x}$	SD
20 m dash — 1 (s)	8.01	1.33	7.05	0.83	6.27	0.95
20 m dash — 2 (s)	7.10	0.75	6.47	0.69	5.80	0.59
20 m dash — 3 (s)	6.55	0.90	5.76	0.52	5.24	0.61
Broad jump — 1 (cm)	42.5	16.3	56.3	16.5	78.5	10.8
Broad jump — 2 (cm)	59.9	19.0	62.4	24.3	89.4	19.9
Broad jump — 3 (cm)	66.4	21.6	85.7	19.2	103.5	18.1
Throwing ball — 1 (m)	2.6	0.7	3.9	1.2	5.9	1.4
Throwing ball — 2 (m)	3.0	1.2	4.5	1.6	6.9	1.8
Throwing ball — 3 (m)	3.6	0.9	5.7	2.0	7.8	1.8

Note: 1,2,3 — number of visits (interval between 1st–2nd visit = 5 ± 1.5 months, 2nd–3rd visit = 6.4 ± 0.5 months). The differences between average values of different age groups, and between average values measured at the occasion of the individual visits 1–3 were all statistically significant.

Compiled from Bénéfice, E., *Early Child Dev. Care,* 61, 81, 1990 and from Bénéfice, E., *Human Growth, Dietary Intake and Other Environmental Influences,* Proc. Symp., 13th ICAES, Mexico City, 1993, Paří́zková , J. and Douglas, P.D., eds., Danone, Paris, 1995, 32.

Senegalese performance in threemotor tasks (Table 7.2) was well below those of the Czech children who weighed 2 to 3 kg more. When the performance was adjusted for a unit of body weight, Czech children still ran faster than

Senegalese children, but the differences tended to diminish. *When the performance in jumping was adjusted for body weight, Senegalese children jumped further than Czech children.* Finally, smaller Senegalese children, after adjusting for body weight, were quite *equal to Czech children in throwing performance.*[25,26]

To our knowledge no other similar measurements of motor skill as related to the nutritional status of preschool children in a Third World country have beenpublished up to now.

D. MUSCLE STRENGTH

Measurement of muscle strength has been more common than testing of other motor faculties. Strength has also been more interesting parameter from the point of view not only actual, but also future work performance level. This is connected with the economic impact of the possibility of child labor and/or future development of labor force in adulthood in Third World countries where malnutrition is usual.

Muscle strength is much more closely related to body size than any other parameter of motor development. This mainly applies to the relationship to *lean body mass* and especially to the *muscles.* Therefore, muscle strength is much more influenced by malnutrition than, for example, speed or skill. In this case, even mild malnutrition, which still does not interfere with speed, skill, or even endurance development, can reduce muscle strength significantly.

1. Turkish Survey

Also Türnagöl et al.[359] measured hand grip strength in preschool children (see Table 7.1d). In this case, too, the average values of *hand grip strength were markedly lower in Ankara children* compared to Prague children. The exact evaluation of the differences is difficult due to the various age groupings in the two samples. There was, however, quite a contrast in muscle strength between preschool children in Turkey and the Czech Republic along with relatively small differences regarding other morphological and functional parameters. Also, in this case, it would be interesting to measure the strength of other muscle groups of the body, which may be more important for daily activities than hand grip. This study of Ankara children continues and further data will reveal more on the possible differences between children with different nutrition.

2. First Senegalese Survey

Bénéfice[25,26] measured longitudinally muscle strength in the above mentioned groups of Senegalese children. The comparison of the results in Senegalese and in other children is not directly possible because quite a different method was used: a special dynamometer, in fact a manometer (Vigorimeter Martin R, Tuttlingen, Germany), was used. The children had to press on a bulb, adjusted to the size of their palm and connected to a manometer; pressure, not force, was assessed. The units were expressed in bars (0.nn bar). The recalculation of the data gained using different methods could give inexact results; however, we can assume *lower values of hand grip strength in Senegalese children.*

A comparison of different measurements showed the usual increase in muscle strength with age. The results were evaluated in a combined group of both boys and girls so sex-linked differences could not be evaluated.

Insufficient muscle mass available for motor performance seemed to be the principle factor limiting the adequate physical achievement in the malnourished children. There are also other hypotheses — reduction in children's habitual physical activity and the neuromotor consequences resulting from preceding severe malnutrition. Therefore, the measurements in Senegalese children from 3 to 6 years of age showed that even a slight degree of malnutrition can affect a child's ability to perform physical work, thus hindering his/her future work output.

3. Tunisian Survey

When muscle strength was tested in youth from poor and well-off families in Tunisia and were compared with Prague children (11 to 12 years) it was shown that *smaller poor children* had significantly less lean body mass, but, for example, *the strength of the extensors of the trunk, flexors and extensors of the elbow, and the extensors of the knee joints was higher than that of their bigger, and fatter peers from well-off families.* (These results are mentioned in spite of age because as far as we know no other study in an African country focused simultaneously on numerous functional variables, i.e., step test, strength of seven muscle groups, vital capacity, forced expiration, performance in 50-m dash, 300-m run, broad jump, along with numerous morphological characteristics including body composition). Hand grip strength and the strength of the plantar and knee flexors were the same in bigger and smaller Tunisian boys. *When muscle strength was related to both total and/or lean body mass, the differences in favor of smaller boys with poorer nutrition were even more apparent: they had always a relatively greater strength compared to bigger Tunisian boys.*

The same also applies for the comparison with bigger Czech boys of the same age. Parallel to that, *smaller Tunisian boys also had better results in the step test,* similarly as smaller south Italian children compared to bigger central Italian children.[104] *The results in sports disciplines, testing of vital capacity, maximum voluntary ventilation, forced expiration, etc. were also better in smaller Tunisian boys compared to bigger ones.*

These results seem to indicate that (1) Hand grip strength might not give exact information on the strength of other muscle groups, and (2) Even in smaller and obviously marginally malnourished children, the absolute values of muscle strength of most important muscle groups on the trunk and on the extremities may be higher than in their bigger peers (in most surveys other muscle groups were not followed). This applies even more when we evaluate muscle strength in relation to total or lean body mass. Last but not least, it is necessary to consider that the *smaller children were from poor families*, had to do *more physical work*, and thus became *more efficient due to adaptation*.

However, all of these results refer to children with marginal malnutrition (which is characterized by normal or only slightly reduced lean, fat free body mass, and obviously unchanged size of vital organs) in prepubertal period, a condition which did not interfere with their spontaneous physical activity and games. This obviously also contributed to the higher level of their physical fitness when compared to the bigger Tunisians and their Czech peers. Moreover, the results of the measurements of muscle strength correlated significantly with other physical performance tests.[233]

4. Second Senegalese Survey

Bénéfice[26] carried out another complex study in Senegalese school children (10 to 12 years of age). Measurements were repeated every 6 months for 2 years.

There were no sex-linked differences in height and weight. Average values of height for age at the beginning of the study decreased from –1.3 z-score to –1.5 z-score. The weight also deteriorated significantly from –1.5 z-score to –1.7 z-score.

Motor performance of Senegalese children was compared with that of African American children from Philadelphia.[205] In the 33-m run, standing broad jump and throwing a softball African American children had a better level of performance. *Senegalese children were lighter than American children or Czech children*; when performance was *adjusted for body weight*, Senegalese children were still slower at running, but they *were significantly superior at the broad jump*. No differences in throwing were found.[26]

Average heart rate at rest and during exercise (another modification of the step test for older children)[26] showed significantly lower values in 12-year-old boys as compared to girls: the cardiorespiratory efficiency at this age was significantly differentiated regarding gender. There were also sex-linked differences in physical activity.[26]

5. Zapotec Survey

Malina et al.[203,204] measured hand grip strength in chronically mild-to-moderately undernourished rural boys in Southern Mexico (Zapotec) aged 9.5 to 14.5 years old. Their height, weight, skinfolds, calculated lean body mass, and hand grip strength (average for right and left hands) were always lower than those of Mexican American boys of the same age. When hand grip strength was related to total body weight, there was no significant difference between Zapotec and Mexican American boys. However, when related to lean, fat-free body mass, the difference was always significant with the exception of the age group of 12.5-year-old boys. Perhaps, this suggests qualitative changes in muscle tissue due to chronic malnutrition in this particular population group which also reduces lean body mass.[203]

In another study, the hand grip strength in Zapotec boys and girls at the age of 6 and 7 years was also investigated. Height and weight were lower in Zapotec children in comparison to Prague children.[256] The BMI was only slightly lower in Zapotec children. Hand grip was, however, markedly lower in Zapotec children. In this case, hand grip strength was the average for the right and left hand. However, even the values of the left hand grip strength in Prague children were much higher than the average value of both hands in Zapotec children. Moreover, in Prague children there were also more marked sex-linked differences at this age period than in Zapotec children where hand grip strength was uniform on a lower level in both boys and girls.

Similar values of averaged hand grip strength of Zapotec children compared to 6- to 7-year-old boys and girls in Prague were found only about 3 to 4 years later in Zapotec boys (i.e., only when they were 3 years older than Prague boys), and slightly sooner in Zapotec girls. In these children, the relative differences in the values of height and weight were greater than those of strength and other functional characteristics of well-off and poor Tunisian and Czech boys,[233] i.e., the difference in dietary intake and degree of malnutrition was also much greater. However, it would also be interesting to compare the strength of other muscle groups, which could not be measured in Zapotec children. As mentioned above, hand grip strength might not be a representative indicator of muscle strength for other muscle groups of the organism.

6. Other Functional and/or Motor Development Surveys

Regarding the level of functional development related to reduced dietary intake, most studies were carried out in school children and adolescents. Eventually, 6-year-old children were also examined; for example, among Ethiopian boys who varied in body weight, physical working capacity (W) at the level of 170 heart rate per minute (PWC_{170}) was related significantly to body size or to nutritional status.[11] In 6-year-old children, the maximal oxygen uptake ($ml \cdot min^{-1} \cdot kg^{-1}$) was lower in severely malnourished children with reduced body mass in comparison to well-fed children.[14] As follows, the *low level of physical performance and fitness in malnourished children results from reduced body mass, especially from reduction of the skeletal muscles.*[73]

Functional consequences of marginal malnutrition in children and youth 6 to 16 years of age were evaluated during a maximal work load on a treadmill. The absolute values of maximal oxygen consumption were reduced in the marginally malnourished boys, who had lower weight for age and height and who were recruited from lower urban and rural social groups in Colombia. However, *when comparing the values of maximal oxygen uptake per kg body weight, boys with lower socioeconomic status and lower body weight for height had higher aerobic power.* This was obviously the reflection of various body compositions, i.e., higher proportion of lean body mass as indicated by smaller skinfold thicknesses.[337,338]

Urban boys always had higher values of maximal oxygen uptake per kg body weight, seemingly due to active sport programs and government sports facilities in the capital of Cali (enabling a higher level of adaptation to work loads), lacking in rural areas. It has been suggested that the urban-rural differences in recreational facilities could have contributed to the lower values of predicted maximal oxygen uptake of rural compared to urban children. This indicates the great importance of early motor stimulation and of an adequate physical activity regimen, in general, which can also (because of adaptation) compensate for certain functional inadequacies of dietary intake and body size.

Another study showed, that *marginal malnutrition did not limit the level of physical activity.*[335,336] Total daily energy expenditure and energy expenditure in physical activity were estimated, in free ranging nutritionally normal and undernourished boys, 6 to 16 years of age, by measuring basal and resting metabolic rates and average heart rate while they were awake during the day. Total energy expenditure increased less with increasing age in undernourished boys, but the increase in energy expenditure due to physical activity was the same in both groups. These observations indicate that the nutritional differences between groups concerning total energy expenditures were due to different body size, and that the *reduced growth and associated economy of energy expenditure in motor activity is sufficient physiological adaptation under conditions of marginal malnutrition.*[338] The same conclusions were observed in a study with normal and undernourished girls. Total daily energy expenditure also measured by means of the sum of heart rate during a certain period of time (calibrated individually), and the energy expended in physical activity did not differ significantly in the two groups characterized by various nutritional status.[335–340]

Davies[73] did not find any urban-rural differences in East African children, but he pointed out that the dividing line between urban and rural areas is often unclear in most areas, not only in Africa. Mentioned values of maximal oxygen uptake in Colombian children were not different from those of European children, but were slightly lower than those in Scandinavian children.[233]

The majority of other data on the influence of nutrition concern body size.[97] Body size may correlate with some of the functional variables,[125] but not with others in children of the same age. Physiological reasons for that still remain to be resolved by further research.

E.   GENERAL CONSIDERATIONS

As follows, most functional measurements were made in older children (school children, adolescents), subjects who are not the focus in this volume. Some of the studies included the oldest age category of children (6 to 7 years old) followed in our studies. We may only speculate that some of the conclusions based on the measurements of older children might also apply to preschool age; this, though, remains to be validated by future research which is still lacking. This seems to result from the difficulties of getting preschool children for functional and motor studies, i.e., normal and healthy children who do not yet need any medical assistance. Therefore, there still remains the problem as to how marginal malnutrition is manifested in preschool children regarding the functional variables mentioned above and whether the symptoms will be similar as in older children. We assume that early diagnosis of functional impairment is of utmost importance because the earlier the intervention, the more feasible any compensation and rehabilitation, including the physical working capacity.

In general, though, marked negative functional consequences especially manifest themselves when the reduction of energy and the individual nutrient intake reaches a certain critical level. It may not be clear as to what conditions the degree of ***marginal nutrition*** still remains within the adaptation limits of the organism (especially when it did not start at the beginning of life) and thus does not last long enough as is the case in younger children. *When lean, fat free body mass, vital organs, and especially important muscle groups are not reduced markedly and mostly fat is decreased, the functional status can be satisfactory or at least acceptable. Weight bearing activities or skill performance seems to be much less affected (if at all) than performance demanding strength and endurance*, which require larger muscle mass and are more dependent on total and lean body mass. A question remains as to whether such a status can be defined as malnutrition. Performance levels in certain tasks (i.e., jumping or strength testing) are equal or even better when adjusted to body weight, as shown in many studies, e.g., in Senegalese or Tunisian children. As shown by the Italian study, the results of the step test, which characterize the cardiorespiratory fitness, were generally better in smaller, marginally malnourished children. Even in industrially developed countries, we can find a number of children who could be defined as marginally malnourished according to a number of parameters mentioned above, and they don't have any functional or health problems.

The manifestations of marginal malnutrition are also modified by possible simultaneous vitamin and mineral deficiencies of a different degree, concerning, for example, iron. There is also evidence that individual functional systems are not impaired by different degrees and different characters of malnutrition in an identical way.

Mild-to-moderate malnutrition, however, is always a *health risk* for a preschool child. The critical limit between marginal, mild, and/or severe malnutrition must be defined as exactly as possible, as mild malnutrition is already a serious survival risk in preschool children in developing countries (e.g., Malawi)[280,281] associated with reduced immunoresistence, etc.

IV. THE INFLUENCE OF SEVERE MALNUTRITION

Many authors followed the impact of extreme malnutrition in children of all ages, including the preschool growth period. The data were recently summarized in an excellent monograph by Waterlow et al.[378] Health status and basic anthropological variables were analyzed. *Functional variables have however been followed mainly under rest conditions*, a state which does not render possible an evaluation of the reaction of the malnourished organism to some degrees of work load. Even if it is hardly feasible to test hungry children in this way, we must bear in mind that *their life often requires physical loads*; thus, more information about their reactions would be certainly desirable.

Obviously, very severe malnutrition interferes substantially with the normal development of the child and leads to deterioration of most systems and functions. The line drawn between marginal, mild-to-moderate, and severe malnutrition may be transient and is not always clear, which can influence various functional systems in a different way. However, when the food intake is severely restricted during longer periods of development, significant functional, metabolic, biochemical, etc., changes occur in all organs and systems (see Waterlow et al. 1992).

Children with severe malnutrition usually have a *lower metabolic rate* than normally nourished children. There are problems how to express the metabolic rate because *the composition of the whole body and of individual tissues is changed.*[378]

Under conditions of severe malnutrition *wasting also occurs in the heart muscle* as shown by autopsy, chest X-rays, and echocardiography. Previous histological studies of the heart showed only nonspecific changes.[378]

Characteristics of the heart muscle in children aged 9.6 to 54 months of age, who suffered from severe protein energy malnutrition, were followed up by various authors.[350,365] Then, the initial heart rate at rest, stroke volume, and cardiac output were reduced. After treatment and recovery, all these variables increased. The cardiac output increased both due to the increase in heart rate and the increase of the cardiac volume. Systemic and pulmonary artery pressure (by cardiac catheterization) was found significantly reduced. The peripheral resistance was increased.[366]

The relationship between heart rate and energy expenditure (kcal/min) is *different in severely malnourished children*: the heart rate is much higher when energy expenditure is not as increased before than after realimentation. As the child recovers, the slope of the regression line becomes steeper, implying a more efficient utilization of energy per heart beat.[334,378] Malnutrition also causes changes in blood volume and hemodynamics, which can be positively changed by realimentation.[364,365]

Though smaller body size does not always interfere with the dynamic performance of an aerobic character and though small individuals may be quite fit during weight bearing activities, *small individuals are at a disadvantage when considering the total work output in physical terms*. Such a work load mainly demands strength (depending on muscle mass and therefore on body size) and endurance. This aspect is mostly important in light of the working efficiency and the economic productivity of a population.

Spurr[335,336] showed that *working capacity related to body weight of Colombian boys who were small for their age was normal,*[335] i.e., their cardiorespiratory fitness was unimpaired. However, no task could be performed continuously at a rate greater than about 40% of their aerobic power (VO₂ max). As also shown by Satyaranayana[315,316], small individuals in India where boys were mostly employed as agricultural laborers were always at a functional disadvantage. A longitudinal study of the same author showed that those *subjects who were small at the age of 5 years were also small adults.*[317] So, the problem perpetuates itself. Small undernourished women also have smaller babies, and the infant mortality rate is also higher than those of larger babies from larger mothers.[206] Overall, then, the problem of low working capacity and productivity starts at the beginning of life.

Another manifestation of severe malnutrition concerning both energy and protein is mild anemia. The ***hemoglobin concentration*** is usually 8 to 10 g/dl. Red cells are of normal size and have a normal or somewhat lower hemoglobin content. The bone marrow may show normal erythropoiesis, or it may be fatty and hypoplastic.[366] Thus, anemia is another factor that limits work performance and physical fitness, causes early fatigue, and limits the level of physical activity.

According to the WHO, about a half of the children under 5 years of age in developing countries are anemic, i.e., hemoglobin is less than 11 g/dl.[78] The principal cause of this anemia is the iron deficiency, which is not always present in protein-energy malnutrition. More important, the connection is indirect, i.e., iron deficiency is the consequence of blood loss from malaria and intestinal parasites. Increased morbidity from these diseases is caused, in part, by suppressed immunoresistency resulting from the lack of energy and high quality protein intake, i.e., this status is finally also the result of malnutrition.

Regarding the ***nervous system***, children from undernourished mothers may be born with ***smaller brains*** as shown in Uganda.[44] Protein energy malnutrition is very dangerous at the period between the tenth and twentieth week of pregnancy, an especially vulnerable period due to rapid growth and multiplication of neuronal cells. This phase is followed by one of slower growth, resulting in the multiplication of glial cells, a phase which extends through the third trimester of pregnancy up until about 6 months of postnatal life.[84] This development varies in different species. According to this theory on vulnerable periods, a protein-energy malnutrition that develops postnatally should have its greatest effect during the second period. Since glial cells are responsible for the production of myelin, it is not surprising that there is evidence of delayed myelin formation in protein energy malnutrition.

In severely malnourished children, some researchers observed a *reduction in conduction velocity in peripheral nerves, both sensory and motor.*[54,126,378] Perhaps the strongest evidence pertains to a decrease in the density of neuronal synapses. A lower synapse to neuron ratio in some regions of the brain is a result of early severe postnatal malnutrition as described by Bedi.[21]

Dobbing[83] concluded that the nerve cell number, which, in any case, may not be significant for mental function, is "out of the reach of malnutrition" in humans, since almost all the adult nerve cells are produced before mid-pregnancy. Adequate quantity and quality of dietary intake during pregnancy, highly desirable, even if there is evidence that the fetus takes all that is necessary from mother. Dobbing claims that not all negative changes are irreversible, and some may be completely reversible, provided that the adequate realimentation is possible (which is not always the case). However, it is not yet known which of these changes caused by dietary intake are significant for higher mental functions, as the mental achievements must be followed up later on in life in the same subjects, who were rarely available.

Among the most important associations of stunting that is well-documented in school-age children is *impaired mental development*.[64-66] This association is not found in children from well-off families, where differences in the height of individual children may be explained by genetic influences. Cravioto and Cravioto[65] have also shown that by the age of ten children who have survived an earlier episode of malnutrition did not reach the same level of competence as those who had not been malnourished.

The level of **spontaneous physical activity** *is, as a rule, reduced to save energy. This low physical activity could be the "first line of defence"* for severely undernourished children.[337-340] Kraut[185] commented that the spontaneous activity of small children can serve as an indicator of the level of nutrition in the particular country: when children are generally inert and inactive, it shows lack of energy and malnutrition of the population.

Some studies in Ugandan children compare their low activity levels to those in European children. These children, in spite of low energy intake, grew normally, i.e., activity was sacrificed to maintain growth[295,378] Similar conclusions were formulated in studies concerning children in Jamaica,[122,213] and Gambia.[192] In Mexico, Chavez and Martinez[51,52] showed that children who received food supplements became more active than those who did not. Their activity was measured using a method that records the number of times the child's foot touches the ground.

In a study in Guatemala, reduction of the energy intake of preschool children from 100 to 80 kcal/kg/day was accompanied by a reduction of expenditure without change in the nitrogen balance or in weight gain.[355] It seems, therefore, that *faced with an inadequate energy intake, the child preserved weight at the expense of physical activity*. This behavior contrasts with that of adults. In young children, physical activity plays a key role in psychological and social development. There is also evidence that it influences the rate of linear growth.[354,357] If so, expenditure on activity should be the key criterion of adequate energy intake at this age, particularly since more activity may be demanded of Third World children than in most industrially developed affluent countries.

Malnourished children admitted to a hospital were much less active even with toys than later, after realimentation. Activity and exploration ratings tested in these children were reduced a lot at the beginning of the treatment for malnutrition than later after rehabilitation. In children over 2 years of age, improvement was usually observed in performance tests of specific cognitive functions and in school achievements.[138] Pollitt et al.[286] have suggested that these improvements are mediated through changes in the child's level of arousal and attention.

As mentioned above, the *level of functional deterioration depends on the degree, sort, and duration of malnutrition*. Many functions of the children were studied, but, in the case of very severe malnutrition, performance tests were usually not applied for obvious reasons.

The transition point where malnutrition is no longer marginal, but severe and eventually irreversible, is interesting not only with regard to the actual functional and working capacity, but also to the future one. Unfit children most often become unfit adults with a lower level of productivity, which is fatal for the whole population or community. When the real optimum of dietary intake cannot be ensured, at least the "minimal optimum" or "optimal minimum" should be provided. This may be favored by certain types of *adequate physical activities which can enable, in realimented children, faster rehabilitation after a malnutrition period*.[354–357]

The effect of exercise on linear growth was investigated in both experimental models with laboratory rats and in preschool children recovering from protein energy malnutrition. Physically active animals grew more in length and weight than their inactive counterparts. Groups of preschoolers recovering from malnutrition were assigned to either an active group (encouraged, but not forced, to participate in games and activities such as walking uphill, climbing, running, etc.; 2.0 BMR) or to a control group (1.7 BMR). With almost identical dietary intakes, weight gain in both groups was practically the same, but the active group grew more in length and in lean body mass.[357]

Malina and Buchang[202] followed up not only marginally but also in severely undernourished children. Absolute values of hand grip strength and motor performance were significantly below those of better-nourished Philadelphia school children. When corrected for body size differences, i.e., *when relating various parameters per unit body height and weight, the rural Zapotec children performed commensurately with their smaller body size in the dash and jump at early ages, but less than expected for their size at the older ages*. Strength per unit body size was slightly, but consistently, smaller in the Zapotec children, while their throwing distance per unit body weight was greater.

Estimated energy, protein, vitamin, and mineral intakes were considerably lower than the recommended dietary intakes for Mexican children. Marked reduction of body size, compared to national standards, was the result. High crude death rates and infant mortality were also apparent in this Zapotec locality, where no change in growth status and secular change in size and sexual maturation over the past 80 years was recorded. In this case excessive malnutrition markedly impaired most of the items of functional capacity and physical performance. Nevertheless, the *throwing performance was better in relation to body size in Zapotec children*. This may be due to a skill development that is not mainly dependent on body size and body mass. Some skill tasks may sometimes be performed even better by children with smaller body size, as shown also in the 11-year-old Tunisian boys with lower values of height and weight.[233] This, though, is an exceptional case in severely malnourished children. However, the transition from marginal to mild-to-moderate to severe malnutrition in the functional parameters is not always clear. As mentioned above, individual items of physical fitness and performance may be influenced in a different degree.

Deterioration of health and function is an unavoidable consequence of extreme malnutrition, which is manifested in all systems; this mainly affects children from Third World countries. However, results of two surveys, HANES I and HANES II,[169] showed lower mean values for growth measures assessed in children living below the poverty threshold. The magnitude of these poverty-associated differences tended to decrease between the times of the HANES I and HANES II surveys, though not sufficiently enough to be statistically significant. These differences in growth were not consistently associated with the differences in dietary intake of energy between poverty groups or surveys. Functional consequences were not followed up.

As mentioned above, muscle weakness results in very limited muscle strength of severely malnourished children. Cardiorespiratory efficiency is also severely limited, especially during physical activity demanding endurance.

Sensomotor development, along with psychological development, is always severely deteriorated. However, in some cases even in severely malnourished children, a certain skill can be sufficiently developed — especially those concerning small muscle groups of the hand. With this faculty children can achieve quite a high level due to adaptation and because it is not very demanding concerning energy needs. For that reason many malnourished children are used as laborers in certain types of manufacturing, in home work, etc.

V. PROBLEMS OF CHILD LABOR

The poorer the country, the larger the number of children who have to perform activities that are an inadequate work load for their age. The age limit for the term "child labor" varies officially in many countries, but the criterion is normally 15 years old. Nevertheless, this age limit is not respected, and many children work under this age.[324] It is obvious that this is an unacceptable phenomenon. Quite often, though, it is not unusual to hear that if the children do not work, they would die of hunger, not only themselves, but their whole family for whom, under conditions of certain countries, this is the only income available.

Different cultures and states define the state of childhood in different ways. The International Labor Office (ILO) sets out minimum ages for work as 14 or 15 years. These limits may be higher for work conditions that jeopardize the health, safety, or morals of the young worker. It was also noted that few children under 5 years of age work. Clearly, then, child labor includes the age group of 5 to 15 years of age. As follows, the problem of child labor also concerns very early periods of life.

Child labor is generally forbidden; nevertheless, it continues to exist for obvious reasons. It is necessary to point out, however, that children in villages or even in cities have always helped their parents by participating in the economic activities of the family, by helping with domestic work, by watching over younger brothers or sisters, by running errands, and so forth. When such activities have not surpassed certain limits of work load or duration, they may be tolerable or when appropriately used, they may even be useful for the education and development of the child, as in exercise.

However, there are some types of child labor that have been defined as exploitative. *Exploitative child labor has been defined by the ILO as any labor that deprives children of any basic need, including health.* Such a definition may be too wide, including most children in developing countries, whether they work officially or not. Some jobs for children have obvious health related problems; while not intrinsically unhealthy, they are simply part of the general environment of poverty.[324]

Certainly, it is necessary to focus on the problems of child labor. The classical epidemiological methods will follow up on the morbidity and mortality associated with the various industries where children work. Perhaps, most child labor is illegal, so exact information on the extent and sort of child labor is very difficult to obtain. Even preschool children have to participate in economic activities in order toearn money for themselves or for their families. Activities like housework, running errands, farm work, or brick carrying may be no exception, even for preschool children.

The influence of these activities are both direct and indirect. *Growth and development may be affected by continuous and thus too demanding rather than unhealthy labor.* **Health effects** are also of **long-term character**. This mainly concerns the labor in sweat shops or in criminal activities. Even when such activities mostly affect older children, the beginning of them may start very young, especially in street children who are abandoned by their parents.

The member states of the WHO, at the historic WHO/UNICEF conference in Alma Ata in 1978, adopted an approach to primary health care through a program called "Health for All by the Year 2000". Although exploitative child labor is not mentioned here, the First World Health Assembly in 1948 adopted a wide-ranging resolution condemning child labor. Until now, very little has happened to prevent this shameful phenomenon.[216] The roots of this problem are of a social, economic, and political character, and as such, they must be solved.[223] Scientific research may eventually help to compensate for the harmful consequences affecting the children and may help to ensure health and fitness later in adulthood, provided that there will be better living conditions.

According to the available literature, except for somatic and possibly psychological assessment, the influence of child labor was not systematically investigated, and there was not even an opportunity for it. (Anybody who could approach such children would, of course, help and not just do research). In general, it is well known that the development of such children is retarded; their health impaired; their immunoresistence reduced, and many die very young when the situation is really bad.

In spite of the fact that children may achieve a relatively high level of ability in some activities (e.g., carpet weaving, where skill and performance of small muscle groups of the hand are mainly involved), the overall result on the health and functional capacity of these children is negative and deteriorating.[400]

Chapter 8

THE DEVELOPMENT OF OBESITY AND ITS INFLUENCE ON THE FUNCTIONAL CAPACITY OF CHILDREN AND YOUTH

I. OBESITY IN YOUNG CHILDREN

Obesity is mainly characterized by the *disproportionate accumulation of depot fat in the organism in relation to all other tissues,* with due consideration to age and sex. Functional capacity and metabolic and biochemical variables also differ in obese subjects including children and youth.[229,231,233,246,264] One of the simplest characteristics is the increased BMI value, which correlates significantly with the percentage of body fat in all age categories of males and females.[243,244] In the adults, a BMI higher than 25 in males and 24 in females is a criterion for being overweight and a BMI of 30 as being obese.

In children, the evaluation of obesity is more difficult because the proportionality of the growing organism changes markedly, and the absolute BMI values considered critical for obesity change throughout the whole period of growth.[299,301,303,306]

Even in children, being overweight and having a high BMI does not always mean excess fatness, i.e., obesity, as shown by densitometry and skinfold thickness measurements.[230,233] Some authors such as Ditschuneit[82] define juvenile obesity as a twofold increase of body fat mass above normal controls and being "overweight" as a 20% increase above the percentiles for body weight and height. A considerable proportion of very fat children may maintain normal weight, and, on the other hand, a considerable proportion of children who are not too overweight may be relatively lean.[229,233] Therefore, the most reliable criterion for obesity is the assessment of the most essential item, the amount of body fat.

Early diagnosis of excess depot fat and its correction is of essential importance: a 40-year weight history and adult morbidity and mortality in a cohort of 504 Swedish overweight children, aged 2 months to 1 year, through adulthood showed that overweight children remained overweight as adults.[81] Subjects who died during the 40-year follow up and those reporting cardiovascular disease were significantly heavier at puberty and in adulthood than healthier subjects. Patients with early onset of obesity displayed a greater frequency and higher levels of emotional distress and psychiatric symptomatology than patients with late onset of obesity.[215]

Studies in Singapore show significantly more severe grades of obesity in Malay preschool children compared to Chinese and Indian children.[296] Ethnicity seems to play an important role in the early development of obesity in the same environment. Lower social class, lower expressive social support, and unmarried status of the caretaker were associated with higher calorie intake and higher weight for height score in children aged 2.5 to 5 years.[124] In northern Italy, parental obesity and birthweight represented major risk factors for obesity among children including those of preschool age.[200]

II. METHODS FOR THE EVALUATION OF DEPOT FAT AND BODY COMPOSITION USED FOR YOUNG CHILDREN

For a long time, ***anthropometric measurements*** remained the most frequently used procedures for the evaluation of the degree of obesity. Since then, the technology has advanced considerably,[375] and many new methods are now available, at least for some richer institutions.

With anthropometry, the protocols are very similar to those used for the studies of normal children and youths. For quite a long time, these criteria have not been accepted generally, and they depended on the local situation in a particular country.

Most commonly, ***body mass index (BMI)*** and its comparison with international and/or national standards are used. The *85th percentile* has been accepted as a criterion for *overweight*, and the *97th percentile* as advanced *obesity*. The absolute BMI values, of course, vary markedly in different growth periods as well as in boys and girls. Up until now there has been no general consensus on the BMI percentile as a criterion for obesity in young children.

Many countries also have standards for other anthropometric characteristics such as ***circumferential*** and ***breadth measures***, ***skinfold thicknesses***, and the percentage of fat and indices (waist/hip ratio, centrality index as mentioned before). Again, similar percentiles for BMI are used for the evaluation of individual anthropometric values that exceed the usual range of these characteristics, qualifying those subjects as obese. Anthropometric measurements are relatively simple, and their validity and reproducibility is great when taken properly. They can also be used in very young subjects and under field conditions. These indices can supplement the evaluation of obesity type.

Densitometry, i.e., ***hydrostatic weighing*** with simultaneous measurements of air in the lungs and respiratory passages[198,233] is simple in principle and reliable, and it has been used for the calibration of nearly all new methods. However, for smaller children, it is usually not feasible because it demands a great degree of cooperation, lack of fear of water, and skill. Our youngest subjects were 6 to 7 years old,[227,229–231,233] and it took a very long time to teach them the procedure in order to obtain reliable data.[233]

Bioimpedance analysis (BIA) is based on the principle of a frequency-dependent impedance to the spread of an applied alternating electrical current develops in biological tissues. At frequencies of between 500 and 800 kHz, the current passes through both intra- and extracellular fluids. Due to the high conductivity of fluids, the fat-free tissues have a far greater conductivity than fat. Two electrodes are fastened, mostly to the hand and foot, and electrical conductivity is measured (l/resistance) as an excitation current is introduced to the subjects. Various prediction equations are used for total body water, depot fat, and fat-free body mass. The results correlate satisfactorily with the results of other methods.[105,156] Bipedal bioimpedance has only become available recently.

There is still a controversy as to how exact the evaluation of body composition by bioimpedance analysis in children can be. The method of BIA is easy, does not require a great deal of active cooperation, and thus is very suitable for children.[134] However, there were doubts as to whether any of the regression equations can give acceptable results on body components in growing children.

Deurenberg et al.[87] used bioelectric impedance simultaneously with densitometry in pubertal children. Goran et al.[134] compared body composition (estimated from total body water measured by $^{18}H_2O$ and using Kushner equation) with bioelectric resistance, which was cross-validated by two independent laboratories in 4- to 6-year-old children. On the basis of these measurements, it was concluded that the bioelectrical impedance may only be an adequate method to assess body composition in epidemiological studies when population-specific prediction formulas are used. This procedure also showed that increased protein intake accelerated catch-up growth in malnourished children and restored the reference body composition in children recovering from malnutrition.[170]

Some authors still claim that BMI or body density gives more exact results for the evaluation of body composition.[87,199] The same applies for the evaluation of body composition using regression equations with skinfold thickness measurements, which gives results with a precision similar to the best fitting equations involving bioimpedance. Children with normal and/or increased body weight were followed up using this method in numerous studies.[358] However, clinical applicability of BIA is still controversial. Further technical improvements will certainly contribute to wider utilization of this method in young children.

Another method highly suitable for children is the *total body conductivity* method *(TOBEC)*. Special apparatuses were developed and used for the youngest infants.[109] This technique, like BIA, is based on the differences in electrical properties of fat and fat-free tissues. The measurement chamber of the TOBEC apparatus consists of a large cylindrical cell. An oscillating electrical current is injected into the cell, inducing an electromagnetic field in the space enclosed by the coil. A meter attached to the system measures the change in coil impedance as the subject passes through the instruments core. The change in impedance is related to the dielectric and conductive properties of the body, and as for BIA, equations for water, fat, and fat-free body mass were developed.[105] As for BIA, the between-day reproducibility of TOBEC measurements in healthy subjects is excellent (2 to 3% for estimates of fat-free mass);[156] correlations with total body water (dilutometry), protein, and fat-free body mass are also excellent.[105]

Body composition can be assessed by measuring total body water, i.e., **dilutometry**. A comparatively safe and valid approach is **deuterium oxide** dilution **(D₂O)** or **tritium** dilution. The latter is a β-emitter and the former a stable isotope. Because deuterium is a stable isotope, it has been used extensively. Orally ingested D_2O is readily absorbed in the gastrointestinal tract and is in equilibrium with body water within a few hours. The equilibrium concentration can be determined in blood, urine, or saliva. About 2% of D_2O exchanges with H^+ in the body, but this slight correction is easily made. Apparently, D_2O is not selectively excreted by the kidneys and is nontoxic in trace amounts. A variety of analytical techniques have been used to measure D_2O concentration, including infrared absorption, falling drop method, freezing point elevation, mass spectrometry, and gas chromatography. Another approach involves exposing the sample to gamma ray irradiation with subsequent measurements of neutron emission. In addition, D_2O doses as low as 10 to 20 g can be used.[105] This method was most widely used for body composition measurements in young children.[74-76]

⁴⁰K whole body counting is generally used to estimate total body potassium. There are different types of whole body counters, e.g., 3π whole body counter containing several plastic scintillators with a varying total volume of a chamber with an efficient iron shielding. This method can be combined with neutron activation analysis. Intracellular potassium concentration is relatively constant and distributed entirely within the fat-free, lean body mass.[105] There is very little potassium outside cells. Therefore, potassium can serve as an indicator of lean body mass.[94] ⁴⁰K spectrometry was used simultaneously with bioelectric impedance and skinfold thickness measurements in subjects 3.9 to 19 years of age.[94]

Computed tomography (CT) represents a major advance in body composition evaluations. The novelty is, in particular, in the use of CT in depicting internal and visceral fat, and subcutaneous fat, along with other tissues. Relatively high radiation exposure of CT does not allow measuring, e.g., very small children, especially in longitudinal studies of growth.[105]

Soft tissues and bone minerals in the skeleton attenuate emitted photons to a different degrees, a property which underlies the **dual photon absorptiometry (DPA)** method. **Dual energy X-ray absorptiometry (DEXA)** as a newer method is faster, requiring 10 to 15 minutes for a whole-body analysis. The relatively low radiation exposure allows repeated studies. The results of DEXA correlated significantly with total carcass chemical analysis in pigs with a weight range of 5 to 16 kg. However, significant differences in the partitioning between bone mineral content, non-bone lean tissue, and body fat compartments were revealed. The influence of these differences in the body composition analyses by DEXA were examined in a group of boys aged 4 to 12 years.[95] Sex-linked differences in body composition were generally evident after puberty as shown by DEXA assessments in subjects 4 to 26 years.[221]

Nuclear magnetic resonance (NMR) shows a promise in the studies of human tissue metabolism. This process of NMR imaging is now also referred to as magnetic resonance imaging (MRI). This method is based on the principle that nuclei containing an odd number of protons or an odd number of neutrons or both have an angular momentum arising from their inherent spin. The utilization of this method for the studies of growth and nutrition problems is still limited, but it is very promising for this research. Magnetic resonance imaging evaluation of adipose tissue and muscle tissue mass was already used in children with growth hormone deficiency, Turner's syndrome, and intrauterine growth retardation treated by growth hormones.[195]

Adipose tissue was measured using magnetic resonance imaging (MRI) in infants,[1] along with total body water and total energy expenditure (stable isotopes). This validation showed a precision of 2%, the same as in adult women. Simultaneous caliper measurements correlated significantly with MRI measurements, enabling the prediction of body fat from skinfolds of infants, with a precision of 5 to 7%.

III. RESULTS OF STUDIES IN DEVELOPING OBESE SUBJECTS

The prevalence of obesity varies in time and in different age categories. The last result of NHANES[188] showed a permanent increase in the average value of BMI in the adult U.S. population, which means that the goals claimed within the framework of the program "Health for All in the Year 2000" will not be fulfilled. Instead of reducing the values of BMI, the very opposite results occurred due to changes in lifestyle of all age categories occurred. This includes nutrition, physical activity, stress management, and many other variables which have an influence on body weight and fatness. In addition, the prevalence of individuals who meet the BMI criteria for obesity have increased significantly by 8%.

A. PREVALENCE OF OBESITY AT AN EARLY AGE

This problem develops from early childhood, reflected not only in an increased fatness, but also in a decreased level of physical fitness of children. This has been best documented by the studies in the U.S. by Rippe et al.[297] Most alarming was the finding that *by the age of 12, 40% of children have at least one major risk factor for heart disease including obesity.* In conjunction with this, it was again pointed out that cardiologists have already been telling us for a long time about the *genesis of atherosclerosis in childhood*. The Bogalusa Heart Study showed that lipids measured in the umbilical cord blood were related to atherosclerotic plaques in the aorta in some of these children who died by accident in their teens,[219] indicating the influence of genetic and prenatal factors.

A similar situation occurs in the U.K. and in many other countries, including the developing industrial nations that include a well-off social strata. There are fewer data on the changes in body weight of Central and Eastern Europe. However, it seems that in all countries with a certain level of industrial development and economic level, the prevalence of obesity is increasing.

During the growth period, the prevalence of overweight and obese children also varies. In our studies of preschool and school children *the prevalence of obesity differed — in preschool age it was rather low (2 to 3%)* and later it increased up to 10 to 15% during the prepubertal and puberal period. It was difficult to compare the prevalence of obesity before BMI was introduced and generally accepted as most countries had different growth grids and different criteria, and there has been little agreement as to when obesity starts. However, some ex post evaluations can be made using height and weight values. As mentioned before, BMI percentiles in Czech children are higher than those in France;[294] regarding secular trends, BMIs of Czech children increased from 1895[209] up until recently.[35,147]

The best predictors of early childhood obesity were a higher fat ratio of the mother before pregnancy, a higher fat ratio of the child at birth, and a higher fat ratio at the age of 1. In addition, maternal age, prolonged breast-feeding, and the late introduction of solid foods seemed to be connected with early obesity.[13] A higher fat ratio at the age 1 year and during pregnancy and delivery complications contributed most to the prediction of obesity in puberty. These observations correspond to the theory of Roland-Cachera et al.,[303] which indicates that the *early rebound of BMI predisposes a child toward later obesity*. Similar conclusions on "critical periods" (including preschool age) for the development of obesity were reported simultaneously by Dietz.[80] Energy intake and expenditure in infants born to lean and overweight mothers can differ.[298]

B. MORPHOLOGICAL CHARACTERISTICS OF OBESITY

As a criterion for children's obesity, +2 SD above the average weight for a given age in the particular country mostly is used. Actually, the 85th percentile of BMI is suggested as a borderline for obesity in children.

Regarding the *percentage of total body fat* there is no general agreement on standard values during the growth period as there are still relatively few data on this variable measured directly by reliable and advanced methods. The critical value for the definition of obesity varies according to factors such as growth period, sex, etc. In The Czech Republic, we are using the average values of the percentage of fat assessed by densitometry[229–233] as a standard for comparison. A measure of +2 SD and/or 85th percentiles of depot fat ratio and/or skinfolds were considered as criteria for the onset of obesity in relation to the percentage of body fat; the critical value varies significantly according to age.

Obese children differ from children with normal weight not only in relation to larger skinfolds, but also with a *different distribution of subcutaneous fat* characterized by *indices*: there is a significant sex-linked difference in the amount of total fat and by its typical gynoid distribution (i.e., relatively more fat on the hips, buttocks, thighs, etc.). This sex-linked difference is absent in the obese even during puberty, when both obese girls and boys have a subcutaneous fat distribution similar to older women.[229–233] Exceptionally, this type of fat distribution can be found in young children.

Other morphological variables are also different in the obese: children and youths usually have **greater lean body mass** and sometimes (especially in individuals who started to be obese quite early in life) *a greater robusticity of the skeleton*, as shown by higher values of breadth measurements.[233] Needless to say, *circumferential measurements are larger*, and waist/hip, as well as waist/thigh ratios, may be different in the obese subjects during growth. In obese prepubertal boys there is also a significantly greater biiliocristal breadth compared to normal lean boys of the same age. The difference was marked even when the biiliocristal breadth was corrected for the thickness of subcutaneous fat in this region. In girls, this difference due to obesity was not apparent.[233]

The measurements of the **heart volume** showed significantly **greater** absolute and relative values in boys 12 to 15 years of age. However, after 3 years, no further increase in heart volume was found in spite of continuing growth and increase in height, weight, lean body mass, etc.[233]

As previously mentioned, the prevalence of more marked obesity in preschool age is much lower than its occurrence later in younger school age and/or in adolescence. Heavier children were also taller and bigger and seemed to be generally more advanced in their development, but not typically obese in the same way as older children or adults.

In Table 8.1 there are data on three groups of preschool children from survey B (6.4 years of age): underweight, average, and overweight to obese. The differences in BMI are apparently similar to the differences in body weight. All circumferential measurements were greatest in the obese and smallest in the underweight. Other morphological variables were not measured in these groups of children.

Japanese children 3 to 6 years old were screened using bioelectrical impedance by Tsukuda et al.[358] The results of the BIA were compared with BMI and percentage of fat ratio in relation to standard weight, and significant correlations were found. Regression equations were also derived. However, it seems that a comparison of data assessed with more exact methods would be necessary to validate the results concerning the amount of body fat in preschool

TABLE 8.1   Anthropometric Variables in Preschool Children with Different Body Weight

		Overweight		Average weight		Underweight	
		x̄	SD	x̄	SD	x̄	SD
Weight (kg)	Boys	28.8	3.9	22.5	2.2	18.5	1.9
	Girls	28.5	3.9	21.9	2.2	17.7	1.7
Height (cm)	Boys	119.5	6.0	118.5	5.3	117.8	6.2
	Girls	118.3	9.9	117.9	5.0	118.1	7.1
BMI (kg/m²)	Boys	20.3	1.1	16.1	0.9	13.3	0.8
	Girls	20.3	1.0	15.7	1.0	12.7	0.9
Circumferences							
Abdomen (cm)	Boys	63.0	6.1	55.4	3.2	52.2	4.4
	Girls	63.6	6.6	54.8	3.5	51.0	5.6
Arm (cm)	Boys	21.5	2.3	18.4	1.3	16.6	1.1
	Girls	21.8	2.1	18.4	1.3	16.6	1.3
Thigh (cm)	Boys	41.3	4.9	35.7	2.6	35.6	2.4
	Girls	43.0	4.3	37.3	2.7	33.6	2.9
Chest (cm)	Boys	65.4	4.6	59.4	2.4	56.0	2.3
	Girls	65.3	4.8	58.0	2.4	54.8	3.0

Adapted from Pařízková, J. and Hainer, V., chapter in *Current Therapy in Sports Medicine-2*, Torg, J.S., Welsh, R.P., and Shephard, R.J., Eds., Dekker, Toronto, 1990, 22.

children. For rapid and safe screening of excess adiposity in preschool children, BIA may be recommended.

More anthropometric variables were also measured in older obese children, before and after reduction treatment. These results were reported previously.[229–233] To our knowledge, there are no results of reducing treatment in preschoolers, but there are some recent studies concerning older children.

C. FOOD INTAKE IN THE OBESE

Food intake was followed either directly by the research team and/or by using diaries completed by kindergarten teachers and parents. There was a very limited opportunity to assess the food intake in the obese preschool children as the prevalence was so low. In our surveys G, H, and J no relationship between the actual dietary intake, on the one hand, and body weight, BMI, and percentage of fat, on the other hand, was found.

In the older children, it was possible to use diaries completed by children who were instructed and supervised. However, the results of the assessments of the *actual dietary intake did not show any significant differences compared to children with normal body weight*; the intake was generally slightly higher than the energy output. The intake of proteins and fats (especially those of animal origin) was somewhat higher than Czech RDAs and much higher than EC or U.S. RDAs. The intake of calcium, fiber, and vitamin C was often lower than the RDAs. Marked intra- and inter-individual variability was found. However, such a type of dietary intake was also found in children who were not obese.[254] So it seems that the actual intake of food is not the main cause of a higher fat ratio in young children.

In markedly obese prepubertal girls in Tunisia, however, an increased food intake was found along with a lower energy output.[264] These girls were obviously in the dynamic phase of obesity, and their food intake was very high (16.2 MJ/day). In chronically obese children and adolescents, though, the food intake might be even lower than in children of normal weight.[233,254]

D. PHYSICAL ACTIVITY IN THE OBESE

Classical observations of Jean Mayer[210] showed that not only *the level of spontaneous physical activity was lower in the obese children*, but that during the same games obese children were much less active than children of normal weight. This was documented by shooting a motion picture of the children. However, upon completing a questionnaire this reduced activity would appear as equal to taking part in the same activity for the same period as normal children.

Physical activity was also followed in other studies: e.g., Huttunen et al.[162] used questionnaires for assessing the history of physical activity of obese and normal children from 5.7 to 16.1 years, which were completed by the children and their parents. There were no significant differences in daily activities between the obese and nonobese children, while the *sport grades at school were lower and participation in the training teams of sports clubs was less frequent among obese than among normal-weight subjects.*

The "fattening of America", which also concerns children, has been explained by a number of authors, e.g., Kuczmarski et al.,[188] by the lack of physical activity. Discretional activities are mostly devoted to TV programs, video games, and films, and very little time is spent on different physical activities and exercise. Even usual everyday activities have become more and more limited because of public transportation, the use of cars, etc.[313]

Blair,[36] who studied the development of risk factors and/or their reduction in adults, showed that even very ordinary activities such as taking a walk, climbing stairs, low-level recreational activities, and house and yard work can make an important contribution to physical fitness and health in sedentary and unfit adult subjects, including reduction of excess fat and cardiovascular risk.

This also applies to children, whose spontaneous activity and need for it is on a much higher level than in adults.

E. FUNCTIONAL CAPACITY
1. Cardiorespiratory Fitness

Generally, it is assumed that obese individuals are clumsy and have a low level of physical fitness. Here again it is *necessary to specify and differentiate what items of physical fitness and functional capacity are most influenced by excess fat deposition.* Finally, there are not many comparable measurements of physical performance in the obese of any age. This mainly applies to children of younger age.

A very negative situation is found in cardiorespiratory fitness evaluated with the help of measurements of maximal oxygen uptake during an increasing work load on a bicycle ergometer, on a treadmill, or during the step test. The oxygen uptake may be normal or even quite high, but related to body weight and/or lean body mass, it is reduced. This corresponds to the general experience that *obese subjects are at a disadvantage, especially in dynamic, weight bearing exercise*. This also concerns endurance. Runners for shorter and longer distances are rarely heavy.

Physical fitness was mostly tested in obese school children and adolescents; e.g., aerobic power, evaluated with the help of the measurements of maximal oxygen uptake, was significantly lower in relation to total and lean body weight. *PWC[170] was also lower in obese children in addition to performance in various sports and disciplines*, especially *running* and *jumping*.[231,233] *Vital capacity and forced expiration*, especially in relative values (per kilograms of total and lean body weight), were also *reduced*. In general, though, *muscle strength was at an adequate level*.[233,246]

Huttunen et al.[162] found a lower level of physical fitness in obese and in normal-weight children 5.7 to 16.1 years old as evaluated by pedalling time in an exercise test. VO_2 max/kg lean body mass was also lower in obese children.

In 5- to 6-year-old children, Gutin et al.[146] showed a *positive relationship between diastolic blood pressure and fatness* and a *negative correlation of diastolic blood pressure and fitness level*, as evaluated by the submaximal treadmill test. The fitness level was inversely related to body fatness for boys and girls, and thus these small children showed risk factors similar to those in adults. We found no relationships between the results of the step test, body weight, BMI, and fatness in 4- to 6-year-old children.[271]

2. Motor Development

The same group of asthenic, normal, and overweight preschool children (see Table 8.1) was also tested in a ***20 m dash***, ***broad jump***, and ***a ball throw***. More marked, significant differences were mainly found for the broad jump and the ball throw (Figures 8.1a, 8.1b, 8.1c, 8.1d). The skinnier children had significantly better results, i.e., they jumped further compared to the overweight children. There was no difference as of yet in the 20 m dash. The differences in dynamic performance usually appear later in school age. Endurance was not tested in this survey.

3. Skill

As to throwing a ball and walking on a horizontal beam, the effect of body weight did not play a part in preschool age; however, in the forward roll there were considerable differences, particularly in girls. Evidently, the influence of different body weight is only manifested in some specific exercises. In selected instances, the ***broad jump*** and the ***forward roll*** (which requires the transfer and manipulation of one's own body weight in space), the negative effect of being overweight is already clear at preschool age. In many other exercises such as walking in a given rhythm, catching a ball, the test of "opening and closing the hands," and laterality, the results were again practically the same as those in normal children.[256] More recent measurements confirmed these trends of physical fitness in obese preschoolers.[254]

4. Muscle Strength and Skill

When considering some positive points of obesity, muscle strength — which depends mainly on body mass — is not influenced by excess fat. The reverse is true — obese subjects usually have increased lean body mass, including muscles. Thus, ***muscle strength*** *in absolute terms (N) is usually greater in obese subjects* than in lean or normal ones. However, in *relation to body weight, muscle strength may be the same or even lower.* By contrast, performance in static exercise is not hampered by excess weight and fat. This is well known from athletics — most representatives of static sport disciplines such as weight lifters and wrestlers of higher weight categories, generally have high fat ratios (but are also very muscular[241,254]). An example are Japanese sumo wrestlers, whose preparation — training and special diet — start during their growth period.

With regard to *skill*, certain activities that demand the coordination of smaller muscle groups of one extremity may be performed without a problem in well-adapted subjects. This applies especially to working skills: many workers performing their special task (mostly of static character) can perform very well. The same applies to static activities in children. When coordination of the whole body is involved in a more dynamic action, the level of performance is usually low, with the exception of special cases of the adapted athletes mentioned above. Within the normal population, a good level of overall skill in the obese is rare.

The development of selected skills and/or strength depends significantly on the beginning of the adaptation process during ontogeny. Subjects who adopted certain skills at a younger age may still preserve them later. As apparent from Figures 8.1a, 8.1b, 8.1c, and 8.1d, being overweight did not interfere with the throwing abilities of preschool children: in this activity muscle strength and coordination of the upper extremities play a decisive role.

5. Biochemical Characteristics

Serum levels of cholesterol were usually higher in obese children, mainly in boys. By contrast, the increase in cholesterol was lower in obese adolescent girls.[233] The same applied to the blood level of triacylglycerols.

The value of nonesterified, *free fatty acids (FFA)* at rest in the serum of obese boys was 1.18 mEq/l of the FFA. There were no differences in the resting values of glucose and EFA among the groups of prepubertal obese and nonobese boys and girls.[233]

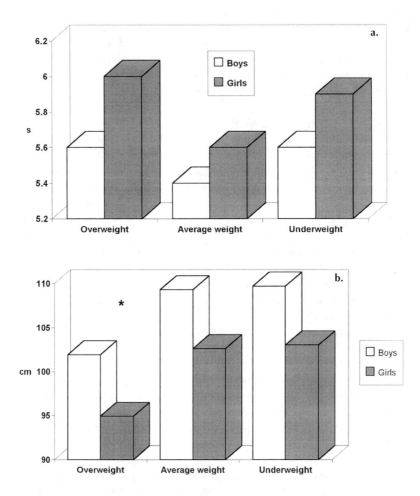

FIGURE 8.1 Comparison of physical performance — 20 m dash **(a)**, broad jump **(b)**, throwing a ball with the right hand **(c)** and throwing a ball with the left hand **(d)** in 6.4 years old boys and girls subdivided according to their weight (survey A).

Under conditions of stress, e.g., work load on a treadmill (maximal work load testing the aerobic power), there was an increase of glycemia during the work load, which continued after 10 minutes recovery. The level of EFA remained the same, decreasing slightly after 10 minutes rest. The FFA level decreased significantly after the maximal work load, remaining the same after 10 minutes rest. There was a significantly negative relationship between the increase of pulse rate during the maximal work load and the change of the FFA level: *the higher the increase of pulse rate during the load (i.e., the lower the level of physical fitness), the greater the decrease of FFA.* This result seems

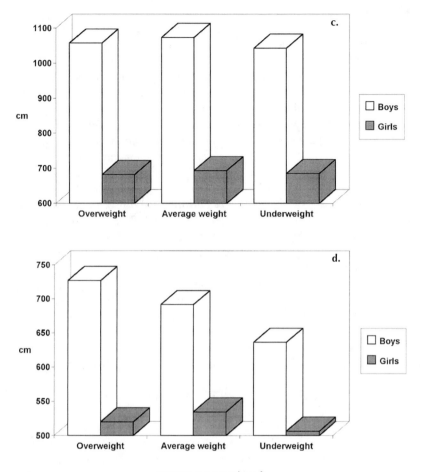

FIGURE 8.1 (continued)

to indicate that a higher fitness level runs parallel to a greater ability to mobilize FFA (which prevents their decline in the blood) as a source of energy.[233]

In preschool children, there was limited opportunity to assess the above blood lipid indicators in the obese, as they are very rare at this age period. However, as mentioned above there was a *significant positive correlation between the percentage of body fat and the blood level of triglycerides* (r = 0.494, 0.02 > *p* > 0.01), and between the *percentage of body fat and the level of blood cholesterol* (r = 0.448, 0.02 > *p* > 0.01) in 52 preschool children with different BMIs and depot fat ratios. It can be assumed that under conditions of a highly increased deposition of body fat the blood lipid indicators would also be higher than those in preschool children of normal weight.

6. Hormonal Variables

Molnar and Porszasz[217] recorded the influence of fasting hyperinsulinaemia on physical fitness in obese children. The hyperinsulinemic obese children had a lower level of physical capacity, in absolute values, when corrected for body weight and lean body mass, than the nonhyperinsulinemic obese children. The exercise period was not significantly different in the two obese subgroups. While *fasting plasma insulin levels* showed a *significantly negative correlation* with *exercise duration and relative physical working capacity in the obese children, the anthropometric parameters did not.*

Gonzales et al.[130] followed the values and their circadian rhythms of insulin and cortisol in obese children and their relationships to anthropometric variables including body fat. *Higher plasma insulin levels were confirmed in obese children.* No correlation between insulin and cortisol values, on the one hand and body fat, on the other hand, were observed. There were some changes in the circadian rhythms of both cortisol and insulin, but they did not have any relationship to the duration of obesity. These studies mostly included school children.

Studies of biochemical and hormonal indicators in very young children with simple obesity are rare. Only recently, in larger studies mainly focused on nutrition problems, were blood lipids examined in larger samples of young children.[141]

IV. THE INFLUENCE OF REDUCING THERAPY

A. PROCEDURES USED TO REDUCE BODY WEIGHT DURING GROWTH

Even under conditions of a desirable lifestyle, when a sudden imbalance occurs, excess fat is laid down e.g., during convalescence after an illness of the child or after an accident. In these situations, physical activity decreases significantly, although food intake may not be reduced: generally, the reverse is true especially when the child is recovering. Then, after a necessary period, it is indispensable to reduce the excess fat in order to prevent development of permanent obesity.

Special outpatient clinics used to exist in The Czech Republic that took care of obese children of all ages. Initial experiences with reducing therapy, based only on limited food intake, did not give good results: using a diet of about 1000 to 1200 kcal, i.e., 4182 to 5000 kJ, children slowed down or even ceased to grow in height, i.e., it was comparable to the onset of stunting due to malnutrition, in spite of a well-balanced, low energy diet. Very low calorie diets in childhood are not recommended.[46,233]

Because of this experience, a comprehensive reduction therapy was developed in the late 1950s, which gave much better results.[233] The following list illustrates some of the steps involved in this type of therapy:

- First, the *diet* was monitored.
- Secondly, an intense but adequate regime of physical activity and *exercise* was implemented.
- Finally, *behavioral intervention*, adapted for children, was also included in the reducing regime.

The *main principle* of this procedure was that the energy balance was corrected using an increased energy output and not by using a reduced energy intake. Of course, the dietary intake was monitored, although children were not left hungry.

This therapy was most effective when children could spend 7 weeks during their holidays in special summer camps for reduction therapy of children. Their monitored dietary intake was on average 1700 kcal, i.e., 7109 kJ/day. All regulations for a reducing diet with a modification for growing children were observed. The intake of high quality protein was at the level of RDAs for this age group or was slightly higher so as to make normal growth and development possible. The intake of fats and sugar was limited. Complex carbohydrates were the most important source of energy, with lots of fruit and vegetables. The diet was palatable, but not excessively attractive. The intake of beverages was limited to tap or mineral water; the intake of sweeter fruit and juices was reduced to a certain amount per day, as children often were thirsty due to exercise, and could get too much energy from sweet beverages. In these camps children of younger school and prepubertal age mostly participated. Thus, the individual food intake varied according to age, sex, and the degree of initial fat ratio.[233]

The greatest stress was put on the physical activity regime and exercise. A very attractive program of sport activities and exercises, adequate for children and youth, was prepared and supervised by specialized physical education teachers. All suitable sports disciplines were included in the daily program, which varied so as to ensure the interest and spontaneous involvement of children. Excursions to interesting places and walks were also on the program. When children claimed they felt too tired, dancing parties and balls were organized. These events were never missed by any of the children.

Very obese children were also treated with special *spa therapy* for several weeks. In the spa *morbidly obese children* could *exercise* at the beginning of treatment in the *swimming pool* which enabled them to develop some skills and endurance under these conditions in which weight-bearing exercise was facilitated by Archimedes' principle. Later on, when some reduction of weight was achieved, children could exercise while lying or sitting on floor mats and then on a bicycle ergometer. Finally, when they were closer to normal weight and acquired some skills they could participate in the general exercise programs for the obese, which were similar to physical education programs for normal children. Other components of the reducing therapy — monitored diet and behavioral intervention — were practically the same as those in the above mentioned summer camps for obese children organized by one of the university children's hospitals.[233]

Behavioral intervention consisted of lessons in healthy nutrition, physical activity and suitable exercises, and the psychological treatment of difficult situations with which obese children may often be faced in school classes or with peer groups.

The greatest advantage of these summer camps was that there were only obese children, so the inhibitions for exercise were absent because all of the children were somewhat clumsy especially in the beginning. During that period, though, most children learned a lot, lost, on the average, 10 to 15% of their initial body weight (which was mostly fat), and improved their physical performance level significantly.

Unfortunately, the situation deteriorated in many of the children when they returned to their normal home life. An increase in body weight that did not correspond to their growth in height occurred. However, after repeated stays in these camps, most of the children improved permanently and almost preserved normal body weight.[233,246] These changes were individual, depending on genetic predispositions (e.g., obesity of the parents and siblings), the situation at home and school, the duration of obesity, and so on. As followed from the life histories of obese children, the reaction to reducing treatment was related to the onset of a high fat ratio and/or obesity — children with a higher birth weight and/or above-average body weight during preschool age had more difficulties losing weight, and most of them regained weight.[233,254]

The treatment of children in the outpatient program of the children's hospital in Prague used the same principles for weight reduction in children, i.e., monitored diet, physical activity regime and exercise, and behavioral intervention. In this case, the results were not as good or as permanent, even when improvement was observed. Everything depended on the family and the ability to adhere to the prescribed regime within the family. Results of Koivisto et al.[184] demonstrated that parental influences on children's eating habits may have implications on special food preferences, which are not always adequate and which may later lead to a higher fat ratio. The situation was also more difficult, especially when there were some normal weight siblings, who all ate at the same table with the family. In this circumstance, it was possible to observe better results, especially in older children and adolescents, who were able to adopt the reducing regime as their own program for which they were personally responsible. With smaller children this was generally impossible.

As follows from the actual trends, it is necessary to consider *ways to influence even slightly overweight young children: the sooner the intervention, the better the results*. Recently, similar reducing procedures with monitored diet and exercise was used more often in school children and adolescents.

B. MORPHOLOGICAL AND FUNCTIONAL CHANGES AFTER REDUCING TREATMENT

Along with the decrease in body weight and BMI, body composition also changed after reducing therapy. Even when exercise and physical activity were included in the reducing program, a small proportion of weight decrement in obese school children was also lean body mass. This was found when using densitometry or when the changes of body composition were assessed by regression equations with skinfold thickness values (derived for our children including obese).[230,233,254]

This decrease in lean body mass was only obvious when the weight reduction was substantial, i.e., in very obese subjects. As mentioned above, very obese children and adolescents are characterized by a greater lean body mass, so a small decrease may be tolerated. This applies especially when no functional deterioration was obvious, and the growth in height continued.[254]

Most of the anthropometric variables diminish too. This mainly applies to circumferential measures or to breadth values, which may be influenced by a layer of fat. For that reason, it was difficult to evaluate the changes, e.g., of the skeleton.

In very young children of preschool age, this therapy has been rarely applied in our country. In overweight children, there has been an effort to reduce the weight increment, along with the further increase in height, so that *the child "grows up" to his/her appropriate BMI*. This trend is often also applied in older children with elevated body weight. It would be difficult, though, to stimulate an adequate BMI when a child is grossly obese.

Nuutinen and Knip[220] studied the ability to predict weight reduction in obese 6- to 15-year-old children. After 1 year of treatment, those who successfully lost weight had a lower body weight, less lean body mass, and lower fasting concentrations of circulating insulin than unsuccessful children. A decrease in the mother's BMI and in documented energy intake over the first year, as well as energy intake at 1 year, were significant predictors of success after 2 years. The combination of these three predictors resulted in correct classification of about 75% of the cases as either successful or unsuccessful weight losers. The preservation of the results of reduction treatment may be difficult, as shown by other studies.[333]

Jirapinyo et al.[167] followed 10 obese children 8 to 13 years old who participated in a 4-week program of weight reduction. A regime of 800 kcal/day and mild exercise were the main features of this program. Mildly and moderately obese children lost more than 5% of their body fat and less than 1% of their lean body mass. Morbidly obese children lost more than 5% of their body fat and lean body mass. It was speculated that for the treatment of morbid obesity, a different sort of treatment must be considered, e.g., spa treatment with exercise in a pool as mentioned above.

Patients from the above mentioned outpatient programs and summer camps were tested using a number methods.[233] First of all, aerobic power was checked *before and after the reduction of excess fat* in the summer camp. Along with somatic changes, the *aerobic power*, characterized by VO_2 max (oxygen uptake during maximal work load), *increased significantly in a group of prepubertal boys* from 38.8 to 40.7 ml · kg⁻¹ · min⁻¹.[246,263] Children were also able to run longer on the treadmill and finish the test after achieving a higher speed, i.e., the whole performance was on a higher level along with a higher level of aerobic power. However, after only 7 weeks of reducing treatment in the summer camp, the VO_2 max in ml · min⁻¹ · kg⁻¹ lean body mass remained the same.

Oxygen uptake and pulse rate during a submaximal work load also decreased significantly after weight and excess fat reduction. The same work load was thus executed more efficiently and economically. Vital capacity and performance in a number of disciplines (running for various distances, jumping, throwing, etc.) improved significantly too. After this summer camp, some children who were not able to run without interruption for 50 or 60 minutes were able to cover this distance in a time comparable to that of the general child population.[233,254]

The results of skill tests also improved significantly, which was due not only to weight reduction, but also to simultaneous adaptation to a number of exercises that were unusual and not feasible for these children before.[233,254]

Along with weight increases, which happened in some children after their return home to their usual way of life, some functional tests also deteriorated. Many of the obese children, though, had the above mentioned treatment in the summer camps repeatedly, and their functional capacity finally improved in spite of temporary fluctuation in their body composition and BMI.[233] However, in 3- to 6-year-old children, there was no opportunity to follow the changes of functional capacity after weight reduction.

Huttunen et al.[162] also found a significantly positive impact of weight reduction on the level of physical fitness and aerobic power. In a group of 6 to 15-year-old children 25 lost weight, and they increased significantly their VO_2 from 44.2 to 47.1 ml · min⁻¹ · kg⁻¹ of lean body mass.

C. CHANGES OF BIOCHEMICAL REACTIONS TO WORK LOAD AFTER REDUCING THERAPY

In prepubertal children, no marked changes were found in rest values of glycemia and EFA after weight reduction. However, the blood FFA level decreased to half of its pretreatment value, i.e., it was 0.613 mEq/l. Moreover, the reaction to a maximal work load was different, i.e., the FFA level remained the same during the load and increased significantly after 10 minutes rest, in spite of the fact that its value was much lower after reducing treatment. The changes in the FFA level seem to indicate that the ability to mobilize and utilize FFA as a source of energy during the work load has markedly improved, for during the work the level of FFA did not decrease as before treatment. By contrast, after the end of the work, the level increased significantly. These results are consistent with the reduction of body fat which was utilized during exercise as fuel for muscle work and was, therefore, the most important part of the treatment.[233,254]

V. GENERAL CONSIDERATIONS: THE VALIDITY OF EXERCISE AND MONITORED DIET AT AN EARLY AGE

Older and newer studies have shown that using a revised energy balance with an energy output increased by exercise and by monitoring the energy intake of an adequate diet is still the best way to improve morphological, functional, metabolic, and biochemical situations of the obese child.[233] The number of studies has recently increased, but they concern mostly school children and adolescents. This is because the more serious degrees of obesity mainly occur during these growth periods.

However, the evidence concerning the early rebound of BMI, observations of increased birth weight, or weight at the age of 1 year as regards the later development of obesity show that *attention to children being overweight and obese and its prevention should be paid very early in life*[74,233,256,296] During puberty many serious problems may appear because of obesity, including psychological ones; reducing treatment is very difficult, often without lasting effects. Weight reduction is generally achieved with a simultaneous decrease of lean body mass. This may not be a great functional harm in very robust and grossly obese subjects, although it is not desirable during this stage of development.

Compared to 20 to 30 years ago, the habitual physical activity of children and youth has decreased considerably. This is basically due to the drastic reduction of walking (to school, for some errands, etc.), the lack of free outdoor games with peers, and so forth. J. Wallace[373] researched this phenomenon in U.K. children, presenting it well in a TV program entitled "Our kids are not all right". The lack of opportunity for the usual levels of physical activity in children is less natural than that of older subjects, having many serious consequences in many respects, including a higher fat ratio, obesity, and a low level of cardiorespiratory fitness.

Therefore, it is essential to provide ample opportunities for a high level of spontaneous physical activity from early childhood. *The child can learn to move and exercise a lot, but he/she can also learn the reverse of this — moving as little as possible.*[182,183] Distraction such as sensationalistic television programs interfere with the above mentioned pedagogic trends. In fact, children spend too much time in front of the television, a situation which is true in the U.S.,[136] as well as in other countries. While watching television, children can actually reduce their metabolic rate when compared to the same conditions without television.[180]

The best guarantee of high spontaneous activity is *early imprinting of proper motor habits*, partiality for and enjoyment of motion, and the cultivation of a need for exercise. This may be ensured not only by teaching, but also by supporting the development of a higher level of fitness which reduces the strain of exercise and renders it enjoyable. All this is essential to the enhancement of natural interest and participation in exercise activities throughout life, which is provided by early intervention. These activities were all quite natural not very long ago.

Chapter **9**

THE INFLUENCE OF ENVIRONMENTAL FACTORS

Environment plays an essential role in human development, depending on genetic predispositions. This problem was analyzed in other documents in greater detail (concerning environmental criteria in environmental epidemiology studies — International Program of Chemical Safety IPCS, WHO, Geneva 1986).[402] In the industrially developed areas, the influence of the environment is mainly related to one's exposure to noxious factors, both outside and inside[23,402]

The interrelationship between the influence of economic and social situations with dietary intake is also evident, both in the industrially developed and in developing countries. Analysis of the influence of environment and its differentiation from hereditary factors is often quite difficult: e.g., the economic situation of the family depends, at least partly, on selected genetic predispositions,the educational level of the parents, the number of children in the family, etc. Up until now, very few studies also focused on the influence of these factors at the level of functional capacity in young children, as related to somatic development. Usually the influence of various environmental factors is mixed, with the differentiation of one particular factor being difficult.

I. THE INFLUENCE OF LIVING CONDITIONS IN THE CAPITAL AND IN OTHER PARTS OF THE COUNTRY

A. SOMATIC DEVELOPMENT AND BODY POSTURE

In survey B of a representative sample of preschool children 6.4 years old (i.e., measured in spring just before entering primary school), we had the opportunity to compare the development of morphological variables, body posture, and motor and sensomotor development in subgroups of children from *Prague*, the capital, on the one hand, and *from all other parts of The Czech Republic*, on the other hand.

The **BMIs** did not differ (Table 9.1), but the average values of *height, weight,* and *circumferential measures* were in almost all cases significantly higher in the children from the capital. In both subgroups of children, there were obvious sex-linked differences — although slight — in the anthropometric

189

TABLE 9.1 Height Weight, and BMI in Preschool Boys and Girls from Prague, and All Other Parts of Czech Republic (Survey B)

Measurement	Prague $\bar{x}$	Prague SD	All other regions $\bar{x}$	All other regions SD
Height (cm)				
Boys	120.3	5.6*	118.5	5.3
Girls	118.4	8.4	117.7	5.2
Weight (kg)				
Boys	22.7	3.3*	22.1	3.2
Girls	22.5	3.4	21.6	3.3
BMI (kg/m²)				
Boys	15.7	1.2	15.7	1.2
Girls	16.1	1.4	15.6	1.3
Circumferences				
Chest (cm)				
Boys	60.1	3.3*	59.2	3.3
Girls	59.2	4.0	57.9	3.7
Abdomen (cm)				
Boys	56.0	5.7*	55.2	4.3
Girls	55.5	5.3	54.8	5.0
Arm (cm)				
Boys	18.3	1.5	18.2	1.7
Girls	18.7	1.9*	18.3	1.8
Thigh (cm)				
Boys	35.1	3.5	35.5	3.5
Girls	37.2	3.8*	37.2	3.6

Note: * $p < 0.05$.

Adapted from Pařízková, J., et al., *Growth, Fitness and Nutrition in Preschool Children,* Charles University, Prague, 1984.

variables, which in this large group were significant. However, all values of body size, BMI, etc. were within the standard reference values of The Czech Republic. Simultaneous assessments by questionnaires also showed a higher economic level in Prague children, in which the per capita income in the family was higher than in other parts of the country. With regard to larger body size in the capital, the impact of increased stimulation of higher nervous activity of children, which accelerates their overall development, was also considered.

A comparison of the results found in Prague children and children from other regions in The Czech Republic (i.e., Bohemia and Moravia) reveals a *clear trend of poorer **body posture** in Prague children.* The depth of the cervical and lumbar lordosis was significantly greater and the average data, i.e., the position of the neck, abdomen, and spinal column indicate a significantly higher ratio of grade 2 and 3 in Prague children.[254,256]

When we evaluated body posture in the individual districts of The Czech Republic, which vary with environmental factors, the comparison showed that, apart from Prague, a relatively poorer posture was recorded in boys and girls from the central Bohemian region. In other parts of the Republic, the highest average values of cervical and lumbar lordosis were rarely found in the remaining regions, i.e., mainly in the south Moravian and north Bohemian regions. Regarding the depth of the cervical and lumbar lordosis, high average values were recorded in the north Moravian Region, where the children also had a more accelerated somatic development. As in Prague, a higher per capita income in the north Bohemian region was recorded. On the whole, the differences among regions were not very marked, although a trend for poorer body posture in children of Prague, or in more industrialized districts such as central and north Bohemia was obvious.[254]

A comparisons of our results with those assembled two decades before revealed that the average value of cervical and lumbar lordosis increased. This may be explained by an accelerated growth rate, along with an increase in bodily dimensions of children of equal age in comparison to then and now. We also must speculate on the possibility of a certain deterioration of body posture, which results from greater weakness of the skeletal muscles. This is more marked in the capital, where the opportunity for games, physical education, and spontaneous exercise is limited. Flabbiness of muscles is manifested most markedly on the abdominal wall where the highest ratio of grade 2 and 3 in the capital was recorded.

B. MOTOR AND SENSOMOTOR DEVELOPMENT

Motor performance was tested using the same protocols as mentioned above (see Appendix 3). The performance level in children from Prague and all of the remaining parts of The Czech Republic was compared in a similar fashion as anthropometric variables and body posture. Performance levels in running, jumping, and throwing a ball with both hands are given in Figures 9.1a through 9.1d. Performance was better in boys,[254,256] and tests characterizing skill showed statistically better results in girls. Only in one (the last) variety of catching a ball (i.e., throwing it vertically above the child, who catches the ball from the air; Appendix 3) were boys slightly better. All of these differences, although small, were statistically significant.[254]

*Comparing the motor performance in children from Prague with those of other regions of Bohemia and Moravia reveals poorer results in Prague boys and girls in **20 m dash*** i.e., a longer time in seconds (Figure 9.1a). Performance in the broad jump was also somewhat worse in Prague children, (although not significantly) despite the fact that Prague children were taller and thus had longer lower extremities (Figure 9.1b). Performance in ***throwing a ball*** *was also significantly worse in Prague* (Figures 9.1c and 9.1d).

In tests of walking on a beam and standing on one leg, there was a certain trend toward better performance in boys and girls from Prague, but the differences

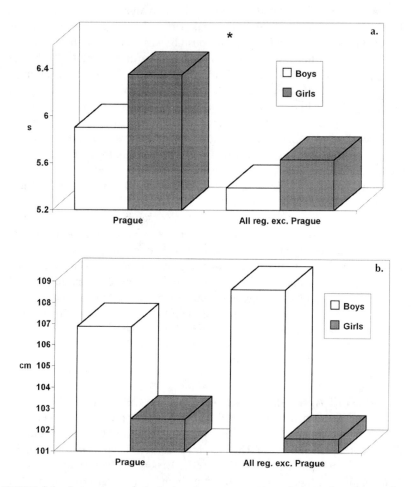

FIGURE 9.1 Comparison of physical performance — 20 m dash (**a**), broad jump (**b**), throwing a ball with the right hand (**c**), and throwing a ball with the left hand (**d**) in 6.4 years old boys and girls living either in the capital of Prague (1.2 million of inhabitants) or in the rest of The Czech Republic (survey A).

were not significant. As to the *forward roll*, performance of *Prague boys* was *significantly poorer*. However, in girls these differences were smaller and not as significant. The other results did not differ significantly.[256]

The evaluation of individual regions showed that the best results in running, jumping, and throwing were recorded in the south Moravian region. A relatively good performance was also recorded in the east Bohemian region. The majority of children examined in these regions were from smaller cities and villages. On the other hand, the poorest performance in these disciplines was recorded not only in Prague, but also (regarding running) in e.g., the

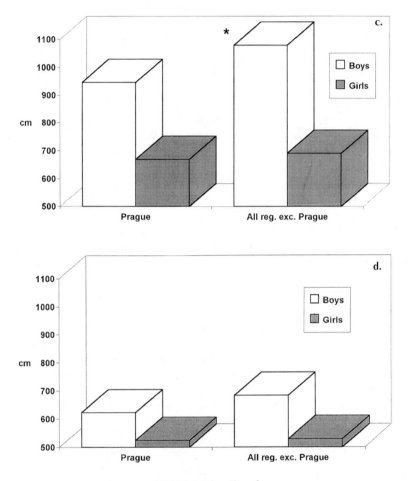

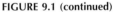

FIGURE 9.1 (continued)

central Bohemian region, which is characterized *inter alia* by a higher level of pollution. The other tests gave varied results.[254]

In Prague and in the other parts of The Czech Republic, the differences in the level of **sensomotor development** are of reverse character: *Prague children have a trend toward better results than children from the other parts of our country.* In four instances, Prague boys did significantly better in the tests of "opening and closing the hands." In all six cases Prague girls performed better.

Prague girls were also significantly better in spatial orientation, and boys did not differ. Prague children were also significantly better in the laterality test.

In the comparison of *sensomotor tests* in individual regions, the results were always the *best in Prague.* Relatively good results were also observed in the north Bohemian region, which is highly industrialized and therefore has the family per capita income that is higher than anywhere else. Better results were observed in the last sub-test of "opening and closing the hands" test, which is the most difficult one. In this case, the performance of north Bohemian boys and girls is better than those of Prague children. The results of children from the other regions were worse, and there are no further differences among these regions.[254]

Similar conclusions can be drawn from the results of tests of *spatial orientation* and *laterality*: the *best results were found in children from Prague* and the North Bohemian region. The differences between other regions were not marked.

In addition, children from the representative sample of survey B were divided into *five categories of cities and localities according to the number of population* so as to show in greater detail the influence of the size of the communities. A total of 11.4% lived in the communities with less than 1000 inhabitants; 32.0% in those with less than 5000 inhabitants; 34.8% in those with less than 20,000 inhabitants; 11.4% in 20,000 to 100,000 inhabitants; and finally 14.2% lived in cities with more than 200,000 inhabitants.

Sociological factors varied according to the size of the community: the lowest per capita income was found in communities with less than 1000 inhabitants. The larger the town, the higher the income was and obviously the higher the living standard of the family was. It may be assumed that this also includes a better dietary intake and higher energy intake. However, these differences may also be due to the fact that in the smallest communities the families were larger, i.e., with more children, compared to families from towns. In small communities, there were also fewer broken families than in larger towns.

Body height was most closely related to the size of the particular locality (Figure 9.2). Body weight and *BMI* did not show as clear a relationship as circumferential measures did. The thigh circumference was, on the contrary, smaller in boys from the largest towns. This seems to be associated with the greater linear constitution of boys in larger towns.

In smaller communities there was a trend toward better body posture and lower values of the depth of the cervical and lumbar lordosis. These differences were most marked when children from smallest communities were compared with children from largest towns and from Prague.

There was a trend toward better *performance* in children from the smallest communities compared to children in largest towns (20 m dash, throwing a ball). Skill and sensomotor tests were accomplished successfully by a some-what greater percentage of children from large towns, however, these differences were not marked and significant.[254,256]

Another study of 200 preschool children from Prague and from a smaller community in an area under the mountains showed worse results in the development of gross motorics in children from the capital.[173]

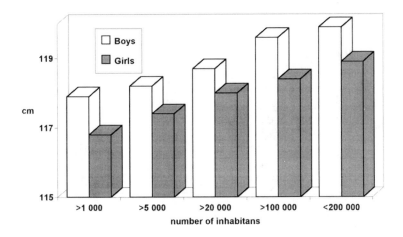

FIGURE 9.2 Comparison of height in boys and girls 6.4 years old from localities with different number of inhabitants (survey A).[254]

C. THE INFLUENCE OF LIFESTYLE ON FOOD INTAKE, BLOOD LIPIDS, AND PERFORMANCE

Another more detailed survey (I) was made separately in groups of pre-school children from a small town in central Bohemia (16,000 inhabitants; Nymburk) and in Prague (survey J; n = 37). Because no significant sex-linked differences were found in any of the variables studied, boys and girls from both Prague and Nymburk were evaluated together. Blood sampling did not permit investigations in larger groups.

Figure 9.3a shows the comparison of **_anthropometric variables_** in both groups. As in other surveys, children from Prague were slightly but significantly taller and heavier than Nymburk children, along with a greater deposition of fat.

Food intake also differed according to locality: the intake of energy, proteins, and fats (total, animal, plant), carbohydrates (Figure 9.3b, 9.3c, 9.3d, 9.3e), minerals, and vitamins (Table 9.2a) was *higher in Prague children.*

Physical performance in the broad jump and in the ball throw was significantly *better* in *Nymburk children* (Table 9.2b), which might be the result of better opportunities for games and spontaneous physical activity in a smaller community compared to a greater urban agglomeration. On the other hand, Prague children of this particular group participated more often in some sort of organized physical education (which was in contrast to the results of representative sample B). Moreover, in this case the results of the 20 m dash were also the same, showing that dynamic performance was not yet influenced by lifestyle at this age (Table 9.2b).[254]

In conjunction with this, the level of serum lipids was also compared. The level of total cholesterol and triglycerides was the same, but the *level of HDL*

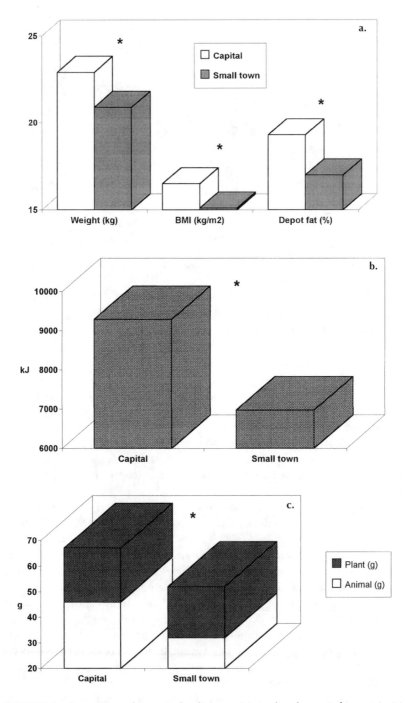

FIGURE 9.3 Comparison of somatic development **(a)**, intake of energy **(b)**, protein **(c)**, fat **(d)**, carbohydrates **(e)**, and blood lipid level **(f)** i.e., total, HDL cholesterol, triglycerides, in a group of preschool children living either in Prague and/or in a small town (survey I).

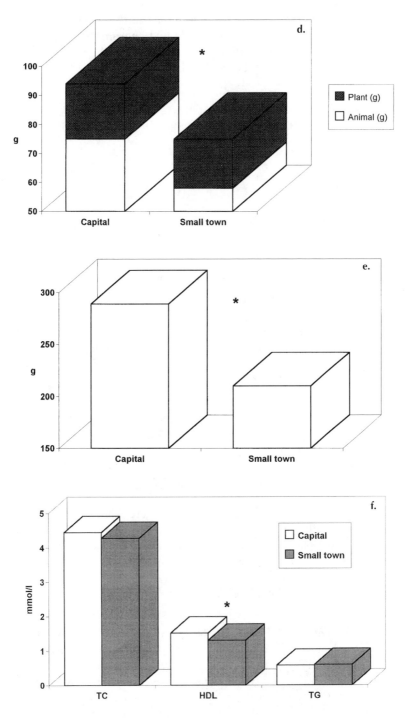

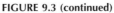

FIGURE 9.3 (continued)

TABLE 9.2a   The Intake of Minerals and Vitamins Per Day in Preschool Children from Different Localities in The Czech Republic (C, Capital; S, Small Town)

	C		S	
	x̄	SD	x̄	SD
Minerals				
Ca (mg)	750	208*	527	215
Fe (mg)	9.6	1.8*	7.3	1.6
Vitamins				
A (μg)	1091	378*	734	240
B_1 (mg)	0.9	0.1*	0.7	0.1
B_2 (mg)	1.2	0.2*	0.8	0.2
PP (mg)	12.0	2.1*	9.4	1.7
C (mg)	68	50**	22	9

Note: $* p < 0.01; ** p < 0.05.$

Modified from Parizkova, J., unpublished data.

TABLE 9.2b   Motor Performance in Preschool Children from Different Localities The Czech Republic (C, Capital; S, Small Town)

	C		S	
	x̄	SD	x̄	SD
20 m dash (s)	5.1	0.6	5.1	0.5
Broad jump (cm)	84	8	97	17
Ball throw (cm)	489	173	632	236

Adapted from Parizkova, J., unpublished data.

was significantly higher in Prague children (Figure 9.3f), with the level of *ApoB* being significantly lower. Obviously, factors other than lifestyle also influenced a more favorable blood lipid spectrum of Prague children.[254]

Results of this particular survey seem to indicate that more exercise in a smaller city can only improve skill, but not dynamic performance, e.g., running. Therefore, serum lipid levels are not more favorable.

D. BODY SIZE AND FUNCTION: IS BIGGER ALSO BETTER?

The accelerated somatic development of Prague children is consistent with the findings in other countries where the *child population from large urban agglomerations attain mostly larger bodily dimensions* at a given age than children from small towns and rural areas. The same applies to children from north Bohemian and north Moravian regions, which have more industry and thus have a higher level of per capita family income. (However, it is important to mention that even the lowest values of factors such as body height, BMI, etc. were still within the values of national standards for height, weight, and BMI. Lower values did not imply retarded development).

Larger bodily dimensions, however, did not ensure better development of other variables, as indicated by the evaluation of body posture or performance in selected disciplines. Among Prague children, there was a much higher percentage of those with poorer body posture than in children from other regions. The more marked cervical and lumbar lordosis could be associated with larger bodily dimensions, while a greater incidence of factors such as flabbiness of the abdominal wall or unequal height of the shoulders is associated with other causes, among them in the first place a reduced muscular tone and general weakness of the skeletal muscles.[265]

As shown by the questionnaires, participation in organized physical education (especially for children together with their mothers and/or fathers, etc.), as well as the opportunity for spontaneous physical activity in Prague, was — in this group of preschool children (survey B) — lower than that of children in other regions of The Czech Republic. Prague children had obviously more favorable prerequisites regarding the development of skill and coordinating abilities as shown by the better results in some sensomotor tests. However, without proper stimulation and ample opportunity for exercise, the potential for the development of higher level of motor abilities was not realized, as seems to be the case in the children from other regions of The Czech Republic. On the other hand, accelerated somatic development cannot be considered an impediment of physical efficiency because children from the north Moravian region, where the somatic development was also accelerated, also had a higher level of performance.[254] *Larger body size alone, though, does not predispose children to a higher level of motor performance.*

A higher level of economics ensured a better quality of dietary intake in Prague children. The opportunity to exercise improved skill in a smaller town, but did not yet improve dynamic performance in running, i.e., cardiorespiratory fitness. Therefore, in spite of higher values of anthropometric variables and increased energy intake, along with a different composition of diet, the blood lipid spectrum was more favorable in Prague children, i.e., HDL level was higher.[254]

II. ECONOMIC LEVEL AND BIRTH RANK

In our studies, the ***economic situation*** was related to the size of the community and to the characteristics of the particular region of The Czech Republic. However, the influence of extreme differences in the economic level of the family could not be demonstrated, but even smaller differences during shorter exposure were obvious.[256]

Children of survey B from the families with the highest average per capita income were the tallest and the heaviest, and also had the highest values of some other anthropometric variables. Children from the families with the lowest per capita income were the smallest. However, all these values were within the range of standard values of The Czech Republic and/or of international standards. Again, BMI did not vary markedly.[254]

The somewhat *smaller bodily dimensions of children from the families with a lower economic standard by far do not imply poorer physical performance*. On the contrary, comparisons showed that the taller and heavier boys from families with the highest economic standard ran worse than boys from families with the lowest income. A similar trend was also found in girls, although in this case the differences were not statistically significant.

There were no significant differences among groups in throwing the ball. Bigger children from better-off families were not predisposed to a higher level of physical fitness and performance in gross motorics tests compared to children with smaller body size.[236,238,265] This applies, however, only within certain limits, in a country without malnutrition and larger differences in body size.

In relation to the influence of **birth rank**, first born children are usually taller and heavier than children born later. Therefore, our representative sample of children 6.4 years of age (survey B) was also examined with this in mind. Somatic, motor, and sensomotor development in groups of children born as first, second — up to the fourth to the fifteenth in the family were compared. It was confirmed that *children born first were taller and heavier*. BMIs did not differ markedly according to birth rank.[254]

When the level of physical performance was compared, boys from the most extremely differing subgroups (i.e., born as the first and/or the fourth to the fifteenth) were roughly equal. Smaller girls born later in the family were significantly better regarding performance than bigger, firstborn girls.

Firstborn children (also often the only children in the family) attended kindergarten more frequently and participated more in organized physical education (special physical education classes of children with mothers and/or fathers, etc.). In these children, there was a trend toward better results in the "open and close the hands" test, along with better results in testing orientation and laterality.[256] However, even under all of these conditions, *these first born children, who seemed to be better predisposed by larger body size and higher level of sensomotor development, did not achieve a higher level of physical performance*.

III. ENVIRONMENT, RISK PREGNANCY, FAMILY CONDITIONS, AND HEALTH

In another similar sample of preschool children aged 4 to 6 years (survey D; n = 9587) the influence of a number of factors was tested including the degree of air and water pollution (as related to the conditions of life in different districts of The Czech Republic), risk pregnancy, birth weight, and health problems at the beginning of life, resulting in the need for regular medical check-ups during the first year. Further aspects were also examined, e.g., the beginning of independent walking of the child, family conditions, and the level of education and the qualifications of the parents.[254]

Table 9.3 shows a relatively high prevalence of risk pregnancies and a prevalence of children who were not really sick, but who had to be checked regularly by a medical doctor to the end of the first year. About 5% of the children wore glasses at preschool age. The results concerning the number of siblings, the duration of attendance at the day care center, and participation in physical education are given in Table 9.3).

TABLE 9.3 Prevalence of Risk Pregnancies, Medical Check-ups of Children Until the First Year of Life, Start of Independent Walking Until the End of First Year, Wearing of Glasses (Percent of Children), then the Number of Siblings, Years in the Day Care Centers and the Number of Hours Per Day Spent there, and the Years of Physical Education (Absolute Values, Years, Hours; Survey D)

		Age (years)					
		4–5		**5–6**		**6–7**	
		Boys	**Girls**	**Boys**	**Girls**	**Boys**	**Girls**
Risk pregnancy %		22.8	28.3	23.0	23.9	23.9	23.5
Medical check-up %		26.0	26.0	21.9	22.6	22.3	22.7
Start of walking %		62.1	64.3	64.6	65.9	61.1	66.1
Glasses %		5.1	4.2	4.8	5.7	6.9	7.2
Number of siblings	$\bar{x}$	0.97	0.99	1.07	1.07	1.12	1.09
	SE	0.01	0.01	0.01	0.01	0.03	0.03
Years in kindergarten	$\bar{x}$	1.91	1.89	2.55	2.52	3.04	3.00
	SE	0.01	0.01	0.01	0.02	0.04	0.04
Hours per day	$\bar{x}$	7.66	7.56	7.44	7.47	7.54	7.47
	SE	0.03	0.03	0.02	0.02	0.05	0.05
Years of physical	$\bar{x}$	1.04	1.02	1.08	1.31	1.32	1.48
education	SE	0.04	0.03	0.03	0.08	0.08	0.06

Pařízková , J., unpublished data.

The children were then evaluated in groups according to the above mentioned variables and were divided in two subgroups according to age, i.e., up to 5 years and older. A subsample of 1005 children was examined by teachers and physical education instructors in greater detail regarding both somatic and motor characteristics mentioned above (see Tables 4.6a, 4.6b, and 9.4; Figures 4.1a and 4.1b).

The analysis of variance and hierarchical loglinear analysis showed that *except for birth weight, the influence of the factors mentioned above were not manifested significantly in the variables assessed at the age of 4 to 6 years.*

TABLE 9.4   **Motor Development in the Subsample of Preschool Children (Survey D; n = 1005)**

		Age (years)					
		4–5		**5–6**		**6–7**	
		Boys	**Girls**	**Boys**	**Girls**	**Boys**	**Girls**
n		138	158	301	267	67	74
20 m dash (s)	$\bar{x}$	6.6	6.9	6.3	6.2	5.7	5.8
	SD	1.8	1.7	1.7	1.6	1.4	1.4
500 m run (s)	$\bar{x}$	219.2	231.3	201.0	208.1	183.3	188.7
	SD	41.1	44.7	47.3	45.7	40.4	32.3
Broad jump (cm)	$\bar{x}$	87.8	84.0	100.4	95.5	110.6	106.2
	SD	17.6	18.3	20.2	19.8	17.0	17.4
Ball throw — right (cm)	$\bar{x}$	618.5	467.3	800.7	600.6	938.9	639.4
	SD	232.2	148.3	308.6	229.5	304.9	146.7
Ball throw — left (cm)	$\bar{x}$	444.3	372.6	560.6	462.2	638.2	523.8
	SD	187.2	122.6	216.9	162.7	239.3	193.6

Modified from Pařízková , J. unpublished data.

However, in survey A occasionally significant positive correlations were found between the period of breastfeeding, the length measurements of the lower extremities, and the circumference of the abdomen and arm. The onset of independent walking correlated significantly with the circumferential measures on the trunk.[256]

IV. BIRTH WEIGHT

Children of survey D were divided into five subgroups according to their birth weight (Table 9.5). Average values of weight, height (Figure 8.4a and 8.4b), z-scores for height and weight, and circumferential measurements (chest, waist, hips; Figures 9.4c, 9.4d, 9.4e) varied significantly according to birth weight, i.e., *children born heavier showed proportionately larger bodily dimensions at the age of 4 to 6 years.* The analysis of this variance showed that the BMI did not differ significantly according to the birth weight category, but only according to age.[251]

Also , in survey A similar results were found, i.e., birth weight correlated significantly positively with the circumferential measurements of the head, chest, abdomen, forearm, thigh, and length of the iliospinale-tibiale in children 3 to 6 years of age.[256]

In spite of more marked morphological differences following different birth weight, the level of *gross motor development was much less influenced at the age of 4 to 6 years.* The analysis of variance only showed significant differences according to birth weight in the *left hand ball throw which was longer in children with a higher birth weight* (Figure 9.4f). Similar differences in the right hand throw were not significant. It was assumed that throw

TABLE 9.5   Birth Weight (g) of Children
Examined at the Age of 4 to 6
Years (Categories 1–5)[251]

Category	Boys			Girls		
	$\bar{x}$	SD	n	$\bar{x}$	SD	n
1	2220	305	33	2111	311	23
2	2925	166	126	2835	153	111
3	3440	141	186	3288	153	220
4	3895	145	136	3741	139	120
5	4519	253	24	5234	189	25

Adapted from Pařízková , J., *Nutrition in Pregnancy and Growth*, S. Karger, Basel, in press.

performance by the right hand could be influenced by previous training. The performance in the 20 m dash, the broad jump and the 500 m run-and-walk were not related to birth weight and actual body weight.[251] The results of the *balance test* (standing on one leg for 10 seconds) were *better in girls born and remaining heavier*. Occasionally a trend appeared toward better results in other skill, sensomotor, laterality, and orientation tests in children with a greater birth weight.[251] There is a question as to whether these differences will not accentuate later on.

V. FAMILY SITUATION

In survey D, the influence of the family situation was also analyzed, first, in the whole sample (boys n = 4822; girls n = 4765), where the level of somatic development was evaluated. Children were subdivided into four subgroups:

1. complete family without any problems (boys 89.9%; girls 90.6%)
2. broken family (divorced or separated parents; boys 6.8%; girls 6.4%),
3. family with a stepfather (boys 3.1%; girls 2.7%)
4. family with a stepmother (boys 0.2%; girls 0.2%).

The parents of our children were young and married for a short amount of time, so the ratio of divorced or separated parents (which is now about 50% in the capital and about 35% in the rest of the country) was low.

First, BMI, the level of height and weight development (expressed as deviation from the 50th percentile), and the proportionality of somatic development were evaluated in the individual subgroups.

When all children were evaluated together, a significant influence of the family situation was apparent in the growth of height and weight: *children from complete families* (subgroup 1), i.e., those with the best family situation *were mostly advanced in growth*. BMI and proportionality were not significantly influenced. When evaluating boys separately, only body weight was

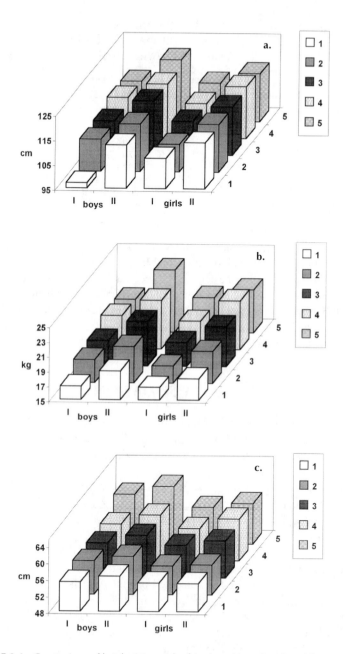

FIGURE 9.4 Comparison of height (**a**), weight (**b**), chest (**c**), waist (**d**) and hip circumferences (**e**), and throwing a ball with left hand (**f**) in younger (I > 5 y) and older (II < 5 y) boys and girls born with different birth weight (five categories; see Table 6.4; survey D).

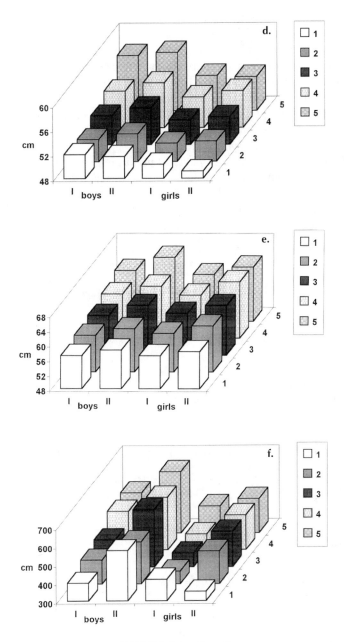

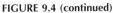

FIGURE 9.4 (continued)

significantly higher in subgroup 1. In girls, only height was significantly highest in subgroup 1.[254]

On the other hand, children of subgroup 4 (stepmother) were always ranked as last; then came the children from families with a stepfather, followed by children from broken families. However, the differences among subgroups 2 to 4 were not significant. As mentioned above, the distribution of children in the individual subgroups was unequal. All of these children, however, were within standard values and norms for The Czech Republic; nevertheless these slight differences were significant.

With regard to the level of ***physical performance***, which could only be followed in a subsample of 1005 children, the influence of the family situation, on the whole, was not significant. *A trend for better results in children from complete families* (subgroup 1) *appeared.*[254] Results in some disciplines (throwing a ball) tended to be better in children with stepfathers, although these differences were not significant.

VI. EDUCATION OF PARENTS

Children of survey D (number of children see above) were also subdivided according to the educational level of fathers and mothers:

1. basic level
2. skilled manual worker
3. high school with higher school certificate
4. university education

Regarding the education of fathers, the percentage of children in the individual subgroups was as follows:

1. boys 5.9%, girls 5.6%
2. boys 55.5%, girls 53.85%
3. boys 23.9%, girls 24.92%
4. boys 14.7%, girls 15.54%

Regarding the educational level of mothers, the percentage of children in subgroups was the following:

1. boys 11.9%, girls 11.9%
2. boys 37.4%, girls 36.5%
3. boys 40.7%, girls 41.3%
4. boys 9.9%, girls 10.3%

Children varied significantly according to the level of education of fathers in BMI, height, and weight: *growth in height and weight was accelerated in subgroup 4 (fathers with the highest level of education)*, and the BMI in this subgroup was the lowest. When evaluating boys and girls separately, the differences were the same (the differences for boys were significant for BMI and height only).

The influence of the educational level of the mother was similar — boys and girls were slightly, but significantly, taller and heavier and had a lower BMI. Growth was accelerated especially *in children with a father from subgroup 4 and mother from subgroup 3*. These results indicate that children of parents with this level of education (which is, however, not related to the economic level in the Czech Republic) are more advanced in height and weight development and are more slender. All variables, however, were within national standards.

Regarding physical performance, the results in the *20 m dash were significantly better in children whose fathers had a higher level of education* (subgroup 4). There was also a trend for better results in the 500 m run and the broad jump in children of the same subgroup. The level of education of mothers did not show any significant influence on the level of physical performance in the subsample of 1005 children of survey D.[254]

VII. HEALTH STATUS OF CHILDREN

The following analysis in survey D concerns the influence of health status and morbidity of children in survey D. Subgroup 1 included children who have been sick rarely or not at all (boys 6.4%, girls 7.4%); subgroup 2 included children who were occasionally sick (boys 85.5%, girls 86.6%); subgroup 3 included children who were sick quite often (boys 5%, girls 4%); and, finally, subgroup 4 included children with some chronic health problems who needed permanent medical check-ups (boys 2.7%, girls 2.0%), but could attend day care centers with other children.

When evaluating all of the children together, no significant differences in growth and BMI were evident. When evaluating boys alone, the BMI was lowest in subgroup 4, compared to subgroups 1, 2, and 3; only subgroup 2 differed significantly from the others. In girls, no differences were observed.

In regard to the level of physical performance, a trend toward better results in subgroups 1 and 2 was not significant because the number of children in subgroups 3 and 4 at individual age levels was too small. It is necessary to stress, though, that in this survey (D) as in other surveys, no children with really serious health handicaps were included.[254]

VIII. GENERAL CONSIDERATIONS

When the whole group of survey D was analyzed globally, *children born with higher birth weight remained bigger, started to walk earlier, had a lower rate of morbidity, showed better results in a few motor and sensomotor tests,* and wore glasses less often. Enrollment in regular physical education was less frequent in children who were born and remained smaller in body size.

Other factors concerning environment, including the conditions of life in different parts and districts of The Czech Republic and/or of the family, did not show any significant influence at this age. Even so it may be speculated that after a longer period of exposure to more polluted air and water (e.g., in the North Bohemian districts), some somatic and functional variables may change later on. However, at preschool age, this was not yet apparent. It is also possible that the individual factors of the environment were not significant enough to change measured parameters, but that some others which we did not evaluate could be influenced significantly.[330,402]

It was surprising to find out that the prevalence of inborn defects did not differ in various regions of The Czech Republic differentiated by the degree of air and water pollution. This mostly concerns the inborn defects that develop during later periods of pregnancy (i.e., defects of brain, which could also be manifested in motor development). Specialists from the Institute of Experimental Medicine of the Czechoslovakian Academy of Sciences (who studied these problems in greater detail) used to explain this by a possible perishing of the imperfect embryo during certain early periods of pregnancy, especially at its initial period. This is not always registered or even correctly recognized, which may apply to the heavily polluted region of northern Bohemia. Babies, in spite of having been born out of risk pregnancies but at full term, were obviously less affected by the environment, and thus no marked deterioration of the somatic and motor development was observed in these children at 4 to 6 years of age. Also, children who should have been followed up until the end of the first year because of some health problems did not show any changes in somatic or motor development at the age of 4 to 6 years.

One of the most dangerous environmental factors is the radiation level. Kozlova (personal communication) followed children from 6 to 17 years in the area of increased radiation (Korosten, Zhitomir district in the Ukraine) before and after the ***Chernobyl disaster***. Her findings confirmed previous observations that small doses of radiation stimulate growth in height and weight of the children. Such a trend, though, does not continue over more than 2 to 3 years, and thereafter a slow-down in the development of the child appears. This was confirmed by longitudinal observation of the same Ukrainian children for 3 years, i.e., from 1990 to 1993.

Long term observations of children exposed to small doses of radiation revealed a higher level of vegetative lability, general weakness, apathy, sleepiness, frequent headaches and colds, and a decreased efficiency and economy of the work of the heart muscle. *The measurements of physical working capacity on the level of the heart rate 170 per minute (PWC$_{170}$) showed a lowered level of functional capacity of children* (Kozlova, personal communication). In a considerable number of children, some deviations in the function of the cardiovascular system were observed, in addition to the enlargement of the lymph nodes and the thyroid gland. The latter becomes more serious with the advancing age of the children. An increased prevalence of thyroid cancer was followed from 1991 by experts of the World Health Organization in the framework of the IPHECA project.

Observations of children after the Chernobyl disaster have continued since 1990. Small doses of radiation seem to have a significant impact on children, which varies according to other interfering factors, including the level of physical activity. Special observations of preschool children have only started recently.

In early childhood, the influence of various stimuli in the environment, which are within the common range and intensity, are usually not yet manifested markedly because of short exposure time. Therefore, the influence of birth weight (which depends, under physiological conditions, on the mother's size and nutritional status as a delayed effect) was more evident (by preserving of bigger body size, better results in few motor and sensomotor tests) than the influence of family lifestyle or in different districts of The Czech Republic, characterized by conditions such as air and water pollution, etc. The same applies to risk pregnancy, family situation, common morbidity, start of independent walking, and the necessity for regular medical check-ups.

Chapter 10

INFLUENCE OF MOTOR STIMULATION, PHYSICAL EDUCATION, AND SPONTANEOUS PHYSICAL ACTIVITY

"Exercise of man ought to begin in the spring of life, i.e., during childhood. All teaching ought to be divided according to the degrees of age, so as not to have something to learn what is not acceptable for understanding"

(J.A. Comenius, 1592–1670)

I. MOTOR DEVELOPMENT AND STIMULATION OF INFANTS

In the complex of all factors that influence the growth and development of children from birth until adulthood, the level of motor stimulation and physical activity is one of the most important. A small child can learn to be active, skillful, and efficient or can learn to become the opposite — unwilling to move, thus remaining clumsy and easily tired. In this respect, early stimulation plays an essential role.

A child learns best through imitation. Therefore, the role of the mother and father and of the whole family is important: children learn to imitate before they know how to act. The example set by those around them can be either encouraging or discouraging.

Development of children in all age categories shows *a large interindividual variability*, as demonstrated by the above mentioned morphological and functional measurements. The level of motor ability is an important indicator for the overall development of the child, as defined and described by a number of authors.[61,182,183,391]

There are two kinds of movement for children: first, **spontaneous movements**, which are made by the child without any external stimulation. Then, there are **directed, learned movements**, adapted to the physiological and functional abilities of the child during individual periods of life. The starting point for directed movements are spontaneous movements.

211

During the first period, a trend has been established to give the child enough room to move, keeping him/her in a free sleeping environment permitting just enough spontaneous movement. Crying is also quite a vigorous physical exercise.

As mentioned before, conditioned reflexes, including motor reactions, can already be elaborated in infants. At the age of 3 to 5 months, a reflex for a conditioned turning of the head to a sound stimulus was elaborated.[224–226] Therefore, the character of stimuli and their eventual regular repetitions during this early period may have an essential importance.

The infant period until the end of the first year is characterized by a marked and fast development, i.e., increase in weight and other bodily dimensions. The nervous system is developing remarkably, and signs of the cerebral cortex activity and of individual senses — sight, hearing, touch — appear. All that a child learns at this time is a starting point for further learning and progress.[182,183]

Some facilitation of motor development in normal healthy children may be introduced. Special activities and games, i.e., a system of motor stimulation of the infant were elaborated to promote motor development of the child by Koch.[182,183] In conjunction with this, it is necessary to point up once more that the influence of motor stimulation and activity in early childhood goes beyond motorics.

There are many inborn reflexes, such as searching, grasping, sucking, swallowing, and crawling. In infant "gymnastics", position reflexes can be used. When an infant is raised, held under the armpits, and bent forward, the head always takes a position facing forward, and the extremities are also raised. This is already apparent during the first month of life. Orientation reflexes also exist, helping the infant become familiar with his/her surroundings.

Education during the *first month* of life aims to facilitate infant contact with the environment. The infant can be taught that certain signals have a certain meaning. Fixation of sight on a certain object can be taught at the age of 1 month. The human voice is the best sound stimulus and should also express some meaningful signal.

Slight signs of contact with the environment at the second and third month are already apparent. When the child lies on his/her back, the upper and lower extremities are bent, fists closed, with the head turned to one side (during the earliest period of life, the activity of flexors prevails). The motions are more fluid and softer.

At the age of *2 to 3 months*, the infant is able to raise the head and to turn it to both sides when lying on its tummy; he/she can also lean with both hands on the ground, and the neck lordosis starts to develop. The infant plays with his/her hands, and observes the surroundings. Visual contact and movement of the neck can be established with the help of a colorful toy. The infant is left free to move spontaneously during more prolonged periods, as well as while bathing in a bathtub. The infant starts to reach for objects, and motions become more intentional. The kicking of the legs is more energetic.

During the second to third month, the infant learns to fix his/her sight on one object and tries to follow it during its movement in all directions. The movement of the eyes is followed by movement of the head. In the second month, the infant starts to seek the source of a certain sound with his/her eyes and eventually finds it. The infant calms down and shows satisfaction when he/she hears the mother's voice, and the infant begins to react to it.

Activities appear that can be considered the ***onset of playing*** (by which we understand a self-satisfying and self-developing activity of the child). Progress in emotional development is manifested by smiling and growling, which enables the development of social contacts. The infant also begins to adapt to the biorhythms of day and night. The greatest progress in motor development is achieved during the second quarter of the first year of life (fourth through sixth month), and this holds the leading position in the overall development of the child. Developmental progress of the infant's personality depends on motorics. Therefore, *parents who stimulate and develop certain activities in their child can observe more progress than the others who do not devote as much attention to their children.*[182,183]

In the ***fourth month***, the infant masters the movements of the head, and is able to bend it back and look up. He/she can hold the head upright and turn it to all sides, raise it when lying on its back, draw the chin to the chest, and look at its feet. There is marked progress in the development of the hands and feet. The development of grasping and manipulation is essential for development of playing and thinking.

At the age of 3 months, the grasp is weakening, but at the age of 4 months, it starts to get strong again: when the infant is offered a finger, he/she can hold it and draw himself/herself to a sitting position. In the beginning, the arms of the infant are erect, i.e., inactive, but later, at the age of 5 months, the child is able to bend the arms and draw his/her head so as to sit up actively. At the age of 6 months, the child is able to draw himself/herself to a sitting position as well as to a standing position. Grasping is so strong that the child can stay in a hanging position or in a standing position on a ladder.[182,183]

When lying on the tummy, a 3-month-old infant can only lean on its hands. Later, he/she can reach for a toy and carry the weight of the head and chest, turning from the back to the tummy and even later, the other way around. Then, some children start to crawl spontaneously. The movements of the feet are mastered last: gross (fourth through fifth month) and finer movements of the legs (sixth month) develop during the second trimester of life. The development of senses is also remarkable at that period; the infant starts to recognize and differentiate faces, objects, voices, etc.

The first signs of play then appear. The child also discovers his/her own body and its individual parts, playing with both hands and feet, and manipulating objects. There is a saying that *"the intelligence of an infant can be recognized by how he/she takes things in the hands".*[182,183]

The manipulation of objects by hand is very important for the development of thinking as the child starts to understand certain relationships between his/her own actions. The emotional status of the child is also more apparent, and some habits can already be introduced.

In the ***third trimester*** (seventh through ninth month) of the first year, the child is growing more independent and starting to understand certain sounds and words. *Motor development is characterized by the development of abilities concerning not only the individual parts but also the whole body.* The main motor abilities that develop are crawling, sitting, standing, and the beginning of walking.

It is essential that the child learn how to crawl before sitting. Children who learn to sit too early often do not crawl at all, and because of too much sitting, their body posture deteriorates. A child who crawls a lot usually starts to stand up earlier. During the fifth month, standing is very uncertain, until the ninth month when the child is able to grasp something from the ground by squatting from the upright position.

The development of fine motorics is related to the development of play, learning, experiences, and thinking.[182,183] Before the fifth month, the child grasps objects with one hand. When offered another object, he/she lets the first one fall down. During the sixth month the child can hold an object with both hands and can switch it from one hand to the other. During the seventh month the child can turn the object around and can hold something in both hands. These manipulations render it possible to acquire various experiences with subjects. Gradually, the movements become more and more precise. The ability not only to grasp, but also to let some object go at the right moment (which is more difficult) are both very important.

Manipulation play is one of the most important self-developmental activities in the third and fourth trimester of life. From non-specific manipulation, the child develops specific manipulation, i.e., when the character of objects is already understood and used specifically. Using an object intentionally can be considered a manifestation of thinking, which shows the understanding of the relationship between things and surrounding phenomena. In addition, children already react to some words, but the development of active speaking is still limited.

The characteristic of motor development during the second half of the first year involves an increasing amount of purposeful movements and actions. Therefore, motor stimulation and play should also be purposeful, which includes achieving some aim, solving some tasks, and overcoming some obstacles. The movements of the hand are more precise, and all actions become more and more meaningful to the development of the whole personality of the child.[182,183] During this period the child also needs more space, more time, and more contact with people and objects.

Let's not forget that the original purpose of a toy is as a substitute, and that the child is longing to get things that are used by adults. It is recommendable to let children play with such things (of course only with those which are not harmful, fragile, or breakable, etc.).

The aim of motor education during this particular period is to develop further the abilities acquired during the previous period. It could be explained as starting the engine of an ancient car, an action which can later happen spontaneously. For this reason, the direct motor stimulation is more limited, and the child is allowed and stimulated to his/her own spontaneous activity. This means letting the child play according to his/her personal liking, with a certain range of purposeful activities.

The infant starts to "think with his/her hands."[182,183] The child plays in many other ways: handling objects, opening drawers, shuffling objects, emptying or filling boxes, etc., displacing objects from one space to the other, placing a stick in a hole in the box, and many other activities are possible.

At the end of the first year of life (tenth to twelfth month) the child has become independent, can already move around a little bit, can handle some objects, and can have some sort of contact with his/her environment. During the twelfth month the child can usually first make his/her independent steps, without being held or leaning on something. *Children who were motorically stimulated start to walk usually during tenth to eleventh month.*

In fine motorics, the child is able to intentionally grasp a selected subject, to adapt the fingers according to its size, and to grasp tiny things with the thumb and index finger. Another change occurs in the ability to let a grasped object go at a specific moment or to place it in a certain place. It is now possible to witness the development of the intellectual abilities of the child, in addition to some experiences which are used in everyday activities.

The development of gross motorics is aimed at overcoming a small obstacle, getting up from the sitting to the standing position or to sit down, and walking without assistance. *It is not recommendable to try to speed up motor development by using babywalkers.* As shown by Crouchman[68] frequent users of the walkers showed a significant delay in the onset of prone locomotion, compared with a low-user and non-user group of babywalkers.

After **9 months**, a baby starts using one object to acquire others; he/she draws a toy with the help of a table cloth. The use of tools is an expression of thinking; it proves that the child understands the relationship between two objects and deliberately uses one to achieve a result with the other. At 9 months, the baby is also capable of solving simple problems of bypassing, e.g., to go around a barrier to reach a toy.

Motor stimulation should be adapted to the character of individual children, to their speed of development, their reactions and so forth. As mentioned above, the goal is not only to *favorize motor development*, but also to *develop the child all-around* — **somatically, intellectually, emotionally, and socially.**[182,183] Joyous goal-oriented play is one of the possible non-verbal stimulating contacts one can have with the child — such as food, emotions, and environmental factors, which help to develop an optimal human being before an intellectual and rational education can take place.

Experiences from other cultural settings, where children live under more natural or even more primitive conditions, showed that children at the beginning of life are motorically more advanced. Later, this acceleration is mostly lost, as the more advanced stimulation and motor education usual in our cultural settings is lacking.

Koch,[182,183] a recognized psychologist who suggested *a special system of motor stimulation*[182,183] followed three groups of stimulated and non-stimulated infants during the first year of life. This project was inspired by two chance discoveries.

In order to give the infant more space for physical activity in the nursery, the infants were placed in higher-than-normal playpens: 6 feet by 4 feet, 2 feet above the floor, with sides 18 inches high, made of crossed bars. Among other things, the infants already learned to crawl by the eighth month and to stand up using the wall of the pen by the ninth month. When they learned this, the infants started to climb up the wall of their pens, so there was a danger of their falling out. At the age of 8 months, they were, therefore, placed on a clean floor. Taking advantage of this situation, we gave the babies a small ladder. Even infants who were not yet able to walk easily climbed up a vertical ladder (of course supervised by an adult). This showed that climbing a ladder was easier for the infant than walking without help.

As there was a desire to rear infants naturally and to make use of their inborn scope for development, a wall with rungs was made accessible to the infants, who first learned to crawl on the floor and then up the ladder. In the end, they walked on the floor without support. Obviously, "normality" of motor development, as perceived in our cultural setting, does not completely correspond to the natural predispositions and abilities of infants. If the infant's feet are left bare, he/she often learns to grasp objects with them, plays with an inflated ball hanging above with hands and feet, then with one hand, one foot, and so forth. If the infant spends all the time with feet wrapped, he/she never touches or feels with his/her feet.[182,183]

These observations led to the conclusions that *not only the development of movements, but also development in general, was strongly influenced by the stimuli the infant received at an early age*, and that a change in the method of stimulation could alter the infant's development. In spite of some ethical reservations, physiological evidence gave support for the practice of adequate motor stimulation during the first year. In addition, the experience from history as well as from some countries of the Third World, gave rise to the "transport hypothesis" (i.e., when the mother carries her baby during her all day activities, the child cannot stay entirely inactive, but has to adapt to the mother's movements, bending, etc., by holding his/her head up, moving trunk and limbs, and holding on with his/her hands and feet. The baby was, therefore, stimulated and activated during long periods to energetic movements). Thus, the infant was equipped with many neuromuscular mechanisms which enabled him/her to perform these movements from the beginning of life.[182,183] Some similar experiences concerning the possible influence of certain customs were mentioned in conjunction with nutritional practices and weaning in Sioux and Yurok Indians.[96]

Infants in our cultural setting are equipped with the same mechanisms. They include the so-called postural reflexes (baby holds the head in the extension of the trunk when you lean him/her forward or to the side) and the grasping reflex (baby holds our hands so firmly that he/she can be lifted up). Carrying the infant around is also a very intensive and natural exercise for him.

II. EXPERIMENTAL OBSERVATIONS ON THE IMPACT OF MOTOR STIMULATION IN INFANTS

The aim of any stimulation, including motor stimulation, is not to speed up development, but rather to render it harmonious and all-around. The child must not be burdened with too many demands, but stimulated by an adequate amount of appropriate factors. However, lack of stimulation and neglect also has unfavorable results. It is known that even the consequences of malnutrition can be at least partly compensated for with proper stimulation of the child,[64] including some motor activities.

Koch[182,183] followed three groups of infants: *the first (I)* consisted of *infants who lived in the Institute for the Care of Mother and Child from birth up to the age of 6 to 7 months.* One specialist devoted himself to each infant every day for a period of wakefulness (about 2 hours), played with him/her to stimulate the movements as described above, and recorded the development from the fourth week to the end of the 6th month.

The *second group (II)* consisted of *infants who lived at home* with their parents and, during their first year, visited the above mentioned Institute regularly once or twice a week, in all, about twenty times. *The parents were shown how to stimulate their babies' movements:* at the same time the infants were examined. The parents then worked with their children at home, as described above. After the first year the parents were not instructed anymore, but the development of children was followed up through their third year.

The third (III) control group consisted of infants who came to one of Prague's children's centers for regular routine pediatric checkups. They lived under normal family conditions *without special stimulation.* Every child was examined once, either in the third, sixth, ninth, or twelfth month of the first year of life. The parents were of all social groups (the population in the Czech Republic has been more homogeneous than in other European countries). They were not informed about the purpose and aims of our study and regarded it as part of the medical checkups.

In all groups, there were both boys and girls. For the presentation of homogeneous data, only **boys** were selected, but *the results of the motor stimulation of girls had the same trend.* Group I consisted of 10 boys, Group II of 20 boys. In Group III there were 10 boys aged 3 months, 13 aged 6 months, 11 aged 9 months, and 15 aged 12 months. The development of head movements, upper limbs, lower limbs, complex locomotion, play, and speech in all children was recorded. Two hundred developmental traits were statistically processed, about 15 each month.

The statistical significance of the differences was evaluated as follows: no infant was able to transfer a toy from one hand to the other in his/her third month. In the ninth month, all children were able to do this. The number of children capable of this task was determined during all measurements and statistically evaluated.

The results of Koch's study[182,183] showed that *the two groups stimulated,* i.e., *Group I and Group II, showed a similar progress of development,* while the non-stimulated *group (III) lagged behind them.* The more complex the testing activities, the more significant were the statistical differences between the stimulated and non-stimulated infants. The differences increased with age and with the complexity of the activity. The infants were mainly stimulated to motor activities, but the difference also appeared in the development of the play and speech.

On the other hand, the *differences between Group I and Group II,* i.e., between infants stimulated in the Institute and at home *decreased with age.* The results of children stimulated in the Institute were, at the beginning, better, which was explained by the fact that they were stimulated by experts. Later on, when the parents got enough experience and practice, this difference disappeared.

The differences in the development of children who were systematically *stimulated at home* (II) and those who were *not stimulated and lived under usual traditional conditions* (III) *were remarkable and gradually increased.* This document emphasizes that intensive early motor stimulation is soundly based and contributes to better infant development.

The differences concerned not only the development of movements, but also overall development, the reason for which is obvious. At first, pure and isolated locomotor stimulation is not possible: when the baby is stimulated to move, the parents or whomever is in close social contact speak and give toys, etc., to him/her. This is so that everything is a complex stimulation, where the locomotor stimulation is stressed because it *also influences the development of speech and thinking.* Thus, the influence of motor stimulation goes beyond motorics only, as in later periods of childhood. The second fact is that parents who succeed in a complex child-rearing method tend to develop their baby in all aspects and deliberately favorize also the other functions.[182,183] Motor stimulation and play, however, make up a complex program on how to treat a child: quite often parents do not really know what to do with their children or how to play with them so as to educate them simultaneously.

It remains an open question whether the higher quality development of a baby, which has been systematically stimulated during the first year of life, is permanent or temporary. The material collected later does seem to indicate that this development is permanent, especially when the children are further systematically stimulated.[182,183] A special experience was also gained by swimming with the children at the beginning of life, a program which was developed by L. Diehm and M. Hoch (Faculties of Physical Education in Cologne, Germany and Prague, The Czech Republic) and which showed also a very favorable influence on the development of children.

Since it was shown that during the first year of life the psychological development can be given an impetus and a direction, this possibility should be studied and developed further. However, there is evidence from other areas of theoretical research, as well as from teaching experiences, which show that early stimulation of any character, which is positive and adequate according to developmental stage and individual characteristics of the organism, gives desirable results and become advantages for the child that can persist after the growth period.

III. TODDLERS

In the *second year*, the main aim of the parents should be to support the natural tendency of toddlers to move spontaneously, to teach the child the changes of attitudes and positions, to protect them from accidents, and to aid in the final development of walking.

In the *third year*, the moving abilities of the upper extremities develop intensively, and locomotion is much more rapid. The main task of the parents is to give an ample opportunity for the child's spontaneous physical activity, to develop his/her ability to run, to jump, to crawl, to play different games, and to teach cultural behavior. The exercise of one parent with the child is a more precise program, as it is already possible to profit from certain motor abilities and previous experiences. Last, but not least, all activities should have an element of play and must be interesting and fun. Under these conditions, the child will persevere more easily in exercise and thus profit from it.

"Aide-moi à faire seul,	"Help me to do by myself,
Ne-fais pas à ma place,	Don't do it in my place
Mais soi présent"	But remain with me"

Maria Montessori

IV. MOTOR DEVELOPMENT AND EDUCATION OF CHILDREN AGED 3 TO 6 YEARS

In the *fourth year* of life the child is overcoming clumsiness, his/her motions become more exact, and his/her ability for intentional activities further increases. Children like rhythmic activities, are more independent, are not afraid to jump from the height of 30 to 40 cm and are able to achieve a certain level of performance. The main goal of motor education is to develop skill, adequate body posture, and a well-balanced gait. It is recommendable to start some sports activities like skiing and swimming. Up until 6 years of age, these abilities improve further.

This period is defined as *"the golden age of motorics;"*[391] it is therefore highly recommendable to make use of tendencies for a high level of spontaneous physical activity and interest in suitable motion games. When proper motor habits and skills are introduced in time and when a certain level of cardiorespiratory efficiency, speed, endurance, and muscle strength is achieved, a good basis for later performance and interest in exercise is created. Relationships between children's and parents' stereotyping of physical activities were analyzed, showing significantly higher scores (Physical Activity Stereotyping Index) for kindergarten and second grade children.[279] The influence of parents and the overall family lifestyle is essential.

The preschool child loves to play, so it is desirable to profit from this by focusing the game on the continuing development of an adequate gait, a fast run, courageous jumps, skillful crawling, throwing, and so forth. *Neglect of motor development, possibly resulting in clumsiness and a low level of fitness, is no means for successful development of other faculties of the child.*

The selection of games depends on the purpose. Nearly all exercise can be turned into play when we give the exercise some attractive name that is interesting for the child, and when we set the rules of the game and, how it will be played: this gives the play some guidelines, however simple.

For some games it is necessary to have more children, sometimes at least three. When the child has no siblings, the parents should participate, which is usually difficult for them because of a time shortage. Only children especially should have the company of other children, which teaches them to adapt to peer partners. At preschool age, the need for the company of children is increasing, and mutual relationships are established among children, based on games. Observations on *how the child plays can help to define his/her personality and how his/her later relationship to other activities will be.*[27–29]

In many countries, organized physical education for preschool children has come to pass more or less recently, either in day care centers or in special ***physical education classes for preschool children along with one of the parent*** (mother, father, grandmother, etc.)[27–29] organized by various sports organizations in individual countries. This was arranged a long time ago in countries such as Spain, France, Germany, the U.S., Italy, Bulgaria, Slovenia, Cuba, and, more recently, Canada, New Zealand, Australia, and many others. However, this sort of physical education mainly exists in individual sports organizations or in selected day care centers and institutions.

In former Czechoslovakia, this type of physical education was introduced in 1964 and developed on a mass scale. This means that organized classes exist in all parts of the country. The initiator was Professor Jana Berdychova (who described her system in her monographs, translated into many languages),[27–29] who received the main credit for the creation and establishment of this system of physical education at an early age. During the more than 30 years of its existence, special physical education classes for preschool children with their mothers or fathers have become an integral part of the general physical education system of The Czech Republic, and the participants also appear in national gymnastic displays, organized at regular intervals.

Under present conditions, this sort of physical education represents the first article of the system of physical education of the national (as well as international) association "Sokol" (the Czech word for Falcon) and of the Association "Sport for all," attached to the Olympic Committee of The Czech Republic. Fortunately, even along with all of the changes occurring in our country, the tradition of physical education for preschool children with one of the parents has been developing further on a massive scale. The results of this system of physical education were presented and analyzed in the last International Seminar "Child-motion-family," sponsored by the Council of Europe in December, 1994 in Prague.

What to Avoid in the Motor Education of Preschoolers.

It should be again pointed up that all physical education in this period of development should be adjusted to the special traits of this stage of child development, keeping in mind the health, physiological, psychological, and social traits of small children.[310] In essence *all activities should be natural and spontaneous*, thus liked by the child. Without spontaneity and the individual involvement of the child, the results of all pedagogical efforts including motor education are always less successful. This can even result in the reverse situation: refusal and negativity of the child and deterioration of his/her potential because of inadequate handling of his/her motor abilities. Overburdening—demanding too much or demanding too little— is also discouraging. This can apply to any other educational effort. Safe conditions for all exercise activities must also be guaranteed.[137]

In motor activities, respecting the spontaneous involvement of the child implies a certain self-regulation, thus avoiding physically overloading the child. When the enthusiasm of the child for some very attractive activity is excessive, though, it is necessary to regulate and influence it. In such a case, the self-regulation is failing. This mainly includes dynamic plays and activities, especially with older peers.

Generally, *static exercises are not recommended for the child*. Overloading of individual joints with static exercises is forbidden. All one-sided activities are also unsuitable, i.e., specialization in one sort of the game or even in the preparation of some sports activities. Unfortunately, certain disciplines in which youngsters mainly win gold medals (gymnastics, figure skating, tennis, etc.) encourage certain parents to introduce training even before their child starts going to primary school. This is nothing new — in ancient times or in the Middle Ages the circus acrobats excessively trained their children "from the cradle"; this was repeated not very long ago in certain countries. This must be avoided in spite of the fact that some individuals will always exist who can overcome it and who can develop a high level of performance without any harmful consequences. For the overall child population, this is not acceptable.

Two extremes seem to exist: *the majority of parents neglect the opportunity to develop the motor abilities of their child properly*, and thus they also miss the opportunity of how to use motor education for the promotion of other faculties of their child. On the other hand, *a small minority tend to burden their child in order to cultivate a sports star as early as possible*, thus to exploiting him or her just like in child labor. Both attitudes are, of course, wrong.

As follows, for the proper education of the child, including motor education, it is necessary to have parents who are well aware of all possibilities on how to prepare their child for their future in an optimal way. It is true that sometimes everything can go very well for the child without a great effort of the parents. The reverse is also true: great care does not always give the best results. When it is too late, though, nothing much can be done. *When parents adequately intervene in all respects including motor stimulation and education, along with other factors such as nutrition, better results can always be expected.*

Mentally retarded children are not the topic of this book, but they are also worth mentioning. In many industrially developed countries, the ratio of handicapped children has increased. Physical education of such individuals can help to compensate, at least in part; we know from the Special Olympics that these individuals are often capable of admirable results of which many healthy people are not able to achieve. The early introduction of some exercises can help these children improve a lot, and the influence of exercises again goes beyond just motorics. Special systems of physical education for the handicapped were suggested and applied[189] in The Czech Republic. We can remember the example of a 3-year-old mongoloid (Down's Syndrome) girl who participated in regular physical education classes with her mother without any problems; her overall situation improved.

V. INFLUENCE OF EXERCISE IN PRESCHOOLERS

A. SOMATIC DEVELOPMENT AND BODY POSTURE

Mean values of height, weight, BMI, and chest circumference in preschool children 6.4 years old (survey B) exercising during different periods of time (0, 1, 2, 3 years) are presented in Table 10.1. *Children who participated for the longest period of time in regular physical education program were the tallest and the heaviest and had the highest values of chest circumference.* The BMIs tended to be the lowest in boys who exercised regularly during the longest period of time, but these differences were slight. In girls there did not seem to be any differentiation of BMI according to the duration of the participation in the physical education program. Other measurements showed significantly higher values of thigh and chest circumference in boys who exercised during the longest period. In girls, these differences were not significant.

Regarding the posture of the neck, abdomen, and spine the results were more favorable for children who took part in regular exercise during the

TABLE 10.1 Anthropometric Variables and Motor Performance in Preschool Boys and Girls Differentiated According to Systematic Participation in Physical Education (2–3 Years) (Survey B; Age 6.4 Years)

Physical education (years)		0		2–3	
		x̄	SD	x̄	SD
Height	Boys	118.6	5.3	120.8	5.1
(cm)	Girls	117.6	5.2	119.0	5.5
Weight	Boys	22.2	3.2	23.6	2.3**
(kg)	Girls	21.6	3.3	22.1	3.6
BMI	Boys	15.8	0.9	15.7	1.0
(kg/m²)	Girls	15.6	1.1	16.6	1.1
Chest	Boys	59.2	3.3	61.0	3.4
(cm)	Girls	57.9	3.7	58.2	4.1
20 m dash	Boys	5.4	1.1	5.5	1.2
(s)	Girls	5.7	1.2	5.7	1.2
Broad jump	Boys	108.0	20.9	119.9	22.3**
(cm)	Girls	100.7	20.4	110.6	18.4
Throwing ball — right	Boys	1060	391	1081	419
(cm)	Girls	676	220	717	240
Throwing ball — left	Boys	672	240	752	302
(cm)	Girls	519	163	551	168

Note: ** $p < 0.02$.

Compiled from Pařízková, J., et al., *Growth, Fitness and Nutrition in Preschool Children,* Charles University, Prague, 1984.

longest period of time. Grade 1 was most frequent in these children, and Grade 2 and Grade 3 were much less frequent. The worst situation was found in children who were completely inactive.

The influence of regular physical education (mostly physical education classes of the child with one of the parents or grandparents) was also analyzed in survey C (Table 10.2) comprised of children 4- to 5, 5- to 6 and 6- to 7 years. For this analysis, children were subdivided according to their participation in organized physical education and according to age. The same trends in somatic development were found: *children enrolled in regular physical education were, as a rule, the tallest and the heaviest, having higher values of circumferential measures* (chest and thigh).[236,238] Due to the smaller number of children in the individual subgroups and their younger age, the differences were less apparent than those in 6.4-year-old children (survey B).[256]

In survey D (boys n = 4822; girls n = 4765), children were subdivided into subgroups according to the enrollment in regular physical education. The subgroups were as follows:

TABLE 10.2   Physical Performance of Preschool Boys and Girls Regularly Enrolled (PE) and not Enrolled (i.e., Control, C) in Physical Education (Survey C)

Age		20 m dash (s)		Broad jump (cm)		Ball throw (cm)			
						Right		Left	
		PE	C	PE	C	PE	C	PE	C
4–5 years									
Boys	x̄	6.2	6.7*	88.1	91.0	655	538**	486	429*
	SD	1.3	1.6	44.0	87.1	281	238	189	170
Girls	x̄	6.4	7.7**	81.4	80.7	472	429*	377	340*
	SD	1.3	1.8	24.4	59.2	163	149	138	127
5–6 years									
Boys	x̄	5.6	6.0	113.6	100.6	880	815	564	556
	SD	1.2	1.5	107.8	38.9	363	344	224	209
Girls	x̄	6.0	6.3*	102.1	95.3	613	582	476	452
	SD	1.4	1.7	65.9	51.7	189	191	165	150
6–7 years									
Boys	x̄	5.5	5.5	118.0	120.4	1095	1054	695	705
	SD	1.4	1.4	61.1	80.4	397	394	255	266
Girls	x̄	5.6	5.7	114.6	105.7	740	697*	563	550
	SD	1.3	2.7	88.8	45.6	228	218	196	252

Note: $* \ p < 0.05$; $** \ p < 0.01$.

Compiled from Pařízková, J., *Principles, practices and application,* Shephard, R.J. and Lavallée, H., Eds., Charles C. Thomas, Springfield, IL, 1978, 238; Pařízková, J. Proc. Int. Symp. Université de Quebec, Oct. 1980; Pařízková , J., *Wld. Rev. Nutrit. Diet.,* 51, 1, 1987.

1. regular exercise once or twice a week
2. occasional exercise
3. no exercise at all
4. limited exercise for health reasons.

The percentage of children in these groups was as follows:

1. boys 11.5%, girls 19.4%
2. boys 7.4%, girls 8.1%
3. boys 80.9%, girls 72.2%
4. boys 0.2%, girls 0.3%

The distribution of children in individual subgroups was unequal. In spite of the opportunity to exercise (especially in classes with parents), participation was low, especially in boys. The majority of children did not take part in any regular exercise. The last group included very few children.[254]

Development of height and weight, BMI, and proportionality of growth was examined in this survey. *Children of subgroup 1 had the significantly lowest values of BMI.* Regarding the height and weight development, no consistent differences among subgroups mentioned above were apparent in this last survey[254] as the groups of exercising children of different ages were small.

B. PHYSICAL PERFORMANCE, SKILL, AND SENSOMOTOR DEVELOPMENT

The influence of physical exercise varied in relation to the results of different disciplines (survey B). There were no significant differences in the 20 m dash (see Table 10.1, Figure 10.1). The broad jump results, however, were *significantly better in children who participated during the longest period in physical education*. In *throwing a ball with the right and left hand, the performance was the best in exercising children*. Children not engaged in regular physical education had the worst physical performance.[256]

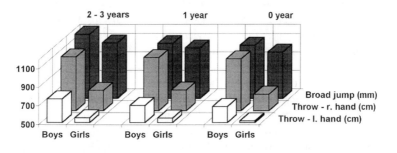

FIGURE 10.1 Physical performance in 6.4-year-old boys and girls enrolled during various periods in regular physical education (survey B).

In tests of skill, children participating regularly for the longest period in physical education were more successful than children who did not participate. The results of tests in the *forward roll, walking on a horizontal beam, and catching a ball were also the best in children who exercised for the longest period of time*. The same applied to the results of testing sensomotor development, i.e., *"open and close the hands"* test. In this case, *significant differences were evident in the most difficult items of this test.*[256]

In survey C, similar results were obtained. Generally, there was always a trend toward better results in children who enrolled regularly in physical education. However, the interindividual variability was again large, and only *in some disciplines were there significantly better results in exercising children* (e.g., 20 m dash and throwing a ball, see Table 10.2).[238]

In survey D the results of physical performance were also analyzed in a subsample of 1005 children subdivided according to the criteria 1 through 4. Again, there was a trend toward better results in all disciplines in the regularly exercising children. *The influence of regular physical education was significant on the results of the 20 m dash, the broad jump, and the ball throw with the right hand, but not with the left one.*[254]

C. VARIABILITY OF THE IMPACT OF EXERCISE IN EARLY LIFE

In contrast to other evaluations, larger bodily dimensions in the exercised children were also associated with an obvious trend toward a higher level of motor performance which was significant in several items.

However, another question appears: the group of children who exercised regularly could have been primarily more advanced in their somatic and motor development and, thus, more interested in physical exercise because it was easier for them. Therefore, they may have adhered to it regularly and for a longer time, and the results of comparison were automatically better for them. Could this be the case?

This problem is apparent in all age categories, including adolescents and adults. It is not possible to pick certain children for exercise and to refuse the others in order to have homogeneous comparable groups for experimental analyses. In everyday life, this is not acceptable with normal healthy children, especially when pedagogues are interested in getting everyone to take part in regular exercise.

However, the differences in body size of exercised and non-exercised children were of similar character as when groups classified according to other criteria, such as urban versus rural children, economic status of the family, birth rank, and so forth, were compared. In contrast with these cases, however, the motor development of exercised children was significantly better. Therefore, we may assume that even when genetic factors played an important role, *the more favorable development of gross motorics in bigger, active children was, in this case, mainly the result of an adaptation to exercise.*

This especially applies to jumping, throwing, and skill tests, as the development of speed does not seem to be influenced by regular exercise. This may also be due to the fact that the physical education classes for preschoolers were more focused on the development of skills, rather than on the development of speed, which does not seem appropriate at this age. Children were always instructed to run to their own liking.

VI. SPONTANEOUS PHYSICAL ACTIVITY, SOMATIC AND FUNCTIONAL DEVELOPMENT, FOOD INTAKE, AND BLOOD LIPIDS

As indicated by serum lipid levels in preschool children in the capitol and in smaller communities, the theoretical opportunity for greater motor activity alone does not always manifest itself in an improved level of morphological, functional, and biochemical variables.

Any sort of adequately increased physical activity under safe conditions seems to be a desirable factor favoring the development of the child. At preschool age, it is difficult to find children who would exercise systematically and long enough to manifest some positive effect. As mentioned above, it was only possible to show the significant influence of exercise on certain aspects of somatic and motor development at the age of 6.4 years (survey B) and only occasionally before this age (survey C and survey D). However, it is of interest to examine the influence of physical activity even earlier.

One of the characteristic features of the individual from the very beginning of life is the level of his/her *spontaneous physical activity*, which varies interindividually. This is even manifested in the framework of the same family. Genetic factors have to be considered among those which can significantly influence motor characteristics. *A great similarity in the motor pattern* of *running* was described by Sklad[332] *in monozygotic twins, where the total volume of physical activity during certain periods of time* (number of paces per day) also varied less than in dizygotic twins.[194] The number of paces per day were shown to be a permanent characteristic of the individual.[121] However, other epigenetic factors have to be considered.

In early childhood, however, the influence of different levels of physical activity is much less apparent because of the child's very short life history. Thus, it is insufficient to draw on the duration of the influence of this particular factor. Some children, however, can spontaneously exercise quite vigorously and on a high level, as was shown by telemetric measurements of the heart rates which could be 210 to 220 beats per minute,[186,187] Generally, it is considered unacceptable to induce over intensive, regular physical exercise at the age of 4 years. Nevertheless, it can be assumed that a high level of spontaneous physical activity at an early age might run parallel to other metabolic characteristics of the individual.

Because it was not possible to find 4- to 5-year-old children who would exercise long and intensively enough on an organized basis, the level of spontaneous physical activity was followed up in a kindergarten in Prague, and children were subdivided according to it.

First, we tried to characterize children by observing them during a period of free play (2 hours in the morning, just after arrival in total during one week). Ten aspects of physical activity levels were followed and registered. We found that children varied quite a lot, and that the results of such a trial assessed during individual days very rarely correlated and then only weakly ($p < 0.30$). It was obvious that such a short period is not representative enough for the evaluation of the level of spontaneous physical activity of the preschool child. In additional methodical experiments we used pedometers, Sport-testers, and heart beat totalizers, which were made for older subjects; these apparatuses did not give reliable results.[254] We had no opportunity to use doubly labeled water.

Therefore, we developed a *special questionnaire* for the kindergarten teachers and parents, which evaluated the *level of spontaneous physical activity during the whole year*. The individual items concerned the initiative in active plays, social contacts in playing and the ability to draw other children into play, the reactivity to both positive and negative orders (i.e., either to move or to stop — this was a particular problem for certain children!), the approximate time spent in action or at rest, the preference of active dynamic games or quiet activities with limited movement, etc. A general evaluation by the teacher was also considered, based on observations during the whole year. The evaluation of this questionnaire rendered the categorization of preschool children possible.[254,270]

This study was undertaken with two kindergarten groups of children from 3 to 5 years of age (n = 22; mean age was 4.7 years) in Prague. Eight of the most active and nine of the most inactive children were selected on the basis of the above mentioned procedure. The rest of the children without any marked trend for either great activity of inactivity were not included in the final evaluations. Somatic development, step test, dietary intake, blood lipids and creatine kinase activity were assessed. Sex-linked differences were not apparent in this group (survey J).

Height, weight, BMI, fat (%), lean body mass (kg) (Table 10.3), circumferential measurements (Figure 10.2a), breadth measures, skinfold thicknesses (Harpenden caliper; Figure 10.2b), and somatotypes (Figure 10.2c) were assessed. As shown by the results, there was a *trend toward lower values of weight, fat, BMI, lean body mass (LBM), and circumferential measurements (with the exception of the thigh) in the active children.* Breadth measures only varied slightly. Skinfold thicknesses measured by a Harpenden caliper also tended to be lower in active children, similarly to the percentage of fat calculated according to the Brook's formula,[42] but the differences were not significant. Ten skinfolds measured by a modified Best caliper[230,233] were also larger in the inactive children.

TABLE 10.3   Anthropometric Variables of Active and Inactive Children (4.9 ± 0.5 Years of Age, Survey J)

	Active		Inactive	
	$\bar{x}$	SD	$\bar{x}$	SD
Height (cm)	109.6	4.4	109.9	6.3
Weight (kg)	18.8	1.7	19.8	3.3
BMI (kg/m^2)	15.7	1.1	16.4	0.9
Fat (%)	14.1	2.4	17.5	4.4
LBM (kg)	15.9	1.7	16.2	2.0

Note: BMI, body mass index; LBM, lean body mass.

Compiled from Parizkova, J. et al, *Human Biol.*, 58, 261, 1986.

Regarding the *somatotype,[154] active children had a lower endomorphic component, the same mesomorphic component, and a higher ectomorphic component* (Figure 10.2c). These differences were not significant. The index LBM/10 cm height was only slightly higher in active children.

The energy and fat intake was somewhat higher than local RDAs. When comparing the food intake with RDAs of the EC and the U.S., energy and protein intakes of the children were higher than the EC[198] and the U.S. RDAs[197] and to the estimated values of energy requirement according to the procedure suggested by WHO[393] (see Table 5.3). *Active children tended to have a higher food intake than inactive children* (Figures 10.2d, 10.2e, 10.2f.), but the differences were not significant. The intake of minerals and vitamins did not differ from the RDAs for this age group.

The results of the step test showed that the work load increased the heart rate by about 40% compared to the initial values. The steady state was established during the second to third minute, and the heart rate returned to resting values during the second to fourth minute of recovery. Boys tended to have slightly, but not significantly, better results, which also applied to the step test index (STI) and cardiac efficiency indexes CEI_1 and CEI_2. Therefore, the results were evaluated together for boys and girls. *Active children tended to have better results in the step test, especially regarding the above mentioned indices, but the differences were not significant.*

Sex linked differences were not apparent; therefore, the average values of serum lipids for both boys and girls together are given. Only *the HDL level was significantly higher in the active children.* The level of LDL tended to be higher in the inactive children (Figure 10.2g).

The average values of creatine kinase activity (CK) in the blood were about half of the values assessed in the adults and were slightly and insignificantly higher in the active children.

Children with highest physical activity tended to have better results in tests for fine motor control, which was manifested mainly in drawing tests and creativity.[207,208,254,270]

VII. GENERAL CONSIDERATIONS

The influence of exercise on preschool age children varied in the individual surveys, which was mainly apparent regarding functional parameters at the age of 6.4 years and only occasionally (and not as markedly) in younger age groups.

The influence of exercise was also differentiated in relation to various motor tasks and tests. There was mostly a trend toward better results in children participating in regular physical education classes for children and their parents. Most often better results in the broad jump were found in our surveys: thus, a *test of jumping seems to be a good approach for the evaluation of motor abilities.*

Although the investigated sample varying in the level of spontaneous physical activity was small (which was due to the striving for a comprehensive

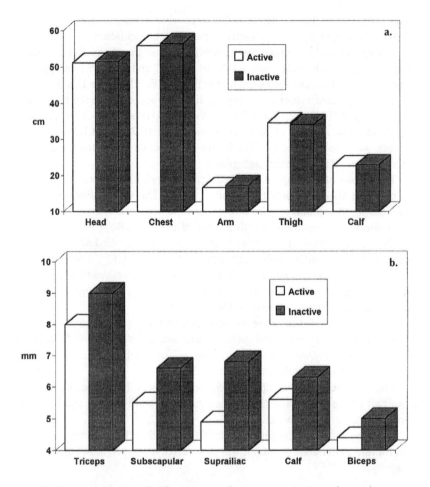

FIGURE 10.2 Comparison of anthropometric characteristics — circumferential measures (a), skinfolds by Harpenden caliper (b), somatotype (c), intake of energy — kJ (d), protein and fat (e) and carbohydrates — g/day (f), and blood lipid level (g), i.e., total, HDL, LDL cholesterol, triglycerides, in 3- to 5-year-old children characterized by a very high and/or low level of spontaneous physical activity (survey J).

methodological approach including blood sampling), anthropometric variables, body composition, cardiorespiratory fitness, dietary intake, psychological development, and the overall lifestyle of the children and their families did not differ significantly from the results in our previous surveys of larger groups of preschool children of the same age.[233,256] Functional parameters, i.e., the reaction to the step test corresponded generally to the results reported before.[256,258,233,254] The same applies to dietary intake, which did not differ from the usually increased values of Czech children, including higher fat intake. Therefore, we can speculate that the results gained in this survey might apply more generally.

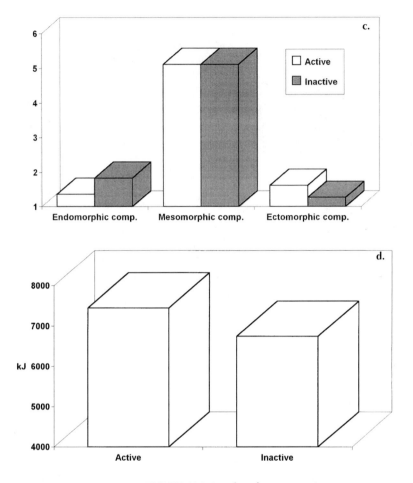

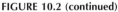

FIGURE 10.2 (continued)

Only a few differences between highly active and inactive children reached the level of statistical significance. However, they had a consistent trend, which was similar to that found in the comparisons of older children and/or adolescents: *highly active children with significantly higher HDL tended to have lower body weight, were less fat and more ectomorphic, had a spontaneously higher energy intake,* and *showed a slightly higher level of cardiorespiratory fitness* (higher values of STI, CEI_1, and CEI_2 indices), and *a higher level of fine motor skills,* along with a trend toward higher CK activity in the blood. In older age categories where the influence of exercise persisted for longer periods of life, these differences were larger and statistically significant, depending on the intensity, character, and duration of increased muscle work and activity.[265]

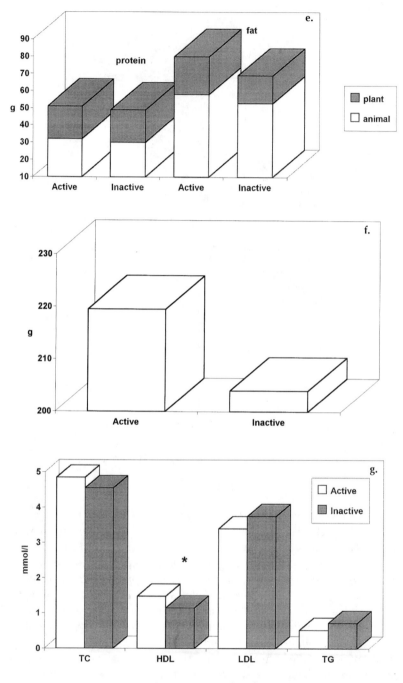

FIGURE 10.2 (continued)

Similar results were later found in another study of U.S. children of the same age.[89] Higher levels of cardiovascular fitness and lower levels of fatness were associated with more favorable serum lipid and lipoprotein levels similarly as in our survey. Physical fitness appeared to have an indirect association with serum lipid and lipoprotein values through its relationship with higher level of physical activity,[139,140] fitness, and a lower deposition of fat. Fitness, activity, and participation in sports activities in preschool children were also analyzed by the American Academy of Pediatrics (1992), because the present situation seems to be unnatural and harmful regarding the actual and future consequences of morphological, functional, metabolical, and biochemical characteristics[139] in the development of preschool children.

As for the aspects of health, the significantly higher level of HDL in the active children is important in regard to the decreased risk of cardiovascular disease morbidity in later age: it was shown that children who had favorable levels of blood lipids at early age generally preserved them later on (Bogalusa study).[219,369-371]

Mentioned data seem to indicate that *a genotype characterized by a high level of spontaneous physical activity* and thus represents a particular "motor individuality" also *has a more favorable spectrum of serum lipids,* namely a higher level of HDL. Such a predisposition may limit the risk of the cardiovascular diseases in later life. Usually this is associated with similar traits in one or both parents. However, *it may be also presumed that the introduction of an active way of life might result in similar favorable changes of serum lipid levels of children.* Therefore, a suitable way of life for the whole family with an adequate diet and a desirable level of physical activity and exercise can contribute to the reduction of this risk in any child. The same applies to the regime of diet and exercise in the kindergartens.

Chapter 11

CRITERIA FOR THE EVALUATION OF MORPHOLOGICAL AND FUNCTIONAL DEVELOPMENT IN PRESCHOOL CHILDREN: RECOMMENDATIONS

I. BODY SIZE AND BODY COMPOSITION

Developing a global definition for the acceptable ranges of body size is a difficult task. The most usual approach includes establishing reference values on the basis of the measurement of a certain population and evaluating average values as norms or, which has become more usual recently, giving percentiles. The 50th percentile is generally accepted as a standard for a population in question. However, what is the *most common or average value in a population does not always translate to the optimal value.*

Body size does not only reflect the level of development and its adequacy, but it also serves as a basis for recommended dietary allowances, especially regarding energy and proteins. There has always been a dilemma concerning the reference standards for the growth of children from industrialized countries — should they be accepted as universally relevant or should local standards be used.[393] Children in many developing countries are already smaller at birth than those in industrialized countries, and they grow at a slower rate during infancy and early childhood. Evidence suggests that in young children these differences are primarily due to environmental factors, including inadequate nutrition, and that genetic and ethnic factors are of lesser importance. Thus, young children of different ethnic groups should be considered as having the same or similar growth potential.

As shown by numerous comparative studies, even a healthy privileged population can show a wide variation in the size of children. Up until now, very limited information concerning the possible relationship of body size to health, well-being, or physiological function was available. However, in some communities where children's growth is severely limited by environmental factors, there is evidence of an association between functional impairment and deficit

235

in linear growth. In such cases, it is necessary to differentiate between the degrees of growth deficit, so as to define health risk.

In studies comparing marginally malnourished and well-nourished children, both during preschool and prepubertal age, it was shown that *larger body size was not a self-evident predisposition for a higher level of functional capacity and physical fitness*. This applied first of all to the level of cardio-respiratory fitness,[104,233] and to factors such as skill. Obviously, when the degree of growth deficit did not trespass certain limits and when they did not reduce to the development of vital organs and tissues, there was no obvious functional deterioration.

The above mentioned studies point up the necessity for the examination of a greater number of characteristics concerning growth and body composition, mainly those which are the markers of functional capacity of the organism and of *"positive health"*. The process of selection and validation of such markers was one of the main aims of our surveys.

Expert consultants of Joint FAO/WHO/UNU[393] felt it was desirable that the growth potential of children should be fully expressed, and that all estimates for requirements such as energy and protein should allow for this. For this reason not only this Expert Committee but also several others recommend that the **reference growth standards** be published for international use by WHO.[376,378] The use of this particular reference population is recommended on the basis of several criteria.

Since then, the average values of height and weight have changed, i.e., increased in the U.S.;[136,188] the higher values of body weight are mainly due to an increasing adiposity of U.S. population, but the reference standards have not been changed up to now.

In epidemiological studies of children who are undernourished, it is conventional to accept −2 SD from the median as the cut-off point between "normal" and "malnourished", corresponding approximately to the third percentile or to 80% of the median for weight and 90% for height. Similarly, +2 SD weight-for-height may be taken as a cut-off point for obesity.[393]

During the last decade, the **body mass index (BMI)** has been used more and more often. Growth grids for BMI[35] were developed as mentioned above[149,301] The values of BMI for 50th percentiles vary with age; generally, BMI increases with age. Its changes during the period of preschool age are relatively small. Percentiles are not the same in all countries, and the optimal, desirable values of BMI for different age categories need validation using additional functional and health variables.

Chest circumference was most often measured along with height and weight. In addition to body composition measurements, it is nowadays also recommended to measure **waist and hip circumferences** and to calculate the **waist/hip ratio**. This ratio may differentiate between different types of obesity — diffuse gynoid, pear-shaped, and/or android, apple-shaped obesity. The latter is connected with a number of pathological changes, such as glucose intolerance, prediabetes and/or even NIDDM, dislipoproteinemia, hypertension, ischemic heart disease, etc.[246] Thus, it may help to define and select, as with indices of fat distribution, individuals at risk for such diseases, merely on the basis of very simple anthropometric measurements. This does not yet seem realistic in young children; however, Bouchard and Johnston[38] already consider *fat distribution in childhoodas a marker of later health risk.*

Circumferential measures of the **head** and **neck** already differentiate boys and girls at a very early age. Circumferences of the **extremities** may also give relevant information on body composition: this applies mainly to arm circumference, which is an important indicator of both muscle and fat development. When the circumference, as well as skinfold, is measured, a net circumference of the muscle mass of the upper arm can be calculated according to the formula:

AMC (mm) = midarm circumference (mm) − (0.314 × triceps skinfold in mm)

(*Note:* AMC, arm muscle circumference).[163]

Thus, it's possible to evaluate the status of the musculature and the nutritional status according to the degree of fat deposition. This parameter was used for the measurements in children of the Third World.

The circumference of the **thigh** is also important in the evaluation of obesity development: the fat layer deposited in the trochanteric region (RTG) correlated best with the total amount of fat. Such measurements were rare, and are not allowed anymore solely for research reasons. However, the circumference of the thigh is considered an important indicator of adiposity. **Waist/thigh ratio** is also calculated and used for the evaluation of the type of fat distribution on the body surface.

Length measures have been mainly used for the evaluation of body proportionality assessments; e.g., index relating sitting/total height make it possible to evaluate the relationship between the length of the trunk and of the lower extremities and how this changes during growth. Other measures on the upper extremity were used for the evaluation of body physique of dancers or athletes specializing in different disciplines. There also appear to be changes during growth and development which are characteristic to individual growth periods.[256]

Breadth measurements of the trunk can help to evaluate body proportionality; this applies especially to the biacromial, biiliocristal and bitrochanteric measures. As shown by our results, at preschool age the proportionality evaluated with the help of indices relating these measures to total height and/or mutually do not change markedly. This occurs later on; indices characterizing relative breadths correlate significantly with body composition.[233]

Breadth measures on the extremities characterize the **robusticity of the skeleton** — bone mass—which changes remarkably during growth. There are also sex-linked differences which are already apparent during preschool age which help to characterize the individual in actual and future development.

In the context of malnutrition and/or obesity, it is important to measure body composition and some indicators of **lean body mass** and *fat* in the body. The assessment of the layer of subcutaneous fat measured as skinfold thickness can give an appropriate answer on body composition, as it is also possible to use certain standard values for individual skinfolds for comparison,[230,233,347] and/or for the calculated percentage of depot fat.[230,233] This is important in light of the great variability of body composition, which can differ even when height, weight, and BMI are the same or very similar. Moreover, a thin child with a low BMI may have quite a lot of fat or vice versa — a child with a high value of BMI and high percentile of BMI can be very lean and have very little fat.

Fat distribution (pattern) calculated as the ratio of individual skinfold thicknesses (subscapular/triceps, or sum of skinfolds on the trunk/sum of skinfolds on the extremities) is actually considered an early marker, already important during growth period for later development, e.g., of diabetes or cardiovascular diseases, later in life.[38] In adults, significant correlations were found for the indices of fat distribution and blood lipid levels.[276]

Many other methods exist for the evaluation of body composition as mentioned in Chapter 7. Under present conditions, anthropometry and bio-impedance analysis (BIA) are used most frequently.

II. FUNCTIONAL MEASUREMENTS: CARDIORESPIRATORY FITNESS

Anthropometric measurements are surely easier than functional evaluation, which has been used less often in very young children. The selection of functional and motor tests, the results of which were presented, are certainly not the only approach. It is necessary to stress that their selection was not accidental, but a result of long testing and trials.[254]

The main consideration in their selection was having tests that would benatural for the children, but at the same time reliable and valid, under conditions of preserving conditions of measurements which should be standardized. All experimental workers were, therefore, trained and tested.

As mentioned in Chapter 6, *physical fitness* and the *functional capacity* of the growing organism *have many facets which may be developed in a synchronic or asynchronic* way. Therefore, the use of a battery of tests is desirable. On the other hand, significant mutual correlations were found; therefore, it was possible to make a selection of some to characterize the level of functional capacity.

With standards and norms, there is a problem similar to the one with morphological development. Obviously, values established in one country cannot always serve as norms in another one or in a different part of the world. Therefore, *data given in this book can serve as a guideline and/or as reference values which should be validated in other countries.*

Whether average values or 50th percentiles are the best criteria is controversial. Let us not forget that the average values of BMI or of total cholesterol values increased in some countries: such values can hardly be considered reference values. The same applies to functional variables, e.g., the aerobic power deteriorated in certain parts of the world that adopted the lifestyle, including diet, normal in industrially developed countries.[327] As in *"positive health"*, *an optimal, not average*, *variable of functional capacity should be used as the criterion and as the goal*. Then, the assessed values should be evaluated considering both average for a given population and the optimal, desirable reference value.

In *cardiorespiratory fitness*, the *step test* (using a mounting step), proved to be a suitable test for young children because it is a natural activity for all children (at least in the industrially developed countries). Even when certain procedures were developed using a modified veloergometer (e.g., stimulating the child by showing a picture which appears and only remains when the child adheres to a special frequency of pedaling, during the necessary period of time), such a test is still less natural because not all children are adapted to cycling; those who have had an opportunity to experience this are at an advantage. Running on a treadmill is also a natural activity, but it may be frightening for 3- to 4-year-old children; 5- to 6-year old children were tested using Balke's walking test. Both of these procedures are much more expensive and difficult to arrange under field conditions. Mounting a step can be fixed much more easily.

The most important criteria for a favorable result in the step test is:

- An increase of the heart rate by about 50% as compared to the rest value
- The establishment of a steady state during the load
- The return of heart rate to the resting value at the end of the recovery period (third to fourth minute of recovery)

The values of cardiac efficiency indices can serve as reference values for the individual age categories, as presented in Figures 6.1a and 6.1b and in Tables 6.1 and 6.3.

III. MOTOR DEVELOPMENT

As mentioned in Chapter 6, motor tests were selected to characterize *speed* (20 m dash), the *explosive strength of the muscles* of the *upper* and *lower extremities* (throwing a ball, broad jump), along with *skill*, and also to characterize endurance (500 m run-and-walk) and hand grip strength. The procedures and results were described in detail in previous chapters. The particular values are given in Table 9.4 and in Figures 6.7a, 6.7b, 6.7c, 6.7d.

The majority of preschool children — at least the older ones — are able to fulfill skill tests such as walking on a beam, standing on one leg, performing a forward roll, walking at a given rhythm, and catching a ball in different ways (Appendix 3). Additional tests such as the sit-and-reach, the shuttle run, and many others, were also used in other studies.[63,222] Reference values for pre-school children are still rare and should be elaborated further in order to eventually become *more culturally specific*. The reference values for muscle strength (which requires special equipment) are presented in Figure 6.5.

IV. SENSOMOTOR DEVELOPMENT

Fine motorics is an important predisposition for many other abilities and skills later in school and elsewhere. Testing of sensomotor development can show the level of development of the child and call attention to the state of the child which may need some assistance. The *"open and close the hands"* test can differentiate individuals on a higher level because only some preschool children are able to fulfill all items of this test before the beginning of school attendance. This test was widely used for U.S., Czech, and other children and gives valid information on the level of development of the child.

Easiest for children is the test of *spatial orientation*; testing of *laterality* gives less satisfactory results, which is partly caused by the fact that this is not yet definitively differentiated before entering primary school.

V. DIETARY INTAKE AND BIOCHEMICAL CHARACTERISTICS

The assessments of dietary intake already has a longer tradition, as described in numerous textbooks. These procedures used in our studies give valuable information; however, personal interviewing by specially trained personnel is preferable whenever possible. Such procedures were used by Gregory et al.[141] in a recent nutritional diet and nutrition survey in the U.K. The same applies to the assessments of biochemical parameters such as serum lipids.[141] In this respect, there are also incomparably better experiences as compared to the evaluation of cardiorespiratory, motor, and sensomotor development in young children.

Chapter 12

SUMMARY OF
EXPERIMENTAL RESULTS

Physical activity and motion, closely interrelated with dietary intake, is not only a basic manifestation of life, but is also a means of significant modification of a number of variables characterizing the organism. This includes morphological, functional, nutritional, biochemical, and motor variables; the opportunity to intervene using both diet and exercise seems to be mostly effective when introduced early in life. The influence of varying degrees and kinds of physical activity can be both positive and negative; the resulting changes also depend on the initial state of the organism in question — age, i.e., ontogenetical stage, and on the duration and kind of physical activity.

I. STUDIES IN THE EXPERIMENTAL MODELS WITH LABORATORY ANIMALS

Results of experimental model studies using laboratory animals showed a significant influence of the change in the physical activity regimes of the pregnant rats, as in the dietary changes at the beginning of life of the offspring (lactation period). As shown by a series of experiments, *the changes in physical activity were closely related to the changes of dietary intake and vice versa; the changes of dietary intake influenced the development of the spontaneous physical activity.*

Rats weaned in large nests (more than 12 pups), i.e., those that had a lower intake of mother's milk, were not only smaller and less fat, but also developed a higher level of spontaneous physical activity in rotation activity cages in contrast to rats weaned in small nests (less than 6 pups). The size of vital organs (heart, adrenals) and, most important muscles was the same. Along with this, there were differences in the parameters of lipid metabolism, i.e., the animals from small nests had higher total lipids and fatty acids concentration in the small intestine of females and a higher synthesis of lipids in the small intestine in both sexes. Cholesterol synthesis in the liver and in the carcass was the same in all groups, but the cholesterogenesis in the liver was higher in the liver of males from large nests. Cholesterogenesis in the carcass was also higher in animals of both sexes from large nests. Apparently, *temporary manipulation of dietary intake early in life influenced body size and*

241

fatness, the level of spontaneous physical activity, and lipid metabolism long after this intervention was made, when the diet was the same in all compared groups. *A higher level of physical activity showed that the functional status of the animals was on a good level* in spite of early marginal malnutrition which resulted in reduced body size.[244,272]

Similar consequences were observed in the animals weaned from 8 pups in one nest; their mothers were fed a reduced protein diet (10%) and a low energy diet during the whole period of lactation, and then the same diet with 5% of protein was used for the animals after weaning (28th day) until the 49th day of life. The offspring spontaneously consumed less of this diet, i.e., their intake of both protein and energy was reduced (REP). Thereafter, REP animals had the same laboratory diet as control animals fed *ad libitum* during all of their life. *Reduced growth, lower depot fat, the same size of vital organs, and better energy economy as characterized by lower food intake/1 g of weight increment during growth period along with significantly higher level of spontaneous physical activity in rotation cages all characterized the animals with reduced protein and energy intake at the beginning of life (REPA).* This was proved by a series of experiments; in addition, some delayed changes in lipid metabolism were also found (higher concentration of lipids, and lower liposynthesis in the liver in REPA animals).[274]

The introduction of a high fat diet early in life (18th to 30th day of life), which was followed with a special regime of self-selected diets (pure starch, fat, casein) significantly changed the free choice of the mentioned dietary components, i.e., temporarily increased the spontaneous intake of fat and later that of protein compared to the animals without a high fat diet early in life. In addition to this, the reduction of body size and depot fat found in the animals living during the whole experimental period on the self-selected diet of pure foodstuffs was prevented by a high fat diet. Therefore, the introduction of a *special diet early in life had a number of significant consequences which only became apparent later in life.*[228]

Increased physical activity, i.e., *the exercise of the rat mother during pregnancy* (mild aerobic exercise, daily run on a treadmill, 15 m/min. for 1 hour) had a *significant impact on lipid metabolism variables in the offspring* which was not revealed in the offspring of control, inactive rat mothers. The cholesterol concentration in the liver was increased in both female and male offspring of the exercised mothers. Significant changes of liposynthesis studied *in vivo* after injection of Na-acetate-1-^{14}C were also observed. *In vitro* study showed lower total lipid and fatty acid concentration in the liver and a higher level of serum free fatty acids in the male offspring of exercised mothers. A higher concentration of cholesterol, a higher synthesis of fatty acids, and a lower cholesterogenesis in the small intestine in male offspring of exercised mothers compared to the offspring of control mothers was also found. As follows, the *daily work load during pregnancy resulted in significant delayed changes of lipid metabolism in the liver and small intestine of the adult offspring.*[244,273]

Exercise during pregnancy also had a significant impact on the cardiac microstructure: *young adult offspring of the exercised mothers had a significantly higher density of muscle fibers and capillaries, a higher capillary to fiber ratio, and a significantly shorter diffusion distance in the heart* compared to offspring of the control, inactive mothers. This influence, which may be physiologically interpreted as positive, was further *amplified by exercise of the offspring during their own postnatal ontogenesis.* However, according to the differences between control offspring of exercised mothers and exercised offspring of control mothers, the influence of exercise during pregnancy seemed to be more important.[232,234,237]

Changes in diet and physical activity early in life are closely interrelated. This is evident from the *elevation of the level of spontaneous physical activity in rats with early marginal protein energy malnutrition (REP)* and/or in rats from large nests which had less milk from their mothers. Such animals are characterized not only by the above mentioned *reduction of body size and fatness*, better energy economy as regards weight increments and elevated physical activity in rotation cages, but also by *a higher resistance of the cardiac muscle against noxious factors*, e.g., isoprenaline which induces experimental cardiac necrosis. Smaller, leaner, and more active animals developed (after the administration of the same dose of isoprenaline) a lower degree of cardiac damage and/or died spontaneously less often than normally *ad libitum* fed animals, which were heavier and fatter, having a lower spontaneous physical activity level in rotation cages.[261]

Apparently, marginally reduced energy and protein intakes early in life, as well as workload during pregnancy, can have positive delayed consequences manifested in the offspring as changes in body size, fatness, the level of spontaneous physical activity, modifications of lipid metabolism, positive changes in the microstructure of the cardiac muscle, and a greater resistance to noxious factors.

II. OBSERVATIONS ON THE INFLUENCE OF MATERNAL NUTRITION ON THE NEWBORN

The follow up of Italian women[6,7] during pregnancy regarding their anthropometric variables, fat pattern, dietary intake, and blood lipids revealed a significant relationship between maternal variables and those in the offspring. Mother to son correlations were found most frequently (birth weight, skinfolds, fat distribution). The mother's weight gain correlated negatively with BMI and skinfolds in sons, and positively with birth weight, BMI, and subscapular skinfolds in daughters. **Fat distribution**, characterized by indices (relating skinfold thicknesses on the trunk and on the extremities, which are considered markers of cardiovascular risk), correlated most closely in mothers and newborn sons;[6,7] even closer correlations were found in mothers and sons 2- to 5-years old. [249]

With maternal diet and cord blood lipids, most relationships were found for total energy intake and energy provided by carbohydrates and for total cholesterol and HDL-cholesterol in sons only; these relationships were significantly negative. *Energy provided by proteins and fats in the maternal diet correlated positively with total cholesterol of the offspring*; when considering sexes separately, though, it was significant in *newborn sons only.* HDL-cholesterol correlated positively with the percentage of energy provided in the maternal diet by fats and negatively with that provided by carbohydrates. Maternal triglycerides correlated positively with cord blood HDL-cholesterol in the joint group of all offspring, but when evaluating sexes separately, the correlation was significant in girls only. Maternal total cholesterol correlated positively with triglycerides and with HDL-cholesterol/total cholesterol ratio in girls only. *In newborns*, only *significant correlation between total cholesterol and fat distribution were found.* All correlations were low, but were mostly highly significant and occurred systematically. The accumulation of weaker, but significantly negative factors affecting the mothers during pregnancy may have undesirable influences on the newborn.[6,7]

These results indicate the importance of the composition of mother's diet regarding blood lipids of the newborn, especially those of sons. Significant relationships between the fat distribution of the mother and the son point up the possibility of a link between maternal nutritional status and markers of cardiovascular risk to that of the offspring, namely that of sons. As indicated by other authors,[219,371] the serum lipid level at birth correlates with the level assessed later and/or with atherosclerotic plaques during the prepubertal period. These results seem to indicate that *the composition of the maternal diet deserves more attention than it had up until now.*

III. MORPHOLOGICAL AND FUNCTIONAL SURVEYS IN PRESCHOOL CHILDREN

Measurements in nine cross-sectional studies, including those of thousands of children in Czech Republic and three longitudinal follow ups made in the 1970s and 1980s, brought more detailed information on somatic, functional, motor, and sensomotor development and on dietary intake and serum lipids of children from 3 to 6 years old. The impact of environmental factors including diet and exercise in preschool age was also investigated. The selection of procedures and methods resulted from previous studies with larger battery of tests.[233,236,238,254,256]

In a group of 238 children, *cross-sectional morphological and functional measurements* in four age subgroups from 3–4 to 6–7 years of age (survey A) and, in 58 children, five *longitudinal* measurements during the same age period (survey E) were made using total and sitting height; weight; body mass index (BMI); length of upper extremity; acromion-radiale; radiale-stylion; length of the lower extremity; bispinale-tibiale; tibiale-sphyrion; breadth measurements on the trunk and extremities (i.e., biacromiale, chest breadth and depth); biiliocristale, hand, wrist, femoral condyles and ankle breadths; and circumferential measurements on head, neck, chest, abdomen, arm, forearm, thigh and calf. In addition to these factors, indices characterizing the body build and proportionality were also evaluated. All variables increased with advancing age, some of them more (weight, length measures), and some very little (head, neck circumferences). ***Head circumferences*** were always *greater in boys*; *length and breadth measures on the trunk and extremities and other circumferences tended to be greater in boys*, but this was mainly significant in the oldest age group (5- to 6- and 6- to 7-year-old children). Interindividual variability was large.

Skinfolds on the cheek, chin, on two sites of the chest, over triceps, biceps, subscapular, abdomen, suprailiac, thigh and calf were measured as a characteristic of body composition using a modified Best caliper;[230,233] skinfolds over triceps, subscapular, suprailiac, calf, biceps were also measured using a Harpenden caliper[247-249] on both sides of the body. *Subcutaneous fat was greater in girls and was the only variable that did not change (in girls) and/or decreased (boys) in children from 3 to 6 years old.* Indices of fat distribution relating to the subscapular and triceps and/or skinfolds measured on the trunk and on the extremities were also evaluated along with ***somatotypes*** (endomorphy, ectomorphy, mesomorphy). These variables were stable at preschool age.[233,256,266] There was a trend toward higher endomorphy in girls and higher ecto- and mesomorphy in boys although the differences were not yet significant.

Body posture, i.e., the position of the neck, back, and abdomen from the side view, the depth of the neck and lumbar lordosis, and the position of the shoulders, scapulae, and spine in the upright and bent forward position from the back view, was also executed. Body posture deteriorated from 3 to 6 years as indicated by both cross-sectional and longitudinal studies.[254,256]

For ***cardiorespiratory fitness***, the ***step test*** was employed (as the only test feasible for 3-year-old girls and boys) in the above mentioned groups, both cross-sectionally and repeatedly in the same children in longitudinal studies. Children mounted a step 25 cm high (oldest children 30 cm) 30 times/min, assisted (but not helped) by a technical assistant; the heart rate was measured during 3 minutes of rest, during 5 minutes of mounting the step, and during 5 minutes of recovery. The average heart rate during all periods of testing decreased with age; a steady state was established during the workload, and the heart rate returned to rest values before the end of the recovery period, indicating that this test was not an excessive strain for preschool children. The cardiac efficiency index (CEI_1, CEI_2) calculated from the values of the heart rate assessed during various phases of the step test revealed *an improvement in the economy of work of the cardiorespiratory system with advancing age of children.* The heart rate was slightly higher in girls. However, though in our groups, these differences did not reach the level of statistical significance.[233,250,254,256,258]

The development of **gross motorics** was tested in an evaluation of performance in a *20 m dash, a broad jump, and a ball throw* with both right and left hands. **Hand grip strength** of the right and left hands was measured using a dynamometer (tensometric principle) specially adapted in our mastery for young children's palms. The performance improved significantly with age. Regarding sex-linked differences *in the tests of gross motorics, those demanding maximal effort were significantly better in boys.*[233,236,238,256]

Skill and **balance** was evaluated using the following tests: walking on a horizontal beam, standing on one leg for 10 seconds, forward roll, walking at a given pace, and catching a ball (five modifications). In skill tests, *girls tended to be better*, manifested in particular in standing on one leg and in the forward roll. Performance in other tests did not differ. The results of these tests also improved significantly with advancing age.[254,256,259]

In several smaller subgroups of children in Prague and Nymburk, the **dietary intake** was assessed repeatedly (entering 7-day records with the help of kindergarten teachers and parents). An *elevated intake of energy, protein, and fat was assessed in* comparison to local recommended dietary allowances (RDAs). The intake of food was even more excessive when compared with RDAs for the U.S. or for the E.C.[398] (which are lower especially for protein). Higher values of BMI were assessed in Czech children already in the preschool period; we might speculate that increased obesity and cardiovascular risk, resulting in a higher morbidity and mortality from cardiovascular disease in the adult Czech population could be, *inter alia,* also due to early overeating.[256] However, marked obesity was not yet apparent in our groups of preschool children.

Assessments in smaller subsamples of preschool children revealed normal levels of **total, HDL-** and **LDL-cholesterol**, and **triglycerides**, which did not correlate with the actual food intake.[249,250,270,271]

Follow ups of height, weight, BMI, circumferential measurements, performance in the 20 m dash, broad jump and throwing a ball, along with skill and sensomotor tests, were repeated in three other cross-sectional surveys (B, boys, n = 2839; girls, n = 2759; C, boys, n = 1848, girls, n = 1864; D in total 9590, subsample 1005) and another longitudinal survey (F, boys n = 367, girls n = 397). Longitudinal observations confirmed the conclusions of cross-sectional surveys.[244,250,254,255,256,258,266–268] *The economic and family situation, education of parents, birth weight of children, the beginning of independent walking* (i.e., whether before or after one year of age), morbidity of children,and the characteristics of the *environment* in different districts of the Czech Republic were evaluated, as in the above mentioned surveys A and E. Additional information on the children's *lifestyle* was also assessed by *questionnaires*, and all children were evaluated globally, as well as in subgroups differentiated according to these characteristics in surveys B, C, and D.

Reference values of the above mentioned variables were established for the individual age groups using cross-sectional data, which were also validated by longitudinal measurements. These data were used repeatedly in the Czech Republic for the evaluation of the level of morphological, functional, motor, and sensomotor development of preschool children. The adequacy of the development from the above mentioned points of view was thus made possible; in special cases, retarded development could also be defined, and/or a talent for special motor activities could be selected. Particular attention was then paid to such children, and pedagogic intervention in groups of individuals was rendered possible. Regarding reference values, the results of the last measurements (survey D) were used.[247]

However, on the basis of the comparisons of repeated measurements in the Czech Republic, as well as on the basis of international comparisons it was recommended that we prepare reference values for morphological, functional, gross, and fine motor variables in individual countries, especially those that vary in geographic, climatic, cultural, social, and economic conditions. In all instances, presented methods and results may serve as guidelines for further research and pedagogic intervention in preschool children, which of course could be supplemented with other innovative ideas.

IV. SURVEYS OF CHILDREN WITH VARIOUS ENVIRONMENTAL CONDITIONS AND DIFFERENT LEVELS OF NUTRITION

A comparison of the results assessed in different parts of the Czech Republic, e.g., when comparing body size and motor performance in the capital and small villages, showed significant differences. *Significantly greater bodily dimensions usual, e.g., in Prague, were not always a predisposition for better physical performance* in subjects of the same age, as shown by comparisons of children from Prague and rural areas, from families with higher and lower income, with children born as first and last in the families, etc. Children most advanced in somatic development, i.e., with largest body size, were not the best in physical performance, in spite of a simultaneously higher level of sensomotor development.[250,256]

Comparison of the results of our measurements with some data on morphological, functional (step test) and motor development in other countries, e.g., different parts of *Italy, Turkey, Estonia,* and *Senegal,* showed some differences among preschool children; e.g., in Italy[104] it was shown that the most important differences were due mainly to social, nutritional, and environmental conditions. Children in areas with similar lifestyles did not differ markedly in morphological and functional parameters. However, *when comparing smaller and leaner children from poor areas of Southern Italy with preschool children from richer Northern Italy, it was revealed that their body size was smaller due to a significantly lower food intake, but the results of the step test, indicating better cardiorespiratory efficiency, were more favorable.*[104] There were only very slight differences between Estonian and Czech children;[222] Turkish children were slightly smaller and less efficient in some functional and motor tests.[359]

The most important differences were found between *Senegalese children*[25,26] on the one hand, and all other children on the other. Their body size was smaller, and their motor performance was also poorer. However, when the *results of performance tests were adjusted to body size, the differences diminished.* In some tests (e.g., the broad jump) the results were even better in Senegalese than in Czech children. The results of the step test differed slightly from the results of Czech children: the heart rate during rest, workload, and recovery were the same for the joint group of all Senegalese children as for Czech girls of the same age. Thus, it was confirmed that in *dynamic, weight bearing physical activities, smaller children with poorer nutrition may not be at such a disadvantage* as compared to their bigger, more abundantly fed peers. This only applies, though, to the *cases of marginal (not severe) malnutrition.* This is still within the adaptation limits of the growing organism and obviously under such conditions does not reduce the size and function of vital organs or diminish lean body mass to a great extent.

However, in this case, performance, which depends more on muscle mass such as *muscle strength, is worse in children with reduced food intake and smaller body size.*[25,26,202–204]

As follows from the literature, *severely malnourished children are functionally and motorically handicapped in all respects.*[378] Functional measurements in severely malnourished children were made mainly under conditions of rest, and not during work loads. Unfortunately, many severely malnourished children have to undergo quite intense workloads, so more knowledge is needed on this issue.

Another extreme, i.e., *obesity* can serve as an example of the undesirable consequences of a food intake which does not correspond to the actual energy needs. *At preschool age, excessive food intake does not yet result in the development of apparent obesity which is usual later in childhood and/or during adolescence;*[233,246,264] we found only 2 to 3% of children are overweight according to our surveys. These children were not only heavier, but also taller and had higher BMI, skinfolds, circumferences, and estimated lean body mass; their physical performance (especially in *jumping, shown to be one of the most relevant motor tests*) was on a lower level compared to their peers with normal or lower BMI. Performance in the 20 m run did not deteriorate. The morphological development in overweight children seemed to be generally accelerated. This does not concern, however, functional development, which revealed already some handicaps compared to children with normal weight. Weight and fat in preschool children were not significantly related to the actual dietary intake.

The low prevalence of marked obesity in preschool age did not allow more opportunities to follow up on further deviations in functional and other variables. However, a s**ignificantly positive correlation between the percent-age of depot fat** (calculated from skinfolds) and **the level of total cholesterol**, as well as that of **triglycerides**,[243,250] revealed that excess fat at preschool age is already a serious health risk in relation to the later development of atherosclerosis and other diseases of the cardiovascular system. The same was found in older children; after reduction of fat and weight with diet and exercise, a decline of total cholesterol was also found, especially in prepubertal boys. As shown by some longitudinal observations, when the dietary intake and the general lifestyle is not modified in a desirable way, children later developed real obesity; this is usually manifested at school age.

Regarding the *influence of environmental factors*, except for the size of the community where the children lived, no marked changes due to environment (air and water pollution, etc. in different areas of The Czech Republic) were found. *Children from Prague or other larger communities were bigger, but their physical performance was generally lower in spite of higher level of sensomotor development.*[233,236,238,256] No differences in somatic and motor development according to risk pregnancy, health status (i.e., indication for regular medical check-ups until the end of the 1st year of life) at the age of 4 to 6 years were found.[251] Regarding the age at the onset of independent walking, some relationships to anthropometric variables were found.[256]

The analysis of the influence of birth weight revealed that *children born heavier started to walk earlier, had higher values of height, weight, and circumferential measures* (average values, z-scores) at the age of 4 to 6 years. They were also *sick less often* and wore glasses less often. BMI did not differ. With motor development, there were only significant differences in throwing a ball with the left hand in both sexes (which was longer in children born heavier), and in some skill tests (better results in the test of standing on one leg in girls).[251]

The influence of the *family situation (i.e., complete or incomplete family) was also significant: children from complete families were more advanced in somatic development*, i.e., had highest values of height and weight, but the BMIs and the level of motor development did not differ. Regarding the education of parents, *children with fathers with the highest level of education* (university level) *were the tallest and the heaviest and more slender; the performance in the 20 m dash was also significantly better.* The education of mothers did not influence motor performance of children. When analysing the influence of both parents, the most favorable results in somatic and motor development were found in children of fathers with a university education and mothers with a high school education.[254]

Common morbidity from normal childhood diseases did not have any significant influence on the child's morphological, functional, and motor development;[254] however, it is necessary to stress that children with more serious health problems were not followed in our surveys.

V. THE INFLUENCE OF EXERCISE

The impact of regular exercise, mainly in the framework of the *system of physical education for the child and the mother* (or father, grandmother, etc.).[27–29] was significant in more of our follow ups. *Children enrolled regularly in physical education* had as a rule significantly *higher values of height, weight, and other morphological characteristics*. Although in contrast to the biggest children, e.g., from the capital or from the families with highest per capita income or born first, *exercised children also had best results in motor performance*. This applied especially to broad jump (surveys A, B, C, and D), but also to the 20 m dash and the ball throw with right hand. As mentioned above, larger body size alone does not guarantee better physical performance which can only be induced with regular longer lasting exercise.[233,238,254,256,250] *The results of skill tests were also the best in exercising children.*

However, better results of physical performance were apparent in older children, after a longer exposure to exercise. When we wanted to examine the possible differences between physically active and inactive children at a younger age, i.e., 4 to 5 years, we had to compare subjects who were spontaneously very active or generally inactive. This differentiation was made possible by a longitudinal follow up of a smaller subgroup of 4.6-year-old children (J) during the whole year by the teachers and the parents, with the help of special questionnaires prepared by us for this purpose. Children who were spontaneously most active during the whole year of observation tended to be taller, heavier, leaner (more mesomorphic), having a slightly higher dietary intake and better results in step test. These differences, however, were not significant. Only the serum level of HDL-cholesterol was significantly higher in very active children compared to inactive ones.[270] Results seem to indicate that a *genotype characterized by high spontaneous physical activity has significantly higher HDL along with a trend for larger body size, less depot fat, higher food intake, higher cardiorespiratory and motor fitness which already manifests itself at preschool age.* It may be assumed that the introduction of adequate exercise in less active preschool children may result in similar favorable characteristics as those in older age.

Thus, exercise and motor stimulation proved to be beneficial for young children and for older ones. Therefore, a system of motor stimulation for infants[182,183] and *special physical education for preschool children and parents was developed and introduced on a massive scale in The Czech Republic for more than 30 years.*[27–29] Similar systems have already been used in many other countries, but they are still less frequent than physical education for school children. Selected activities and exercises were described for systematic physical education in young children.[27–29,182,183] It was revealed that such a system during infancy has already had a positive influence on child development, manifested not only in motor, but also in social and psychological development.[182,183] As described above, the influence of exercise on preschool children was also found to be beneficial, provided it was individually adjusted and it only included exercises suitable for this early period of growth.

Chapter 13

PERSPECTIVES: PHYSICAL ACTIVITY, EARLY PREVENTION OF DISEASES, AND THE DEVELOPMENT OF POSITIVE HEALTH

"It is not a soul, it is not a body, that we are training up, but a man, and we ought not to divide him"

Montaigne, 1888

Life and motion cannot be separated — motor activity and exercise can be used as a part of general education, which goes beyond motorics. The close relationship between diet and physical activity links both of these factors, and an adequate manipulation of both at an early age in a mutual relationship (which implies energy balance and turnover) has a decisive influence on the individual, not only now, but also later on because of delayed consequences.

To start with, the fetal period was proven to be essential from more than one points of view: the relationship between maternal diet and cord blood lipids shows the importance of the composition of the diet of the future mother during her pregnancy. The same applies to the relationship of fat patterns in the mother and newborn son, indicating the genetic conditioning of this marker and a possible health risk at the very beginning of life.

All potentials of the human organism should develop in mutual harmony from the earliest periods of life. When we also include the criterion of "positive health," requiring mainly a high level of cardiorespiratory fitness and resistance to noxious environmental factors as well long life expectancy in full activity, we must develop more objective evaluation criteria. The endeavor to "achieve the maximal growth potential", which up to now was mostly identified with the achievement of greater body size, should be further specified. As repeated many times, all children in the world have the right to reach the highest level of potential, including body size — provided enough food is available. *Under conditions of the real world, it does not seem wise to consider body size as a priority, but rather the level of positive health, physical as well as overall fitness, and thus also the economic productivity.*

Therefore, *additional reference values of functional, motor, metabolic, and health variables are needed for the characterization of the growing organism at an early age.* This might render a more exact evaluation of the level of development possible and in time may also give the information as to whether the child is developing in an adequate way or not. The disclosure of more discreet deviations from the desirable development, which might later become a more serious health risk, has become an essential issue in the appraisal of child development. Measuring body size is the first, most important approximation, but it is necessary to know more if at all possible.

The selection of characteristics of the functional and motor development in early life used in our studies is only a modest addition which should be developed further. With the help of the above mentioned measurements, we were able e.g., to reveal relationships between slightly increased and differently distributed depot fat and serum lipids in young children (and their possible consequences). We also demonstrated the influence of the composition of the diet during pregnancy on serum lipids in newborns, especially sons. We tried to analyze the inconsistencies between body size and certain functional parameters relating mainly to cardiorespiratory fitness (which concerns both overfed or underfed growing individuals) or inconsistencies between the level of somatic, sensomotor, and gross motor development under conditions of insufficient motor stimulation. Attention should also be paid to problems of deteriorating body posture before the child enters primary school and to many other issues which seem to be relevant in relation to future health development.

Reservations regarding the actual recommended dietary allowances (RDAs), which are now considered too high (especially those for The Czech Republic) for generally hypokinetic young children, do not imply the promotion of very low food intake and/or the promotion of an inadequately intense work load. *Under conditions of industrially developed countries the dietary intake of children has reached levels that do not correspond to real needs of the young child.* The increasing prevalence of obesity, dyslipoproteinemias, disorders of carbohydrate metabolism, and so on stimulates an earlier onset of cardiovascular diseases, precipitates the development of atherosclerosis in genetically predisposed individuals, and can precondition even normal children to pathological problems later in life.

To recommend more modest nutrition still contradicts family customs in most industrially developed countries. However, the example set by long-lastingg populations, as well as the results of experimental models, seem to indicate that such an adjustment would be useful. "Has malnutrition only bad consequences? What is the definition of health?" were the questions posed by G. Fanconi,[102] who showed a number of advantages to adequately lower food intake.

The population explosion and the occasional lack of resources results not only from the *number of inhabitants in the actual world, but also from their size:* all of these together require more and more resources. The definition of some "optimal minimum" or "minimal optimum" of diet seems to be justified, for not enough food is available under present conditions in all parts of the world. Even under adverse circumstances, adequate manipulation of reduced dietary intake can ultimately result in at least an acceptable development of the growing child. As indicated by the assessments in children from developing countries, under conditions of *"marginal malnutrition"* (by which we can understand *smaller body size and reduced fat deposition,* with *preserved size and function of vital organs and essential muscle groups) a better level of cardiovascular fitness can be achieved.* Moreover, there seems to be evidence that such a physical status used to be *natural not very long ago*when motion and greater physical work loads were a much more integral part of life.

In spite of the fact that it is impossible to directly apply the conclusions from animal studies to humans, there seems to be corresponding evidence from a number of experimental models. The importance of the level of physical activity during pregnancy or of certain dietary modifications, including a more modest intake of protein and energy at the beginning of life, was shown to have positive results on the later development of spontaneous physical activity, on changes in body composition or certain characteristics of lipid metabolism, as well as on cardiac microstructure, resistance to noxious substances inducing the development of cardiac necrosis, etc. The experience with high RDAs for protein and fats (which are mostly exceeded) in the Czech Republic result not only in higher BMI in early childhood, but also might contribute to higher morbidity and mortality from atherosclerosis and other cardiovascular diseases, especially in Eastern Europe. Recent trends toward improving these conditions run parallel to certain adjustments in the diet.

For physiological reasons, *during growth it is much more justifiable to adjust the energy balance and turnover by increasing energy output* — mainly by increased physical activity — rather than to reduce the food intake corresponding to reduced energy output, as this is associated with risks of inbalance and deficiencies of some essentialdietary ingredients. The definition of a reduced, but fully adequate, diet for young growing children in practical life would be very difficult. *The influence of inadequately increased food intake is not manifested immediately, but seems to be a predisposition for later obesity, dyslipoproteinemias, etc., thus increasing the health risk in later life.* Therefore, even if modifications of the actual diet are needed, the main adjustment concerns the general lifestyle with much *more activity and exercise.*

The growth of children in long lived populations, e.g., in Caucasus, is slower; sexual maturation occurs later, and the growth period is longer than elsewhere. People are characterized by more marked development of lean body mass — especially muscles — and a low fat ratio. They also have an active lifestyle until advanced age. There are certainly other factors that influence the lifespan of these people; however, they may serve as a model for our lifestyle.

Promotion of a higher level of physical activity and exercise in early life seems to be justified or even self-evident. *Unfortunately, in industrially developed countries, most parents stop being interested in further motor development when their child is able to walk unassisted.* This is just the moment, though, when motor abilities could be developed to a higher level, which is also a predisposition for a higher level of fitness and functional capacity later in life. Well-developed motor abilities are a predisposition for more intense involvement in physical exercise, which becomes more enjoyable because it is less straining. This also encourages children to remain active throughout life.

It is a great mistake to leave the development of motor abilities to chance. Many parents think that with further growth the child will automatically learn new skills, and that all necessary motor abilities will develop without any assistance. This does not apply to any other faculty, and it is also not true for motor development — at least not in every child. Along with motor skills and other improvements of the functional capacity, the child also acquires other faculties — courage, readiness, independence, proper attitude to unknown situations, and so forth. Of course, it is necessary to supervise children, not leaving them unattended in an unsafe situation. All the above mentioned qualities are not only advantageous for the children, but also for their parents.

Slight retardation in motor development does not translate to a great handicap. It is a warning, though, for the parents not to neglect this aspect of education, but to make an effort to improve the situation.

Motor stimulation at early age can support and improve the development of children in relation to functional, motor, and work performance,*which may apply even under conditions of reduced dietary intake*; motor stimulation may also have, under special conditions, an anabolic influence on the growing child (provided it is adequate according to the developmental stage). This may be a supporting factor in the development and rehabilitation of populations with limited resources.

Some of the main issues on the program of international congresses on nutrition during the last decades focused on two problems: on the one hand, the consequences of lack of food and eventually on child labor, especially in children of the Third World countries. On the other hand, the consequences of excess eating along with hypokinesia, which belong to the most important pathogenetic factors of the diseases which are the main killers in the industrially developed countries, was also a main focus. The importance of early intervention regarding diet and physical activity regime in young children is now recognized. Many of these changes could be made by returning to old customs of a more modest diet and an ample opportunity for play and exercise in early life. Education, in any respect, has to be individualized and adjusted to the particular character of the child: as J.A. Comenius reminds us[57–59] "some need a bridle, the others spurs ..." The same applies to motor education; an individual approach is needed, created to a child's particular predisposition and liking.

Therefore, it is necessary to find ways that can help children cope with actual health problems and, even under adverse conditions of any kind, to achieve optimal results regarding overall fitness, high economic production, high resistance to noxious factors and long life expectancy, in full and ample activity. Early intervention in physical activity, dietary regimens, and functional development can improve our perspectives, under both conditions of abundance and of scarcity.

> "The hope of universal reform of the world depends entirely on the first stage of education. Our nature — in body, mind, morals, pursuits, conversation, and gesture — is conditioned by our earliest education and training of adolescence that follows it. If this is right and aims at high standards of truth and goodness, those who had the advantage of it must exceed the others ..."

J.A. Comenius, Pampaedia, 1640

Appendix 1

BODY POSTURE

Name:	Date of birth:		Date of examination:	
View from profile				
	1	2		3
Neck (axis)	vertical	slightly bent forward		markedly bent forward
Outline of back (s-shaped curvature)	slight	increased		very marked
Scapulae	adjacent, not protruding	slightly protruding		protruding
Abdomen (xiphoid process)	does not proceed	proceeds can be drawn in		bulged, relaxed, flaccid, abnormally large
Depth of cervical lordosis (cm): Depth of lumbar lordosis (cm):				
View from back				
	1	2		3
Shoulders	equal height	one shoulder slightly higher (+1 cm–2 cm)		considerably higher (>+2 cm)
Scapulae (inner margins)	parallel	diverging and protruding slightly		asymmetrical protruding very
Course of spine Back Straight Deep forward bend (outline of back)	identical to string of plummet symmetrical	deviates slightly from string of plummet slightly assymmetrical		deviates considerably from string of plummet very asymmetrical

Appendix 2

STEP TEST

Name:	Date of birth:		Date of examination:		Weight:

	Rest ($\overline{X}$)	Work load (A)	Recovery (B)	
Heart rate:	☐☐☐	☐☐☐☐☐	☐☐☐☐☐	HR/min.
Minutes:	1 2 3	1 2 3 4 5	1 2 3 4 5	
	$\overline{X}$ (Σ/3)	A(Σ)	B (Σ)	

HR = mean heart per minute at rest

HR_{wr} = sum of heart beats during work (A) and recovery (B)

$HR_P = HR_{WR} - 10 \times HR \; \overline{X}$

$CEI_1 = Kpm/HR_{WR}$ Kpm = weight of the child × 150 × height of the step (25 cm)
(150 = 30 mounts during 5 minutes of work load)

$CEI_2 = Kpm/HRp$

$HR_R = B - 5 \times HR \; \overline{X}$

Index = 30,000/Σ 2nd + 3rd + 5th minute of B
(Brouha)

Appendix 3

MOTOR PERFORMANCE

Name:	Date of birth:	Date of examination:
Dash 20 m from high start ....s	**Standing broad jump** ....cm	

Throwing
   right hand ....cm
   right hand ....cm
	left hand ....cm
	left hand ....cm
		(1)
		(2)

Crossing horizontal beam	yes	no
Standing on one leg (10 seconds)	yes	no

Forward roll
perfect turning on shoulders straight
correct but small deviation of
  direction
incorrect turning on back of head
Impaired direction, incorrect
  procedure
not properly "followed", deviation,
  incorrect
	5
	4
	
	3
	2
	
	1	

Walking at a given speed, rhythm	yes	no

Catching ball:
  1. Child throws ball on ground and
     after the ball strikes the ground,
     the child
	catches	does not catch the ball

2. The adult throws the ball two
     steps in front of the child; after
     it strikes the ground the child
	catches	does not catch the ball

3. The same, but catching with one hand (the palm upwards)	catches	does not catch the ball

4. The adult throws the ball above
     the child who is supposed to
     catch it in the air
	catches	does not catch the ball

Note: The evaluation of tests with two grades (yes = 1, no = 2) gives the average numbers which by values exceeding 1 define also the percentage of subjects not fulfilling the test (2).

SENSOMOTOR TESTS

Opening and closing the hands	1	2
1. Both hands are opened and closed simultaneously	yes	no
2. One hand opens continuously, the other remains closed	yes	no
3. Same with other hand	yes	no
4. One hand opens and closes, the other hand opens and closes	yes	no
5. Alternate opening and closing hands: one hand opens, the other closes etc.	yes	no
6. Consecutive opening and closing of hands: one opens, the other one closes	yes	no
Spatial orientation		
1. Point hand downwards	yes	no
2. Point hand upwards	yes	no
Laterality		
1. Show your left hand	yes	no
2. Show your right hand	yes	no
3. Show with your left hand your right knee	yes	no
Special comments		
1. Child wears spectacles	yes	no
2. Other abnormalities	yes	no

REFERENCES

1. **Ahlgren-Olhager, E., Thoumas, C.-A., Wigström, L., and Forsum, E.,** Description, evaluation and application of a method based on magnetic resonance imaging to measure adipose tissue volume and total body fat of infants, in *The 6th European Congress on Obesity,* Abstract Book, *Int. J. Obes.,* 19 (Suppl. 2), 1995, 42.

2. **Akerblom, H. K., Viikari, M., Uhari, M., et al.,** Multicenter study of atherosclerosis precursors in Finnish children: report of two pilot studies, in *Children and Sport,* Ilmarinen, J. and Valimäki, I., Eds., Springer, Heidelberg, 1984, 219.

3. **Akerblom, H., Viikari, J., Räsanen, L., Kuusela, V., Uhari, M., and Lautala, P.,** Cardiovascular risk in young Finns. Results from the second follow-up-study, *Ann. Med.,* 21, 223, 1989.

4. **Alberti-Fidanza, A., Ekokobe, E., Fruttini, D., and Genipi, L.,** Anthropometric measurements, food habits, food preferences and aversions, and physical activity in a group of Cameroon and Italian children, in *Proc. Symp. Human Growth, Dietary Intake and Other Environmental Influences,* 13th ICAES (Int. Congr. Anthrop. Ethnol. Sci.), Mexico City, 1993, Pařízková, J. and Douglas, P. D., Eds., Danone, Paris, 1995, 27.

5. **Alberti-Fidanza, A. and Fidanza, F.,** A nutrition study involving a group of pregnant women in Assisi, Italy. I. Anthropometry, dietary intake and nutrition knowledge, practices and attitudes, *Int. J. Vit. Nutr. Res.,* 56, 373, 1986.

6. **Alberti-Fidanza, A., Pařízková, J., and Fruttini, D.,** Relationships between mother's and newborn's nutritional and blood lipid variables, *Eur. J. Clin. Nutr.,* 49, 289, 1995.

7. **Alberti-Fidanza, A., Pařízková, J., and Fruttini, D.,** Changes in anthropometric variables and fat pattern during pregnancy and their relationship to newborn values, in press.

8. **Albertson, A. M., Tobelman, R. C., Engström, A., and Asp, E. H.,** Nutrient intakes of 2- to 10-year-old American children: 10-year trends, *J. Am. Diet. Assoc.,* 92, 1492, 1992.

9. **Allix, E.,** *Étude sur la Physiologie de la Première Enfance,* Paris, 1867.

10. **Amador, M., Flores, P., and Pena, M.,** Normocaloric diet and exercise: a good choice for treating obese adolescents, *Acta Pediatr. Hung.,* 30, 123, 1990.

11. **Areskog, N. H., Selinus, R., and Vahlquist, A.,** Physical working capacity and nutritional status in Ethiopian male children and young adults, *Am. J. Clin. Nutr.,* 22, 471, 1969.

12. **Arshavskyi, I. A.,** *Developmental Physiology,* Medicina, Moscow, 1967 (in Russian).

13. **Bal, L., Smirnova, S., and Zaborskis, A.,** "Pro" and "con" of early obesity prevention in children population, in 7th Int. Congress on Obesity, Toronto, Canada 1994, *Int. J. Obesity* 18 (Suppl. 2), 15, 1994.

14. **Barac-Nieto, M., Spurr, G. B., and Reina, J. C.,** Marginal malnutrition in school-aged Colombian boys: body composition and maximal oxygen consumption, *Am. J. Clin. Nutr.,* 39, 830, 1984.

15. **Baranowski, T., Bryna, G. T., Harrison, J. A., and Rassin, D. K.,** Height, infant feeding and cardiovascular functioning among 3 and 4 year old children in three ethnic groups, *J. Clin. Epidemiol.,* 42, 513, 1992.

16. **Bar-Or, O.,** *Pediatric Sports Medicine,* Springer-Verlag, New York, 1983.

17. **Barker, D. J. P.,** The fetal and infant origin of adult disease, *Br. Med. J.,* 301, 1111, 1990.

18. **Barker, D. J. P.,** *Fetal and infant origin of adult disease,* British Medical Journal Publishing Group, London, 1992.

19. **Basch, C. E., Zybert, P., and Shea, S.,** 5-A-DAY: dietary behavior and the fruit and vegetable intake of Latino children, *Am. J. Public Health,* 84, 814, 1994.

20. **Beaton, G. H.,** Small but healthy? Are we asking the right question?, *Eur. J. Clin. Nutr.,* 43, 563, 1989.

21. **Bedi, K. S.,** Lasting neuroanatomical changes following undernutrition during early life, in *Early Nutrition and Later Development,* Dobbing, J., Ed., Academic Press, London, 1987, 1.

22. **Bellu, R., Ortisi, M. T., and Giovanini, M.,** Determination of intra- and inter-individual variability and its effect on the number of days required to assess the usual intake of a 1-year-old infant population, *Pediatr. Perinat. Epidemiol.,* 9, 1, 1995.

23. **Bencko, V.,** Health risk of indoor air pollutants: a Central European perspective, *Indoor Environ.,* 3, 213, 1994.

24. **Benedict F. G. and Talbot, F. B.,** *Metabolism and growth from birth to puberty,* Washington, D.C., Carnegie Institute, Publ. No. 302, 1921.

25. **Bénéfice, E.,** Motor skills of mild-malnourished compared with normal preschool Senegalese children, *Early Child Dev. Care,* 61, 81, 1990.

26. **Bénéfice, E.,** Fitness of healthy Senegalese children living in Sahelian environment, in *Human Growth, Dietary Intake and Other Environmental Influences,* Proc. Symp., 13th ICAES (Int. Congr. Anthropological Ethnology Sci.), Mexico 1993, Pařízková, J. and Douglas, P. D., Eds., Danone, Paris, 1995, 32.

27. **Berdychová, J.,** *Mother, Father Exercise with Me,* Olympia, Prague, 1969 (in Czech; then also in German — Südwest Verlag, München 1975; Polish — Warszawa 1972; Serbian-Beograd 1973; Russian — Moscow 1975; Spanish — Havana 1976; Japanese — 1979; Bulgarian — Sofia 1974; Slovak — Bratislava 1970 and 1985).

28. **Berdychová, J.,** *Mother, Father Exercise with Me — At Home, in the Open Air, in Sokol,* Sokolvzlet, Prague, 1993 (in Czech).

29. **Berdychová, J.,** *So as Our Children Grow Up Healthy,* Olympia, Prague 1978 (in Czech).

30. **Best, W. R.,** An improved caliper for measurement of skinfold thickness, *J. Lab. Clin. Med.,* 43, 967, 1954.

31. **Birch, L. L., Johnson, S. L., Andresen, G., Peters, J. C., and Schulte, M. C.,** The variability of young children's energy intake, *N. Engl. J. Med.,* 324, 232, 1991.

32. **Black, A. E., Billewicz, W. Z., and Thomson, A.,** The diets of preschool children in Newcastle-upon-Tyne 1968–1971, *Br. J. Nutr.,* 35, 105, 1976.

33. **Black, A. E., Cole, T. J., Wiles, S. J., and White, F.,** Daily variation in food intake of infants from 2 to 18 months, *Hum. Nutr. Appl. Nutr.,* 37A, 448, 1983.

34. **Blade, B. L., Dudman, N. P., Wilcken, D. E.,** Screening for familial hypercholesterolemia in 5000 neonates: a recall study, *Pediatr. Res.,* 23, 500, 1988.

35. **Bláha P.,** *W/H² Body Mass Index of the Current Czechoslovak Population Between the Ages of 3 to 70,* Institute of Sports Medicine, Prague, 1991.

36. **Blair, S. N., Kohl, H. W., Gordon, N. F., and Paffenberger, R. S.,** How much physical activity is good for health?, *Annu. Rev. Publ. Health,* 13, 9, 1992.

37. **Bleyl, D. W. and Przibylski, H.,** Diaplacental transition of selected fatty acids in the rat, *Nahrung,* 35, 107, 1991.

38. **Bouchard C. and Johnston F. E., Eds.,** *Fat distribution during growth and later health outcomes,* Alan R. Liss, New York, 1988.

39. **Bouchard, C., Perussé, L., Leblanc, C., Tremblay, A., and Theriault, G.,** Inheritance of the amount and distribution of human body fat, *Int. J. Obes.,* 12, 205, 1988.

40. **Bouchard, C., Tremblay, A., Després, J. P., Theriault, G., Nadeau, A., Lupien, P. J., Moorjani, S., Prudhomme, D., and Fourrier, G.,** The response to exercise with constant energy intake in identical twins, *Obesity Res.,* 2, 400, 1994.

41. **Boyd E.,** in *Growth Including Reproduction and Morphological Development,* Altman P.L. and Dittmer D.S., Eds., *Federation of American Societies for Experimental Biology,* Washington, D.C., 1962, 346.

42. **Brook, C. G. D.,** Determination of body composition of children from skinfold measurements, *Arch. Dis. Child.,* 46, 182, 1975.

43. **Brown, J. E. and Tieman, P.,** Effect of income and WIC on the dietary intake of preschoolers: results of a preliminary study, *J. Am. Diet. Assoc.,* 86, 1189, 1986.

44. **Brown, R. E.,** Organ weight in malnutrition with special reference to brain weight, *Dev. Med. Child Neurol.,* 8, 512, 1966.

45. **Brožek, J.,** From QUACK stick to a compositional assessment of man's nutritional status, in *Nutrition and Malnutrition, Identification and Measurement,* Roche, A. F. and Falkner, F., Eds., *Advances in Experimental Medicine and Biology,* Vol. 49, Plenum Press, New York, 1974, 151.

46. **Canadian Task Force on the Periodic Health Association,** Periodic health examination, 1994 update. I. Obesity in childhood, *Can. Med. Assoc. J.,* 150, 871, 1994.

47. **Carter J. E. L. and Heath B. H.,** *Somatotyping — Development and Applications,* Cambridge University Press, Cambridge, 1990.

48. **Cashdan, E.,** A sensitive period for learning about food, *Hum. Nature,* 5, 279, 1994.

49. **Čermák, J.,** Möglichkeit der Wertung der Funktionstüchtigkeit des Kreislaufsystems der Schuljugend mit Hilfe der eigenen Modifikation des Step teste mit durchlaufender Messung der Pulsfrequenz, *Schweiz. Z. Sport Med.,* 7, 1, 1969.

50. **Čermák, J., Pařízková, J., Venclík, Z., and Mařaková, A.,** Reaction of the circulatory system of preschool children to a work load of medium intensity as related to the degree of somatic development, *Physiol. Bohemoslov.,* 22, 377, 1973.

51. **Chavez, A. and Martinez, C.,** School performance of supplemented and unsupplemented children from a poor rural area, in *Nutrition in Health and Disease, an International Development,* Harper, A.E. and Davis, G.K., Eds., Alan R. Liss, New York, 1981, 393.

52. **Chavez, A. and Martinez, C.,** Behavioral measurements of activity in children and their relation to food intake in a poor community, in *Energy Intake and Activity,* Pollitt, E. and Amante, P., Eds., Alan R. Liss, New York, 1984, 303.

53. **Chinn, S. and Rona, R. J.,** Trends in weight-for-height and triceps skinfold thickness for English and Scottish children, *Paediatr. Perinat. Epidemiol.,* 8, 90, 1994.

54. **Chopra, J. S., Upinder, K., et al.,** Effect of protein-energy malnutrition on peripheral nerves: electrophysiological and histopathological study, *Brain,* 109, 307, 1986.

55. **Clapp, J. F., Capekess, E. L.,** Neonatal morphometrics after endurance exercise during pregnancy, *Am. J. Obstet. Gynec.,* 163, 1805, 1990.

56. **Clugston, G. A. and Garlick, P. J.,** The response of whole-body protein turnover to feeding in obese subjects given a protein-free, low-energy diet for three weeks, *Hum. Nutr. Clin. Nutr.,* 36, 391, 1982.

57. **Comenius, J. A.,** *Novissima linguarum methodus (1646),* Opera omnia, Akademia, Prague 1959, 91.

58. **Comenius, J. A.,** Schola Infantiae (1632), in *School of Infancy,* (1650–4), chap. 5 (translated by Will S. Monroe), Boston, 1983.

59. **Comenius, J. A.,** School of birth, in *Panpaedia, or Universal Education* (1650), chap. 8, Buckland Publications, Dover, U.K., 1956, 103.

60. **Conning, D., Ed.,** *Early Diet, Later Consequences,* Proc. 13th Brit. Nutr. Foundation Annual Conference, 14 June, 1991, British Nutritional Foundation, London, 1991.

61. **Cooper, K. H.,** *Kid Fitness. The Complete Shape-up Program From Birth Through High School,* Bantan Books, New York, 1991.

62. **Cratty, B. J.,** *Perceptual and Motor Development in Infants and Children,* Prentice-Hall, Englewood Cliffs, NJ, 1986.

63. **Cratty, B. J., Cortinas, D., and Kelly, J.,** *The Motor Abilities of Elementary School Children,* unpublished monograph, Perceptual Learning Laboratory, UCLA, Los Angeles, CA, 1973.

64. **Cravioto, J. and Arrieta, R.,** *Nutrición, Desarrollo Mental, Conducta y Aprendizaje. Sistema Nacional para el Desarrollo Integral de la Familía (DIF),* Instituto Nacional de Ciencias y Tecnologias — DIF, Centro Colaborador de la Organizacion Mundial de la Salud en Crecimiento y Desarrollo, Impresiones Modernas, S. A. Mexico, 1985.

65. **Cravioto, J. and Cravioto, P.,** Some long-term psychologic consequences of malnutrition, *Ann. Nestle,* 48, 93, 1990.

66. **Cravioto, J. and DeLicardie, E. R.,** Malnutrition in early childhood and some of its later effects at individual and community levels, *Food Nutr.,* 2, 2, 1976.

67. **Croft, J. B., Cresanta, L., Webber, L. S., Srinivasan, S. R., Freedman, D. S., Burke, G. L., and Berenson, G. S.,** Cardiovascular risk in parents of children with extreme lipoprotein cholesterol level: the Bogalusa Heart Study, *South. Med. J.,* 81, 341, 1988.

68. **Crouchman, M.,** The effect of babywalkers on early locomotor development, *Dev. Med. Child. Neurol.,* 28, 757, 1986.

69. **Cunnane S. C. and Chen, Y. Z.,** Triacylglycerol: an important pool of essential fatty acids during early postnatal development of rat, *Am. J. Physiol.,* 262, R8, 1992.

70. **Dancis, R.,** Transfer of free fatty acids across human placenta, in *Early Diabetes in Early Life,* Camerini-Davalos, R. A. and Cole, H. S., Eds., Academic Press, New York, 1975, 233.

71. **Darvay, S., Agfalvi, R., and Bodanszky, H.,** A longitudinal study of the growth of low birth weight infants (from births to 3 years), in *Growth and Ontogenetial Development in Man IV.,* Hajniš, K., Ed., Charles University, Prague, 1994, 25.

72. **Dauncey, M. J.,** Activity and energy expenditure, *Can. J. Physiol. Pharmacol.,* 68, 17, 1990.

73. **Davies, C. T. M.,** Physiological response to exercise in East African children. I. Normal values for rural and urban boys and girls aged 7–15 years, *Environ. Child Health,* June, 110, 1973.

74. **Davies, K. and Christoffel, K. K.,** Obesity in preschool and school-age children. Treatment early and often may be best, *Arch. Pediatr. Adolesc. Med.,* 148, 125, 1994.

75. **Davies, P. S. W., Coward, W. A., Gregory, J., White, A., and Mills, A.,** Total energy expenditure and energy intake in the pre-school child: a comparison, *Br. J. Nutr.,* 72, 13, 1994.

76. **Davies, P. S. W., Gregory, J., and White, A.,** Energy expenditure in children 1.5 to 4.5 years: a comparison with current recommendations for energy intake, *Eur. J. Clin. Nutr.,* 49, 360, 1995a.

77. **Davies, P. S. W., Gregory, J., and White, A.,** Physical activity and body fatness in preschool children, *Int. J. Obes.,* 19, 6, 1995b.

78. **DeMayer, E. and Adiels-Tegman, O.,** The prevalence of anemia in the world, *W.H.O. Statistical Q.,* 38, 302, 1985.

79. **DeToni, G., Aicardi, G., Bulgarelli, R., Dalla Volta A., DeToni, E., and Gobessi, I.,** *Auxologia,* Vol. 2, *Auxologia Postnatale Fisiologica,* Edizioni Minerva Medica, Stabilimento di Saluzzo, 1968.

80. **Dietz, W. H.,** Critical periods in childhood for the development of obesity, *Am. J. Clin. Nutr.,* 59, 955, 1994.

81. **DiPietro, L., Mossberg, H. O., and Stunkard, A. J.,** A 40-year history of overweight children in Stockholm: life-time overweight, morbidity and mortality, *Int. J. Obes. Relat. Metab. Disord.,* 18, 585, 1994.

82. **Ditschuneit, H.,** Obesity and related disorders, in *Obesity in Europe 1991, Proc. 3rd Eur. Congr. Obesity,* Ailhaud, G., Guy-Grand, B., Lafonta, M., and Ricquier, D., Eds., John Libbey, London, 1992, 191.

83. **Dobbing, J.,** Early nutrition and later achievement, *Proc. Nutr. Soc.,* 49, 103, 1990.

84. **Dobbing, J. and Sands, J.,** Quantitative growth and development of human brain, *Arch. Dis. Childhood,* 48, 757, 1973.

85. **Doležaļ A. and Gutwirt, J., Eds.,** *Antropologia Maternitatis,* Proc. Conf., Prague, 1975, Universitas Carolina Pragensis, 1977.

86. **Donker, G. A., Goff, D. C. Jr., Ragan, J. D., Killinger, R. B., Harrist, R. B., and Labarthe, D. R.,** Factors associated with serum cholesterol level in a pediatric practice. Cholesterol screening in a pediatric practice, *Ann. Epidemiol.,* 3, 49, 1993.

87. **Duerenberg, P., Smit, H. E., and Kusters, C. S.,** Is the bioelectrical impedance method suitable for epidemiological field studies?, *Eur. J. Clin. Nutr.,* 43, 647, 1989.

88. **DuRant, R. H., Baranowski, T., Johnson, M., and Thompson, W. O.,** The relationship among television watching, physical activity, and body composition of young children, *Pediatrics,* 94, 449, 1994.

89. **DuRant, R. H., Baranowski, T., Rhodes, T., Gutin, B., Thompson, W. O., Carroll, R., Puhl, J., and Greaves, K. A.,** Association among serum lipid and lipoprotein concentrations and physical activity, physical fitness, and body composition in young children, *J. Pediatr. .,* 123, 185, 1993a.

90. **DuRant, R. H., Baranowski, T., Puhl, J., Rhodes, T., Davis, H., Greaves, K. A., and Thompson, W. O.,** Evaluation of the children's activity rating scale (CARS) in young children, *Med. Sci. Sports Exerc.,* 25, 1415, 1993b.

91. **Durnin, J. V. A. G., Lonergan, M. E., Good, J., and Ewan, A.,** A cross-sectional nutritional and anthropometric study with an interval of 7 years on 611 young adolescent children. *Br. J. Nutr.,* 32, 169, 1974.

92. **Durnin, J. V. G. A.,** Energy balance in childhood and adolescence, *Proc. Nutr. Soc.,* 43, 271, 1984.

93. **Elcarte-Lopez, R., Villa-Elizaga, I., Sada-Goni, J., Gasco-Eguiluz, M., Oyar-Irigoyen, M., Sola-Mateos, A., Garcia Ibero, C., Elcarte-Lopez, T., Ferrer, G., and Fontaneda-Estibaliz, A.,** A study from Navara. Hiperlipidemias. Average scores and percentage of lipids and lipoproteins in a population of children and adolescents. Correlation with anthropometric parameters, *An. Esp. Pediatr.,* 38, 307, 1993 (in Spanish).

94. **Ellis, K. J. and Shypailo, R. J.,** Whole body potassium measurements independent of body size, *Basic Life Sci.,* 60, 371, 1993.

95. **Ellis, K. J., Shypailo, R. J., Pratt, J. A., and Pond, W. G.,** Accuracy of dual-energy X-ray absorptiometry for body-composition measurements in children, *Am. J. Clin. Nutr.,* 60, 660, 1994.

96. **Erikson, E. H.,** *Childhood and Society,* W.W. Norton, New York, 1950, 117.

97. **Eveleth, P. B. and Tanner, J. M.,** *Worldwide Variation in Human Growth.,* 2nd ed., Cambridge University Press, Cambridge, 1990.

98. **Falkner, F. and Tanner, J. M., Eds.,** *Human Growth. II. Postnatal Growth,* Plenum Press, New York, 1979.

99. **Faltová, E. and Pařízková, J.,** Effect of age, body weight and body fat on experimental cardiac necrosis, *Physiol. Bohemoslov.,* 19, 275, 1970.

100. **Faltová, E. and Pařízková, J., Mráz, M., Šedivý, J., and Špátová, M.,** Influence of motor activity on the development of isoprenaline induced heart lesions, *Physiol. Bohemoslov.,* 32, 203, 1983.

101. **Faltová, E., Mráz, M., Pařízková, J., and Šedivý, J.,** Physical activity of different intensities and the development of myocardial resistance to injury, *Physiol. Bohemoslov.,* 34, 289, 1985.

102. **Fanconi, G.,** Has malnutrition only bad consequences? What is the definition of health?, in *Protein-Calorie Malnutrition,* von Muralt, A., Ed., Nestle Foundation, Springer Verlag, Berlin, 1969, 57.

103. **FAO/WHO ad hoc,** *Expert Committee Report on Energy and Protein Requirements,* FAO Meet. Rep. Ser. No. 257, Her Majesty's Stationary Office, London, 1973.

104. **Ferro-Luzzi, A., D'Amicis, A., Ferrini, A. M., and Maiale, G.,** Nutrition, environment and physical performance of preschool children in Italy, in *Nutritional Aspects of Physical Performance,* Somogyi, C. and deWijn, JF., Eds., S. Karger, Basel, 1977, 85.

105. **Fidanza, F.,** *Nutritional Status Assessment,* A Manual for Population Studies, Fidanza, F., Ed., Chapman & Hall, London, 1991.

106. **Fidanza F. and Versiglioni N.,** Tabelle di Compositione degli Alimenti, Idelson, Napoli, Italy, 1989.

107. **Field, C. R., Freundt-Thurne, J., and Schoeller, D. A.,** Total body water measured by [18]O dilution and bioelectrical impedance in well and malnourished children, *Pediatr. Res.,* 27, 98, 1990.

108. **Figueroa-Colon, R., et al.** Childhood obesity: nature versus nurture, *Pediatr. Adolesc. Med.,* 2, 1, 1992.

109. **Fiorotto, M. and Klish, W. J.,** Total body conductivity measurements in the neonate, *Clin. Perinatol.,* 18, 611, 1991.

110. **Firouzbakhsh, S., Mathis, R. K., Dorchester, W. L., Oseas, R. S., Groncy, P. K., Grant, K. E., and Finkelstein. J. Z.,** Measured resting energy expenditure in children, *J. Pediatr. Gastroenterol. Nutr.,* 16, 136, 1993.

111. **Fomon, S. J., Haschke, F., Ziegler, E. E., and Nelson, S. E.,** Body composition of reference children from birth to age of 10 years, *Am. J. Clin. Nutr.,* 35 (Suppl. 5), 1169, 1982.

112. **Fontvieille, A. M., Harper, I. T., Ferraro, R. T., Spraul, M., and Ravussin, E.,** Daily energy expenditure by five-year-old children, measured by labelled water, *J. Pediatr.,* 123, 200, 1993.

113. **Fox, P. T., Elston, M. D., and Waterlow, J. C.,** Pre-school child survey, in *Sub-Committee on Nutritional Surveillance: Second Report,* Her Majesty's Stationery Office, Dept. Health and Social Security, Report of Health and Social Subjects 21, London, 1981, 64.

114. **Fraňková, S.,** Behavioral responses of rats to early overnutrition, *Nutr. Metabol.,* 12, 228, 1970.

115. **Fraňková, S.,** Lasting effects of early malnutrition on children's behaviour, *Bibl. Nutr. Dieta,* 31, 40, 1982.

116. **Fraňková, S.,** Nutrition and behavior: animals (other than primates), in *CRC Handbook of Nutritional Requirements in a Functional Context,* vol. II, Rechcigl, M., Ed., 1981, 479.

117. **Fraňková, S. and Barnes, R. H.,** Influence of malnutrition in early life on exploratory behavior of rats, *J. Nutr.,* 96, 477, 1968.

118. **Fuertez-Dominguez, A., el-Musa-Munir, M., and Perez Gonzales, J. M.,** Feeding and growth during the first year of life, *Ann. Esp. Pediatr.,* 32, 427, 1990.

119. **Gage, T. B. and O'Connor, K.,** Nutrition and the variation in level and age patterns of mortality, *Hum. Biol.,* 66, 77, 1994.

120. **Galloway, R. and Anderson, M. A.,** Prepregnancy nutritional status and its impact on birthweight, *SCN News,* United Nations, No. 11, 1994, 6.

121. **Gapon, A. Ya.,** Investigation of habitual physical activity in mental workers, in *Physical Activity in Man and Hypokinesia,* Slonim, A. D. and Smirnov, K. M., Eds., Academy of Sciences, Siberian Dept., Novosibirsk, 1972, 46 (in Russian).

122. **Gardner, J. M. and Grantham-McGregor, S. M.,** Physical activity, undernutrition and child development, *Proc. Nutr. Soc.,* 53, 241, 1994.

123. **Garn, S. M.,** The earlier gain and later loss of cortical bone, in *Nutritional Perspectives,* Charles C Thomas, Springfield, IL, 1970.

124. **Gerald, L. B., Andersson, A., Johnson, G. D., Hoff, C., and Trimm, R. F.,** Social class, social support and obesity risk in children, *Child Care Health Dev.,* 20, 145, 1994.

125. **Ghesquiere, J. and D'Hulst, C.,** Growth, stature and fitness of children in tropical areas, in *Capacity for Work in the Tropics,* Collins, K. and Roberts, D., Eds., Cambridge University Press, Cambridge, 1988, 165.

126. **Ghosh, S., Vaid, K., et al.,** Effect of degree and duration of PEM on peripheral nerves in children, *J. Neurol. Neurosurg. Psychiatr.,* 42, 760, 1979.

127. **Ginzburg, B. E. and Zetterstrom, R.,** Serum cholesterol concentrations in early infancy, *Acta Pediatr. Scand.,* 69, 581, 1980.

128. **Gobedzhishvili, M. S., Kondrateva I. I., and Abdushelishvili, G. V.,** Daily energy consumption, physiological standards of energy requirement and energy value of food rations for children in boarding schools of the Georgian SSR, *Vopr. Pitaniya,* 4, 37, 1990 (in Russian).

129. **Godfrey, S. and Baum, J. D.,** *Clinical paediatric physiology,* Blackwell Scientific, Oxford, 1979.

130. **Gonzales-Moran, I., Sarria-Chueca, A., Bueno-Sanchez, M., and Abos-Olivarez, M. D.,** Estudie de ritmos circadianos de cortisol e insulina en la obesidad nutricional infantil, *An. Esp. Pediatr.,* 30, 79, 1989.

131. **Gopalan, C.,** "Small is healthy?" For the poor, not for the rich, *Nutr. Found. India Bull.,* October 1983.

132. **Gopalan, C.,** Maternal health, fertility control and child nutrition, *Nutr. Found. India Bull.,* 6, 1, 1985.

133. **Goran, M. I., Carpenter, W. H., and Poehlman, E. T.,** Total energy expenditure in 4- to 6-year-old children, *Am. J. Physiol.,* 264, E706, 1993.

134. **Goran, M. I., Kaskoun, M. C., Carpenter, W. H., Poehlmann, E. T., Ravussin, E., and Fontveille, A. M.,** Estimating body composition of young children by using bioelectrical resistance, *J. Appl. Physiol.,* 75, 1776, 1993.

135. **Goran, M. I., Kaskoun, M., and Johnson, R.,** Determinants of resting energy expenditure in young children, *J. Pediatr.,* 125, 362, 1994.

136. **Gortmaker, S. L., Dietz, W. H., and Cheung, W. Y.,** Inactivity, diet, and the fattening of America, *J. Am. Diet. Assoc.,* 90, 1247, 1990.

137. **Gould, J. H. and DeJong, A. R.,** Injuries to children involving home exercise equipment, *Arch. Pediat. Adolesc. Med.,* 148, 110, 1994.

138. **Grantham-McGregor, S. M.,** The effect of malnutrition on mental development, in *Protein Energy Malnutrition,* Waterlow, J. C., Ed., Edward Arnold, London, 1992, 344.

139. **Greaves, K. A. and Thompson, W. O.,** Evaluation of the children's activity rating scale (CARS) in young children, *Med. Sci. Sports,* 25, 1415, 1993.

140. **Greaves, K. A.,** Lipids and lipoproteins in a triethnic sample of 5- to 6-year-old Type A or Type B children, *Behav. Med.,* 16, 133, 1990.

141. **Gregory, J. R., Collins, D. L., Davies, P. S. W., Hughes, J. M., and Clarke, P. C.,** *National Diet and Nutrition Survey: children aged 1 1/2 to 4 1/2 years,* Vol. 1, *Report of the Diet and Nutrition Survey,* HMSO, London, 1995.

142. **Griffiths, M. and Payne, P. R.,** Energy expenditure in small children of obese and non-obese parents, *Nature (London),* 260, 698, 1976.

143. **Griffiths, M., Payne, P. R., Stunkard, A. J., Rivers, J. P. W., and Cox, M.,** Metabolic rate and physical development in children at risk of obesity, *Lancet,* 336, 76, 1990.

144. **Guminskyi, A. A., Elizarova, O. S., Zhurkova, N. N., Zolotayko, G. A., and Novozhilova, A. D.,** On functional acceleration of actual youth, *Pediyatriya,* No. 3., 10, 1972 (in Russian).

145. **Guo, S. S., Roche, A. F., Chumlea, W. C., Gardner, J. D., and Siervogel, R. M.,** The predictive value of childhood body mass index values for overweight at age 35y, *Am. J. Clin. Nutr.,* 59, 810, 1994.

146. **Gutin, B., Basch, C., Shea, S., Contento, I., DeLozier, M., Rips, J., Irigoyen, M., and Zybert, P.,** Blood pressure, fitness, and fatness in 5- to 6-year-old children, *JAMA,* 264, 1123 1990.

147. **Hajniš, K.,** Die neue Wachstumsnorm der tschechischen und slowakischen Kinder und Jugendlichen, *Antrop. Anz.,* 51, 207, 1993.

148. **Hambidge, K. M., Hambidge, C., Jacobs, M., and Baum J. D.,** Low levels of zinc in hair, anorexia, poor growth, and hypogensia in children, *Pediatr. Res.,* 6, 868, 1972.

149. **Hammer, L. D., Kraemer H. C., Wilson, D. M., Ritter, P. L., Dornbusch, S. M.,** Standardized percentile curves of body mass index for children and adolescents, *Am. J. Dis. Child.,* 145, 259, 1991.

150. **Harbottle, L. and Duggan, M. B.,** Daily variation in food and nutrient intakes of Asian children in Sheffield, *Eur. J. Clin. Nutr.,* 48, 566, 1994.

151. **Hardy, S. C. and Kleinman, R. E.,** Fat and cholesterol in the diet of infants and young children: implications for growth, development, and long-term health, *J. Pediatr.,* 125, S69, 1994.

152. **Haschke, F., Fomon, S. J., and Ziegler, E. E.,** Body composition of a nine-year-old reference boy, *Pediatr. Res.,* 15, 847, 1981.

153. **Hausman, D. B., Seerley, R. W., and Martin, R. J.,** Effect of excess dietary fat during the third trimester of pregnancy on maternal, placental and fetal metabolism in the pig, *Biol. Neonate,* 59, 257, 1991.

154. **Heath, B. H. and Carter, J. E. L.,** A modified somatotype method, *Am. J. Phys. Anthrop.,* 24, 87, 1967.

155. **Hejda, S.,** *Dietary Intake and Nutritional Status of Old People,* State Health Editing House (SZN), Prague, 1967 (in Czech).

156. **Heymsfield, S.,** Body composition methodology. 2.4. Advanced methods, in *Nutritional Status Assessment, A Manual for Population Studies,* Fidanza, F., Ed., Chapman & Hall, London, 1991, 83.

157. **Higginbotham, J. C., Baranowski, T., Carroll, R. M., Hills, A. P., and Parker, A. W.,** Obesity management via diet and exercise intervention, *Child Care Health Dev.,* 14, 409, 1988.

158. **Hiremagalur, B. K., Vadlamudi, S., Johanning, G. L., and Patel, M. S.,** Long-term effects of feeding high carbohydrate diet in pre-weaning period by gastrostomy: a new rat model for obesity, *J. Obesity,* 17, 495, 1993.

159. **Holt, T. L., Cui, C., Thomas, B. J., Ward, L. C., Quirk, P. C., Crawford, D., and Shephard, R. W.,** Clinical applicability of bioelectric impedance to measure body composition in health and disease, *Nutrition,* 10, 221, 1994.

160. **Honda M., Lowy C., and Thomas, C. R.,** The effects of maternal diabetes on placental transfer of essential and non-essential fatty acids in the rat. *Diabetes Res.,* 15, 47, 1990.

161. **Hunt, S. M. and Groff, J. L.,** *Advanced Nutrition and Human Metabolism,* West Publishing, St Paul, 1990.

162. **Huttunen, N. P., Knip, M., and Paavilainen, T.,** Physical activity and fitness in obese children, *Int. J. Obes.,* 10, 519, 1986.

163. **Imbembo, A. L. and Walser, M.,** Nutritional assessment, in *Nutritional Management, The John Hopkins Hospital Handbook,* Walser, M., Imbembo, A. L., Margolis, S., and Elfert, G. A., Eds, W. B. Saunders, Philadelphia, 1984, 18.

164. **Jackson, A. A. and Forrester, T.,** Human requirements for protein, amino acids and nitrogen: the role of urea salvage in adaptation to low intake, in *Nestle Foundation, Annual Report 1993,* Lausanne, Switzerland, 1993, 58.

165. **Jackson, A.,** How can early diet influence later disease?, in *Tomorrow's Nutrition,* Ashwell, M., Ed., The British Nutrition Foundation Nutrition Bulletin, Vol. 17 (Suppl. 1), 1992, 23.

166. **James, W. P. T. and Schofield, E. C.,** *Human energy requirements. A Manual for Planners and Nutritionists.* Oxford University Press, Oxford, 1990.

167. **Jirapinyo, P., Wongarn, R., Limsathayourat, N., and Limpwong, V.,** Compartmental change after weight reduction in childhood obesity, *J. Med. Assoc. Thai,* 75, 240, 1992.

168. **Johnson, R. K., Guthrie, H., Smiciklas-Wright, H., and Wang, M. Q.,** Characterizing nutrient intakes of children by sociodemographic factors, *Public Health Rep.,* 109, 414, 1994.

169. **Jones, D. Y., Nesheim, M. C., and Habicht, J. P.,** Influences in child growth associated with poverty in the 1970's: an examination of HANES I and HANES II, cross-sectional US national surveys, *Am. J. Clin. Nutr.,* 42, 714, 1985.

170. **Kabir, I., Malek, M. A., Rahman, M. M., Khaled, M. A., and Mahalanabis, D.,** Changes in body composition of malnourished children after dietary supplementation as measured by bioelectrical impedance, *Am. J. Clin. Nutr.,* 59, 5, 1994.

171. **Kajaba, I., Budlovský, J., Dvorský, A., Hruškovič, I., Hejda, S., Turek, B., Ošancová, K., and Jodl, J.,** New recommended dietary allowances for Czechoslovak population, *Čas. Lék. Čes.,* 131, 198, 1992 (in Czech).

172. **Kaplowitz, H. J., Wild, K. A., Mueller, W. H., Decker, M., Tanner, J. M.,** Serial and parent-child changes in components of body fat distribution and fatness in children from the London Longitudinal Growth study, ages two to eighteen years, *Hum. Biol.,* 60, 739, 1988.

173. **Karniková, R.,** Motor development of rural and Prague preschool children, in *Motor Development and Problems of Early Specialization in Preschool Age,* Methodical Bulletin of Czechoslavak Sport Assoc., Pařízková, J., Ed., Prague, 1983 (in Czech).

174. **Kaskoun, M. C., Johnson, R. K., and Goran, M. I.,** Comparison of energy intake by semiquantitative food-frequency questionnaire with total energy expenditure by the doubly labelled water method in young children, *Am. J. Clin. Nutr.,* 60, 43, 1994.

175. **Kent, G.,** Nutrition and Human Rights, *SCN News,* United Nations Administrative Committee on Coordination — Subcommittee on Nutrition, No. 10, 1993, 9.

176. **Kesteloot, H., Claes, J., and Dodion-Fransen,** *J. Eur. J. Cardiol. (abstr. from Excerpta Med.),* 2/3: 285, 1975.

177. **King, J. C., Bronstein, M. N., Fitch, L., and Wieninger, J.,** Nutrient utilization during pregnancy, *World Rev. Nutr. Diet.,* 52, 71, 1987.

178. **Kimm, S. Y., Gergen, P. J., Malloy, M., Dresser, C., and Carroll, M.,** Dietary pattern in U.S. children: implications for disease prevention, *Prev. Med.,* 19, 432, 1990.

179. **Kisteneva, G. S., Ladodo, K. S., and Stepanova, T. N.,** The energy expenditures of children of preschool age, *Vopr. Pitan.,* 6, 34, 1990 (in Russian).

180. **Klesges, R. C., Shelton, M. L., and Klesges, L. M.,** Effects of television on metabolic rate: potential implications for childhood obesity, *Pediatrics,* 91, 281, 1993.

181. **Knopp, H., Bergelin, O., Wahl, P. W., and Walden, C. E.,** Relationships of infant birth size to maternal lipoproteins, apoproteins, fuels, hormones, clinical chemistries and body weight at 36 weeks gestation, *Diabetes,* 34, 1985.

182. **Koch, J.,** *The Education of the Infant in the Family,* Avicenum, Prague, 1977 (in Czech).

183. **Koch, J.,** *Total baby development,* Wallaby Pocket Books, New York, 1978.

184. **Koivisto, U. K., Fellenius, J., and Sjöden, P. O.,** Relationships between parental mealtime practices and children's food intake, *Appetite,* 22, 245, 1994.

185. **Kraut, H.,** Food intake as a factor of production, in *Alimentation et Travail,* 1st Symp. Int. Vitell, France, 1971, Débry, G. and Blayer, R., Eds., Masson, Paris 1972, 216.

186. **Kučera, M., Berdychová, J., Javůrek, J., Pařízková, J., and Zika, K.,** Somatic development of children in early years of life, in *Report on State Plane of Research,* Fac. Pediatrics, Charles University, Prague, 1975.

187. **Kučera, M.,** The importance of physical activity of preschool children, Int. Seminar *"Child-Motion-Family",* Council of Europe, Czech Sports Organization, Prague 1994, in press.

188. **Kuczmarski, R. J., Flegal, K. M., Campbell, S. M., and Johnson, C. L.,** Increasing prevalence of overweight among U.S. adults, *JAMA,* 272, 205, 1994.

189. **Kvapilík, J. and Černá, M.,** *Physical activity of mentally retarded,* National Center of Health Promotion, Prague, 1992 (in Czech).

190. **Lawrence, M., Coward, W. A., Lawrence, F., Cole, C., and Whitehead, R.,** Fat gain during pregnancy in rural African women: the effect of season and dietary status, *Am. J. Clin. Nutr.,* 45, 1442, 1987.

191. **Lawrence, M., Killop, F. M., and Durnin, J. V. A. G.,** Women who gain more fat during pregnancy may not have bigger babies: implications for recommended weight gain during pregnancy, *Obstet. Gynecol.,* 98, 254, 1991.

192. **Lawrence, M. and Lawrence, F., et al.,** A comparison of physical activity in Gambian and U.K. children aged 6–18 months, *Eur. J. Clin. Nutr.,* 45, 243, 1991.

193. **Lechtig, A. and Klein, R. E.,** Prenatal nutrition and birth weight: is there a casual association? in *Maternal Nutrition in Pregnancy. Eating for Two?,* Dobbing, J., Ed., Academic Press, New York 1981, 131.

194. **Ledovskaya, N. M.,** Experiences in the assessment of physical activity in twins, in *Physical Activity in Man and Hypokinesia,* Slonim, A., D., and Smirnov, K. M., Eds., Academy of Sciences of USSR, Siberian Dept., Institute of Physiology, Novosibirsk, 1972, 30 (in Russian).

195. **Leger, J., Carel, C., Legrand, I., Paulsen, A., Hassan, M., and Czernichow, P.,** Magnetic resonance imaging evaluation of adipose tissue and muscle tissue mass in children with growth hormone (GH) deficiency, Turner's syndrome, and intrauterine growth retardation during the first year of treatment with GH, *J. Clin. Endocrinol. Metab.,* 78, 904, 1994.

196. **Livingstone, M. B. E., Davies, P. S. W., Prentice, A. M., et al.,** Comparisons of simultaneous measures of energy intake and expenditure in children and adolescents, *Proc. Nutr. Soc.,* 50, 15 A, 1991.

197. LSRO Life Sciences Research Office (LSRO), *Effect of Dietary Factors on Skeletal Integrity in Adults: Calcium, Phosphorus, Vitamin D and Protein,* Federation of American Societies for Experimental Biology, Bethesda, Md., 1981.

198. **Lohmann, T. G.,** *Advances in Body Composition,* Current Issues in Exercise Science, Human Kinetics Publishers, Champaign, IL, 1992.

199. **Lukaski, H. C., Bolonchuk, W. W., Hall, C. B., and Siders, A.,** Validation of tetrapolar bioelectrical impedance method to assess human body composition, *J. Appl. Physiol.,* 60, 1327, 1986.

200. **Maffeis, C., Micciolo, R., Must, A., Zaffanello, M., and Pinelli, L.,** Parental and perinatal factors associated with childhood obesity, *Int. J. Obes. Relat. Metab. Disord.,* 18, 301, 1994.

201. **Magalhaes, L. C., Koomar, J. A., and Cermak, S. A.,** Bilateral coordination in 5- to 9-year-old children: a pilot study, *Am. J. Occup. Ther.,* 43, 437, 1989.

202. **Malina, R. M., and Bushang, P. H.,** Growth, strength and motor performance of Zapotec children, Oaxaca, Mexico, *Hum. Biol.,* 57, 163, 1985.

203. **Malina, R. M., Little, B. B., and Buschang, P. H.,** Estimated body composition and strength of chronically mild-to-moderately undernourished rural boys in Southern Mexico, in *Human Growth, Physical Fitness and Nutrition,* Shephard, R.J. and Pařízková, J., Eds., Medicine and Sport Science, Vol. 31, S. Karger, Basel, 1991, 119.

204. **Malina, R. M., Little, B. B., and Buschang, P. H.,** Muscular strength in Zapotec children and adults, in *Human Growth, Dietary Intake and Other Environmental Influences,* Proc. Symp., 13th ICAES (Int. Congr. Anthropological Ethnology Sci.), Mexico City 1993, Danone, Paris, 1995, 17.

205. **Malina, R. M. and Roche, A. F.,** *Manual of Physical Status and Performance,* Vol. 2, *Physical Performance,* Plenum Press, New York, 1983.

206. **Martorell, R.,** Body size, adaptation and function, *Hum. Organ.,* 48, 15, 1989.

207. **Matějíček ,Z. and Strnadová, M.,** *Psychodiagnostic and Didactic Tests,* Bratislava, 1974 (in Czech).

208. **Matějíček, Z. and Vágnerová, M.,** The knowledge test for preschool children, *A Manual — Psychodiagnostic and Didactic Tests,* Bratislava, 1976 (in Czech).

209. **Matiegka, J.,** *Somatology of school children,* Czechoslovak Academy of Sciences and Arts (CAVU), 1929 (in Czech).

210. **Mayer, J.,** *Overweight, Causes, Cost and Control,* Englewood Cliffs, N.J., Prentice-Hall, 1968.

211. **McArdle, W. D., Katch, F. I., and Katch, V. L.,** *Exercise Physiology, Energy, Nutrition and Human Performance,* 3rd ed., Lea & Febiger, Philadelphia/London, 1991.

212. **McCance, R. A. and Widdowson, E. M.,** The determinants and form, *Proc. R. Soc. London,* 185, 1, 1974.

213. **Meeks-Gardner, J. M., Grantham-McGregor, S. M., et al.,** Dietary intake and observed activity of stunted and non-stunted children in Kingston, Jamaica. II. observed activity, *Eur. J. Clin. Nutr.,* 44, 585, 1990.

214. **Miklashevskaya, N.,** Growth processes in children and adolescents of the longevity populations, in *Growth and Ontogenetic Development of Man, IV,* Hajniš, K., Ed., Charles University, Prague, 1994, 175.

215. **Mills, J. K. and Andrianopoulos, G. D.,** The relationship between childhood onset of obesity and psychopathology in adulthood, *J. Psychol.,* 127, 547, 1993.

216. **Naidu, U. S. and Kapadia, K. R., Eds.,** *Child Labor and Health, Problems and Prospects,* Tata Institute of Social Sciences, Bombay, India, 1985.

217. **Molnar, D. and Porszasz, J.,** The effect of fasting hyperinsulinaemia on physical fitness in obese children. *Eur. J. Pediatr.,* 149, 570, 1990.

218. **Neumann, C. G. and Harrison, G. G.,** *Onset and Evolution of Stunting in Infants and Children.* Examples from the Human Nutrition Collaborative Research Support Program, Kenya and Egypt studies, *Eur. J. Clin. Nutr.,* 48 (Suppl. 1), S90, 1994.

219. **Newman, W. P. III., Freedman, D. S., Voors, A. W., Gard, P. D., Srinivasan, S. R., Cresanta, J. L., Williamson, G. D., Webber, L. S. and Berenson, G. S.,** Relation of serum lipoprotein levels and systolic blood pressure to early atherosclerosis: the Bogalusa Heart Study, *N. Engl. J. Med.,* 314, 138, 1986.

220. **Nuutinen, O. and Knip, M.,** Prediction of weight reduction in obese children, *Eur. J. Clin. Nutr.,* 46, 785, 1992.

221. **Ogle, G. D., Allen, J. R., Humphries, I. R. J., Lu, Pei Wen, Briody, J. N., Morley, K., Howman-Giles, R., and Cowell, C. T.,** Body-composition assessment by dual-energy X-ray absorptiometry in subjects aged 4–26 y, *Am. J. Clin. Nutr.,* 61, 746, 1995.

222. **Oja, L. and Jürimae, T.,** Assessment of motor ability in 4- to 5-year old children, in press.

223. **Onyango, P. and Kayongo-Male, D.,** *Child labor and health,* Proc. 1st Natl. Workshop on Child Labor and Health, Nairobi, Kenya, Dec. 2–3, 1982, *Transafrican J. Hist.* and *J. East. Afr. Res. Dev.,* University of Nairobi, 1983.

224. **Papousek, H.,** Conditioned head rotation reflexes in the first months of life, *Acta Pediatr.,* 50, 565, 1961.

225. **Papousek, H. and Papousek, M.,** Cognitive aspects of preverbal social interaction between human infants and adults, in *Parental-Infant Interaction,* O'Connor, M., Ed., Elsevier, Amsterdam, 1975, 241.

226. **Papousek, H. and Papousek, M.,** Early ontogeny of human social interaction: its biological roots and social dimensions, in *Human Ethology,* Van Granach, M., Poppa, K., Lepenies, W., and Ploog, D., Eds., Cambridge University Press, Cambridge, 1979, 456.

227. **Pařízková, J.,** The assessment of lean body mass in adolescents by hydrostatic weighing, *Cs. Fysiol.,* 8, 426, 1959 (in Czech).

228. **Pařízková, J.,** Effet sur la croissance du jeune rat d'un régime librement choisi comparé a un régime gras, *Nutr. Dieta,* 3, 236, 1961.

229. **Pařízková, J.,** Age trends in fatness in normal and obese children, *J. Appl. Physiol.,* 16, 1734, 1961.

230. **Pařízková, J.,** Total body fat and skinfold thickness in children, *Metabolism,* 10, 794, 1961.

231. **Pařízková, J.,** The impact of age, diet and exercise on man's body composition, *Ann. N.Y. Acad. Aci.,* 110, 661, 1963.

232. **Pařízková, J.,** Impact of daily work-load during pregnancy on the microstructure of the rat heart in male offspring, *Eur. J. Appl. Physiol.,* 34, 323, 1975.

233. **Pařízková, J.,** *Body Fat and Physical Fitness. Body Composition and Lipid Metabolism in Different Regimes of Physical Activity,* Martinus Nijhoff B.V./Medical Division, The Hague, 1977.

234. **Pařízková, J.,** The impact of daily work load during pregnancy and/or postnatal life on the heart microstructure of rat male offspring, *Basic Res. Cardiol.,* 73, 433, 1978.

235. **Pařízková, J.,** Body composition and lipid metabolism in relation to nutrition and exercise, in *Nutrition, Physical Fitness and Health,* Pařízková, J. and Rogozkin, V. A., Eds., University Park Press, Baltimore, 1978, 61.

236. **Pařízková, J.,** The impact of ecological factors and physical activity on the somatic and motor development of preschool children, in *Physical Fitness Assessment. Principles, Practices and Applications,* R.J. Shephard and Lavallée, H., Eds., Charles C Thomas, Springfield, IL, 1978, 238.

237. **Pařízková, J.,** Cardiac microstructure in female and male offspring of exercised rat mothers, *Acta Anat.,* 105, 382, 1979.

238. **Pařízková, J.,** Nutrition and metabolic factors as related to growth, and physical activity of preschool children, in *Child Growth and Development,* Proc. Int. Symp., Université du Québec, October 1980, Lavallée, H. and Shephard, R.J., Eds., Université du Québec a Trois Rivières, 1980, 141.

239. **Pařízková, J.,** Nutrition and work performance, in *Critical Reviews in Tropical Medicine,* Vol. 1, Chandra, R.K., Ed., Plenum Press, New York, 1982, 307.

240. **Pařízková, J.,** Adaptation of functional capacity and exercise, in *Nutritional Adaptation in Man,* Blaxter, K. and Waterlow, J.C., Eds., John Libbey, London, 1985, 127.

241. **Pařízková, J.,** Body composition and nutrition of different types of athletes, in *Proc. 13th Int. Congr. Nutr.,* Taylor, T.G. and Jenkins, N.K., Eds., John Libbey, London, 1986, 309.

242. **Pařízková, J.,** Growth, functional capacity and physical fitness in normal and malnourished children, *World Rev. Nutr. Diet.,* 51, 1, 1987.

243. **Pařízková, J.,** Age-dependent changes in dietary intake related to work output, physical fitness, and body composition, *Am. J. Clin. Nutr.,* 49, 962, 1989.

244. **Pařízková, J.,** Nutritional individuality and physical performance in different periods of life, in *International Perspectives in Exercise Physiology,* Nazar, K., Terjung, R. L., Kaciuba-Uscilko, H., and Budohoski, L., Eds., Human Kinetics Books, Champaign, IL, 1989, 104.

245. **Pařízková, J.,** Human growth, physical fitness and nutrition under various environmental conditions, in *Human Growth, Physical Fitness and Nutrition,* Shephard R.J. and Pařízková, J., Eds., Medicine and Sport Science, Vol. 31, S. Karger, Basel, 1991, 1.

246. **Pařízková, J.,** Obesity and its treatment by exercise, in *Nutrition and Fitness in Health and Disease,* Simopoulos A., Ed., *World Rev. Nutr. Diet.,* S. Karger, Basel 1993, 78.

247. **Pařízková, J.,** The impact of environment on somatic and motor development of preschool children, in *World-Wide Variation in Physical Fitness,* Claessens, A.L., Lefevre, J., and Vanden Eynde, B., Institute of Physical Education, Katholieke Universiteit, Leuven, Belgium, 1993, 131.

248. **Pařízková, J.,** Food choices in Czechoslovakia, *Appetite,* 21, 299, 1993.

249. **Pařízková, J.,** Changes in approach to the measurement of body composition, in *Proc. Int. Symp., Body Composition Techniques and Assessment in Health and Disease,* Soc. Study Hum. Biol., Cambridge, 1993, Cambridge Univ. Press, Cambridge, 1995, 222.

250. **Pařízková, J.,** Nutrition and physical performance during growth, in *Proc. 15th Int. Congr. Nutr. Symp. Nutrition and Physical Performance,* Adelaide, Australia, Sept. 26–Oct. 1, 1993, Smith and Gordon, London 1994.

251. **Pařízková, J.,** The relationship of nutritional status and functional development in preschool age, in *Proc. Annu. Symp. (33rd Meeting), European Academy of Nutritional Science, Nutrition in Pregnancy and Growth,* Milano, June 1–2, 1994, S. Karger, Basel, in press.

252. **Pařízková, J.,** Somatic and motor development in preschool age, and the impact of regular exercise, in *Proc. Int. Symp. Child-Motion-Family,* Dec. 1994, Council of Europe — Czech Sport Organization, Prague, in press, 1995.

253. **Pařízková, J.,** Dietary intake and physical activity as preventive measures during early growth, Workshop 9, in 7th European Nutrition Conference, *Over and Undernutrition in Europe, FENS,* Vienna, May 24–28, 1995, Book of Abstracts, WS 38, 10, 1995.

254. **Pařízková, J.,** unpublished data.

255. **Pařízková, J. and Adamec, A.,** Longitudinal study of anthropometric, skinfold, work and motor characteristics of boys and girls, three to six years of age, *Am. J. Phys. Anthrop.,* 50, 387, 1980.

256. **Pařízková, J., Adamec, A., Berdychová, J., Čermák, J., Horná, J., and Teplý, Z.,** *Growth, Fitness and Nutrition in Preschool Children,* Charles University, Prague, 1984.

257. **Pařízková, J., Bunc, V., and Halíčková L.,** Relation of working energy output to basal metabolic rate and body size in different age groups, *Human Nutr. Clin. Nutr.,* 38C, 233, 1984.

258. **Pařízková, J., Čermák, J., and Horná, J.,** Sex differences in somatic and functional characteristics of preschool children, *Hum. Biol.,* 49, 437, 1977.

259. **Pařízková, J. and Douglas, P. D.,** Eds., *Human Growth, Dietary Intake and Other Environmental Influences.* Proceedings of a Symposium, the 13th Int. Congress Anthropological Ethnology Sciences, Mexico City 1993. Danone, Paris 1995, 1, 2.

260. **Pařízková, J. and Faltová, E.,** Physical activity, body fat and experimental cardiac necrosis, *Br. J. Nutr.,* 3, 24, 1970.

261. **Pařízková, J., Faltová, E., Mráz, M., and Špatová, M.,** Growth, food intake, motor activity and experimental cardiac necrosis in early malnourished male rats, *Ann. Nutr. Metab.,* 26, 121, 1982.

262. **Pařízková, J., Fraňková, S., Špatová, M., and Petrásek, R.,** Spontaneous motor activity, energy cost of growth and lipid metabolism in the liver in male rats with early protein energy malnutrition, *Baroda J. Nutr.,* 7, 49, 1980.

263. **Pařízková, J. and Hainer, V.,** Exercise in growing and adult obese individuals, in *Current Therapy in Sports Medicine-2,* Torg, J.S., Welsh, R.P. and Shephard, R.J., Eds., H.B.C. Decker, Inc, Toronto, 1990, 22.

264. **Pařízková, J., Hainer, V., Štich, L., Kunešová, M., and Ksantini, M.,** Physiological capabilities of obese individuals and implications for exercise, in *Exercise and Obesity,* Wahlquist, M. and Hills, A.P., Eds., Smith-Gordon, London, 1995, 131.

265. **Pařízková, J. and Heller, J.,** Relationship of dietary intake to work output and physical performance in Czechoslovak adolescents adapted to various work loads, in *Human Growth, Physical Fitness and Nutrition, Medicine and Sport Science, Vol. 31,* Shephard, R.J. and Pařízková, J., Eds., S. Karger, Basel, 1991, 156.

266. **Pařízková, J., Juřinová, I., and Adamec, A.,** Individual stability of motor development and somatotype in preschool age, *Humanbiol. Budapest.,* 16, 113, 1985 (in Czech).

267. **Pařízková, J. and Kábele, J.,** Somatic and psychological development, performance and fitness, body posture and food intake in the relationship to physical activity regime of preschool children, *Acta Univ. Carol. Gymnica,* 21, 55, 1985.

268. **Pařízková, J. and Kábele, J.,** Longitudinal study of somatic, motor and psychological development in preschool boys and girls, *Coll. Anthropol.,* 12, 67, 1988.

269. **Pařízková, J. and Lát, J.,** Growth, body composition and excitability in male rats with increased or decreased motor activity in early ontogeny, in *Physical Fitness,* Seliger, V., Ed., Universita Karlova, Prague, 1973, 304.

270. **Pařízková, J., Macková, E., Kábele, J., Macková, J., and Škopková, M.,** Body composition, food intake, cardiorespiratory fitness, blood lipids and psychological development in highly active and inactive preschool children, *Hum. Biol.,* 58, 261, 1986.

271. **Pařízková, J., Macková, E., Macková, J., and Škopková, M.,** Blood lipids as related to food intake, body composition, and cardiorespiratory efficiency in preschool children, *J. Pediatr. Gastroenterol. Nutr.,* 5, 295, 1986.

272. **Pařízková, J. and Petrásek, R.,** Impact of early nutrition on later development of spontaneous physical activity and lipid metabolism, *Nutr. Metab.,* 23, 266, 1979.

273. **Pařízková, J. and Petrásek, R.,** The impact of daily work load during pregnancy on lipid metabolism in the liver of the offspring, *Eur. J. Appl. Physiol.,* 39, 81, 1978.

274. **Pařízková, J., Petrásek, R., and Frankova, S.,** The impact of reduced energy and protein intake at the beginning of life on growth, spontaneous motor activity and lipid metabolism in male rats, *Ind. J. Nutr. Dietet.,* 16, 412, 1979.

275. **Pařízková, J. and Staňková, L.,** Influence of physical activity on a treadmill on the metabolism of adipose tissue in rats, *Br. J. Nutr.,* 18, 325, 1964.

276. **Pařízková, J., Vetvička, J., Poušek, L., and Liška, O.,** Relationship of cardiorespiratory indicators, blood lipids, amount and distribution of adipose tissue in middle-aged men, *Čas. Lek. Cek,* 134, 404, 1995 (in Czech).

277. **Pařízková, J., Wachtlová, M., and Soukupová, M.,** The impact of different motor activity on body composition, density of capillaries and fibres in the heart, and soleus muscle, and cell's migration *in vitro* in male rats, *Int. Z. Angew. Physiol.,* 30, 207, 1972.

278. **Pavlovic, M.,** Dietary changes in preschool children's social nutrition for the early prevention of cardiovascular diseases, Workshop 9, in Seventh European Nutrition Conference, *Over- and Undernutrition in Europe,* Vienna, May 24–28, 1995, Book of Abstracts WS 50, 13, 1995.

279. **Pellett, T. L. and Ignico, A. A.,** Relationship between children's and parents' stereotyping of physical activities, *Percept. Mot. Skills,* 77, 1283, 1993.

280. **Pelletier, D. L.,** The relationship between child anthropometry and mortality in developing countries: implications for policy, programs and future research, *J. Nutr.,* 124, 2047S, 1994.

281. **Pelletier, D. L., Low, J. W., Johnson, F. C., and Msukwa, L. A.,** Child anthropometry and mortality in Malawi: testing for effect modification by age and length of follow-up and confounding by socioeconomic factors, *J. Nutr.,* 124, 2082S, 1994.

282. **Percy, P., Vilbergsson, G., Percy, A., and Mansson, J. E.,** The fatty acid composition of placenta in intrauterine growth retardation, *Biochim. Biophys. Acta,* 1084, 173, 1991.

283. **Pike, R. L. and Brown, M. L.,** *Nutrition — An Integrated Approach,* 3rd ed., John Wiley & Sons, New York, 1984, 832.

284. **Pistulková, H., Poledne, R., Kaucká, J., Škodová, Z., Petržilková, Z., Paclt, M., Valenta, Z., Grafnetter, D., and Pisa, Z.,** Cholesterolemia in school-age children and hypercholesterolemia aggregation in the family, *Cor Vasa.,* 33, 139, 1991.

285. **Pitkin, R. M.,** Assessment of nutritional status of mother, fetus and newborn, *Am. J. Clin. Nutr.,* 34, 658, 1981.

286. **Pollitt, E., Sacco-Pollit, C., et al.,** Iron deficiency and behavioral development in infants and preschool children, *Am. J. Clin. Nutr.,* 43, 555, 1986.

287. **Politt, E.,** Poverty and child development: relevance of research in developing countries to the United States, *Child Dev.,* 65, 283, 1994.

288. **Prentice, A. M., Ed.,** *The doubly labelled water method for measuring energy expenditure. International Dietary Intake Consultative Group,* Technical Recommendations For Human Applications, Vienna, IAEA/IDECG NAHRES 4, 1990.

289. **Prentice, A. M., Lucas, A., Vasquez-Velasquez, L., Davies, P. S. W., and Whitehead, R. G.,** Are current guidelines for young children a prescription for overeating?, *Lancet,* ii, 1066, 1988.

290. **Prokopec, M.,** New anthropometric data of the CSSR population, *Acta Facult. Rer. Natur. Univ. Comenianae Anthropologica,* 22, 187, 1976.

291. **Prokopec, M.,** The trend of development of children population in ČSR over the last 30 years, *Čs. Hyg.,* 31, 541, 1986 (in Czech).

292. **Prokopec, M., Titlbachová, S., Dutková, L., and Zlámalová, H.,** Development of height and weight of Czech children since 1951 up to 1981, *Anthropologie,* 24, 217, 1986.

293. **Prokopec, M. and Bellisle, F.,** Body mass index variation from birth to adulthood in Czech youths, *Acta Med. Auxol.,* 24, 87, 1992.

294. **Prokopec, M. and Bellisle, F.,** Adiposity in Czech children followed from 1 month of age to adulthood: analysis of individual BMI patterns, *Ann. Hum. Biol.,* 20, 517, 1993.

295. **Ratishouser, I. H. E. and Whitehouse, R. G.,** Energy intake and expenditure in 1–3 year old Ugandan children living in a rural environment, *Brit. J. Nutr.,* 28, 145, 1972.

296. **Ray, R., Lim, L. H., and Ling, S. L.,** Obesity in preschool children: an intervention program in primary health care in Singapore, *Ann. Acad. Med. Singapore,* 23, 335, 1994.

297. **Rippe, J. M., Blair, S. N., Freedson, P., Micheli, L. J., Morrow, J. R., Pate, R., Plowman, S., and Rowland, T.,** Childhood health and fitness in the United States: current status and future challenges, Part I (p. 97) and II (p. 171) of a *Round Table Discussion at the American College of Sports Medicine,* Orlando, Florida, May, 1991.

298. **Roberts, S. B., Savage, J., Coward, W. A., Chew, B., and Lucas, A.,** Energy expenditure and intake in infants born to lean and overweight mothers, *New Engl. J. Med.,* 318, 461, 1988.

299. **Roland-Cachera, M. F.,** Prediction of adult body composition from infant & childhood measurements, in Proc. Symp. *Body Composition Techniques and Assessment in Health and Disease,* Soc. Study Hum. Biol., Cambridge, 1993, Cambridge University Press, Cambridge, 1995, 100.

300. **Roland-Cachera, M. F., Bellisle, F.,** No correlation between adiposity and food intake: why are working class children fatter?, *Am. J. Clin. Nutr.,* 44, 779, 1986.

301. **Roland-Cachera, M. F., Bellisle, F., Deheeger, M., Guilloud-Bataille, M., Pequignot, F., and Sempé, M.,** Adiposity development and prediction during growth in humans: a two decade follow-up study, in *Obesity in Europe 88,* John Libbey, London, 1988, 73.

302. **Roland-Cachera, M. F., Bellisle, F., Deheeger, M., Pequignot, F., and Sempé, M.,** Influence of body fat distribution during childhood on body fat distribution in adulthood: a two decade follow-up study, *Int. J. Obes.*, 14, 473, 1990.

303. **Roland-Cachera, M. F., Bellisle, F., Sempé, M., Guillaud-Bataille, M., and Patois, E.,** Adiposity rebound in children: a simple indicator for predicting obesity, *Am. J. Clin. Nutr.*, 39, 129, 1984.

304. **Roland-Cachera, M. F., Bellisle, F., Tichet, J., Chantrel, A. M., Guilloud-Bataille, M., Vol, S., and Péquignot, G.,** Relationship between adiposity and food intake: an example of pseudocontradictory results obtained in case-control versus between-population studies, *Int. J. Epidemiol.*, 19, 571, 1990.

305. **Roland-Cachera, F. M., Cole, T., Sempé, M., Tichet, J., Rossignol, C. and Charraud, A.,** Variations in body mass index in the French population from 0 to 87 years, in *Obesity in Europe 91,* Ailhaud, G. A., et al. Eds., John Libey, London, 1991, 113.

306. **Roland-Cachera, M. F., Deheeger, M., Avons, P., Guillaud-Bataille, M., Patois, E., and Sempé, M.,** Tracking obesity patterns from 1 month to adulthood, *Ann. Hum. Biol.*, 14, 219, 1987.

307. **Roland-Cachera, M. F., Deheeger, M., and Bellisle, F.,** Early nutrition and later outcomes, in *The 6th European Congress on Obesity,* Abstract Book, *Int. J. Obes.*, 19, Suppl. 2, 1995, 11.

308. **Ross, M. H.,** Nutrition, disease and length of life, in *Diet and Bodily Constitution,* CIBA Foundation, Study Group No. 17, Wolstenholme, G.E.W. and O'Connor, M., Eds., J. & A. Churchill, London, 1964, 90.

309. **Ross, M. H., Lustbader, E., and Bras, G.,** Dietary practices and growth responses as predictors of longevity, *Nature (London),* 262, 548, 1976.

310. **Rowland, T. W.,** *Exercise and Children's Health,* Human Kinetics Books, Champaign, IL, 1990, 47.

311. **Rush, D., Sloan, N. L., Leighton, J., Alvir, J. M., Horvitz, D. G., Burleigh, Seaver, W., Garbowski, G. C., Johnson, S. S., Kulka, R. A., Mimi Holt, A. B., Devore, J. W., Lynch, J. T., Woodside, M. B., and Shanklin, D. S.,** Longitudinal study of pregnant women, *Am. J. Clin. Nutr.,* (Suppl.), 48, 439, 1988.

312. **Ruwe, P. J., Wolverton, C. K. , White, M. E., and Ramsey, T. G.,** Effect of maternal fasting on fetal and placental lipid metabolism in swine, *J. Anim. Sci.,* 69, 1935, 1991.

313. **Sandler, R. B., Slemenda, C. W., La Porte, R. F., Cauley, A., Schlicker, S. A., Borra, S. T., and Regan, C.,** The weight and fitness status of United States children. *Nutr. Rev.,* 52, 11, 1994.

314. **Satyaranayana, K., Prasanna Krishna, T., and Narasinga Rao, B. S.,** Effect of early childhood undernutrition and child labour on growth and adult nutritional status of rural Indian boys around Hydarabad, *Hum. Nutr. Clin. Nutr.,* 40C, 131, 1985.

315. **Satyaranayana, K., Naidu, A. N., and Narasinga Rao, B. S.,** Nutritional deprivation in childhood and the body size, activity and physical work capacity of young boys, *Am. J. Clin. Nutr.,* 32, 1769, 1979.

316. **Satyaranayana, K., Nadamuni Naidu, A., and Narasinga Rao, B. S.,** Agricultural employment, wage earnings and nutritional status of teenage rural Hydarabad boys, *Ind. J. Nutr. Diet.,* 17, 281, 1980.

317. **Satyaranayana, K., Prasanna Krishna, T., Bannerji, D., and Narasinga Rao, B. S.,** Social epidemiology of nutrition in the Ranga Reddy District of India and its implications for human resources development, in *Human Growth, Physical Fitness and Nutrition,* Shephard, R.J. and Pařízková, J., Eds., Medicine and Sport Science, Vol. 31, S. Karger, Basel, 1991, 33.

318. **Schlicker, S. A., Borra, S. T., and Regan, C.,** The weight status and fitness of United States children, *Nutr. Rev.,* 52, 11, 1994.

319. **Schürch, B. and Scrimshaw, N. S.,** *Chronic energy deficiency: Consequences and Related Issues,* International Dietary Energy Consultancy Group, IDECG Meeting, Aug. 3–7, 1987, Guatemala City, Nestle Foundation, Lausanne, Switzerland 1987.

320. **Schramm, M. M., Baresi, M. I., and Kriska, A. M.,** Postmenopausal bone density and milk consumption in childhood and adolescence, *Am. J. Clin. Nutr.,* 42, 270, 1985.

321. **Scrimshaw, N. S.,** Nutrition prospects for the 1990th, *Annu. Rev. Public Health,* 11, 53, 1990.

322. **Seckler, D.,** Small but healthy: a basic hypothesis of the theory, measurement and policy of malnutrition, in *New Concepts in Nutrition and Their Implications for Policy,* Sukhatme, P. V., Ed., ??.

323. **Seitz, P. F. D.,** The effects of infantile experiences upon adult behavior in animal subjects: I. Effects of litter size during infancy upon adult behavior in the rat, *Am. J. Psychiatr.,* 110, 916, 1954.

324. **Shah, P. M. (Ed.),** *Child Labour: A Threat to Health and Development,* 2nd ed., Defense for Children International, Geneva, Switzerland, 1985.

325. **Shea, S., Basch, C. E., Gutin, B., Stein, A. D., Contento, I. R., Irigoyen, M., and Zybert, P.,** The rate of increase in blood pressure in children 5 years of age is related to changes in aerobic fitness and body mass index, *Pediatrics,* 94, 465, 1994.

326. **Shea, S., Basch, C. E., Stein, A. D., Contento, I. R., Irigoyen, M., and Zybert, P.,** Is there a relationship between dietary fat and stature or growth of children three to five years of age?, *Pediatrics,* 92, 579, 1993.

327. **Shephard, R. J.,** Somatic growth and physical performance in Canada, in *Human Growth, Physical Fitness and Nutrition,* Medicine and Sports Science, Vol. 31, Shephard, R.J., and Pařízková, J., Eds., S. Karger, Basel, 1991, 133.

328. **Seliger, V.,** Survey of the physical fitness of the inhabitants of Czechoslovakia, in *Human Adaptability,* Weiner, J.S., Ed., Taylor & Francis, London, 1977, 88.

329. **Siervogel, R. M., Roche, A. F., Guo, S. M., Mukherjee, D., and Chumlea, W. C.,** Patterns of change in weight/stature^2 from 2 to 18 years: findings from long-term serial data for children in the Fels longitudinal growth study, *Int. J. Obes.,* 15, 479, 1991.

330. **Siniarska, A.,** Biological development of children and youth from selected regions of Poland in relationship to family conditions and biological indicators of parents. Studies in human ecology (Suppl. 1) *Polish Studies in Human Ecology,* Wolanski, N., Ed., Institute of Ecology Publishing Office, Dziekanow Lesny, 1994, 89 (in Polish).

331. **Skinner, J. S.,** *Exercise testing and exercise prescription for special cases.* Theoretical basis and clinical application, Lea & Febiger, Philadelphia, 1987.

332. **Sklad, M.,** Similarity of movements in twins, *Wychowanie Fiz. Sport,* 3, 119, 1972.

333. **Sothern, M., Suskind, R., von Almen, K., Schumacher, H., Schultz, S., De Leon, E., Gastanaduy, A., McMasters, P., Farris, R., and Udall, J.,** One year results of four phase treatment program for childhood obesity, in 7th Int. Congress on Obesity, Toronto, Canada, 1994, *Int. J. Obes.,* 18 (Suppl. 2), 17.

334. **Spady, D. W. and Payne, P. R.,** Energy balance during recovery from malnutrition, *Am. J. Clin. Nutr.,* 29, 1073, 1976.

335. **Spurr, G. B.,** Body size, physical work capacity and productivity in hard work: is bigger better?, in *Linear Growth Retardation in Less Developed Countries,* Waterlow, J.C., Ed., Nestle Nutrition, Vevey, Raven Press, New York, 1988, 215.

336. **Spurr, G. B., Barac-Nieto, M., Reina, J. C., and Ramirez, R.,** Marginal malnutrition in school-aged Colombian boys: efficiency of treadmill walking in submaximal exercise, *Am. J. Clin.,* 39, 452, 1984.

337. **Spurr, G. B., Reina, J. C., Barac-Nieto, M., and Maksud, M. G.,** Maximum oxygen consumption of nutritionally normal white, Mestizo, and black Colombian boys 6–16 years of age, *Hum. Biol.,* 54, 553, 1982.

338. **Spurr, G., Reina, J. C., Dahners, H. W., and Barac-Nieto, M.,** Marginal malnutrition in school-aged Colombian boys: functional consequences in maximum exercise. *Am. J. Clin. Nutr.,* 37, 834, 1983b.

339. **Spurr, G. B. and Reina, J. C.,** Energy expenditure/basal metabolic rate ratios in normal and marginally undernourished Colombian children 6–16 years of age, *Eur. J. Clin. Nutr.,* 43, 515, 1989.

340. **Spurr, G. B., Reina, J. C., and Hoffmann, R. G.,** Basal metabolic rate of Colombian children 2–16 years of age: ethnicity and nutritional status, *Am. J. Clin. Nutr.,* 56, 623, 1992.

341. **Stephen, A. M. and Sieber, G. M.,** Trends in individual fat consumption in the U.K. 1900–1985, *Br. J. Nutr.,* 71, 775, 1994.

342. **Stephenson, T. J., Stammers, J. P., and Hull, D.,** Effects of altering umbilical flow and umbilical free fatty acids concentration on transfer of free fatty acids across the rabbit placenta, *J. Dev. Physiol.,* 15, 221, 1991.

343. **Sylvén, Ch., Jansson, E., and Olin, Ch.,** Human myocardial and skeletal muscle enzyme activities: creatine kinase and its isoenzyme MR as related to citrate synthetase and muscle fibre types, *Clin. Physiol.,* 3, 461, 1983.

344. **Suzuki, S., Oshima, S., Tsuji, E., Tsuji, K., and Ohto, F.,** Interrelationships between nutrition, physical activity, and physical fitness, in *Nutrition, Physical Fitness and Health,* Pařízková, J. and Rogozkin, V.A., Eds., Int. Ser. Sports Sci., Vol. 7, University Park Press, Baltimore, 1978, 167.

345. **Szabo, A. J., Oppermann, W., Hannover, B., Guggliucci, C., and Szabo, O.,** Fetal adipose tissue development. Relationship to maternal free fatty acid levels, in *Early Diabetes in Early Life,* Camerini-Davalos, R.A. and Cole, H.S., Eds., Academic Press, New York, 1975, 17.

346. **Taggart, N., Holliday, R. M., Billewicz, W. Z., Hutten, F. E., and Thomson, A. M.,** Changes in skinfolds during pregnancy, *Br. J. Nutr.,* 21, 439, 1967.

347. **Tanner, J. M.,** *Growth at Adolescence,* 2nd ed., Blackwell Scientific, Oxford, 1962.

348. **Tanner, J. M., Whitehouse, R. H., and Takaishi, M.,** Standards from birth to maturity of height, weight, height velocity and weight velocity: British children 1965, *Arch. Dis. Children* I, 41, 454; II, 41, 613, 1966.

349. **Tanner, J. M., Whitehouse, R. H., et al.,** Standards for children's height at ages 2–9 years allowing for heights of parents, *Arch. Dis. Child,* 45, 755, 1970.

350. **Tanman, B.,** Changes of cardiac output and total body oxygen consumption in protein-calorie malnourished infants, in *Proc. 13th Int. Congr. Pediatrics,* Wiener Medical Academie, Vienna, 1971, 407.

351. **Thomas, C., Evans, J. L., and Lowy, C.,** The effect of alloxan induced diabetes in the rabbit on placental transfer of glucose and non-esterified fatty acids, *Diabetes Res.,* 11, 55, 1989.

352. **Thompson, F. E. and Dennison, B. A.,** Dietary sources of fats and cholesterol in U.S. children aged 2 through 5 years, *Am. J. Public Health,* 84, 799, 1994.

353. **Thulin, A. J., Allee, G. L., Harmon, D. L., and Davis, D. L.,** Utero-placental transfer of octanoic, palmitic and linoleic acids during late gestation in gilts, *J. Anim. Sci.,* 67, 738, 1989.

354. **Torún, B.,** Role of energy metabolism in regulation of protein requirements, in *Proc. 13th Int. Congr. of Nutrition,* John Libbey, London, 1986, 414.

355. **Torún, B.,** Physiological measurements of physical activity among children under free-living conditions, in *Energy Intake and Activity,* Pollitt, E., and Amante, P., Eds., Alan R. Liss, Inc. (for the United Nations University), New York, 1984, 159.

356. **Torún, B., Chew, F., and Mendoza, R. D.,** Energy cost of activities of pre-school children, *Nutr. Res.,* 3, 401, 1983.

357. **Torún, B. and Viteri, F. E.,** Influence of exercise on linear growth, *Eur. J. Clin. Nutr.,* 48 (Suppl. 1), S186, 1994.

358. **Tsukuda, T., Hanaki, K., Ohzeki, T., Ohtahara, H., Urashima, H., and Shiraki, K.,** Obesity in young children aged 3 to 6 years can be easily screened by measurement of bioelectrical impedance, 7th Int. Congress on Obesity, 1994, Toronto, Canada, *Int. J. Obes.,* 18 (Suppl. 2), 9, 1994.

359. **Türnagöl, H. H., Aritan, G., Yerlisu, T., Turker, F., and Türnagöl, P.,** A preliminary study on growth and physical fitness in preschool children in Ankara, in Proceedings of the Symposium *Human Growth, Dietary Intake and Other Environmental Influences*, 13th ICAES (Int. Congr. Anthropological Ethnology, Sci.), Mexico City, 1993, Pařízková, J. and Douglas, P.D., Eds., Danone, Paris, 1995, 8.

360. **Uemura, K. and Piša, Z.,** Trends in cardiovascular disease mortality in industrialized countries since 1950, *World Health Statistics Quarterly,* 41, 155, 1988.

361. **Underwood, P. B., Kesler, K. F., O'Lane, et al.,** Parental smoking empirically related to pregnancy outcome, *Obstet. Gynecol.,* 29, 1, 1967.

362. U.S. Public Health Service, Physical activity in children, *Am. Fam. Physician,* 59, 1285, 1994.

363. **Vettorazzi, C., Molina, S., Grazioso, C., Mazariegos, M., Siu, M. L., and Solomons, W.,** Bioelectrical impedance indices in protein-energy malnourished children as an indicator of total body water status, *Basic Life Sci.,* 55, 45, 1990.

364. **Viart, P.,** Blood volume changes during treatment of protein-calorie malnutrition, *Am. J. Clin. Nutr.,* 30, 349, 1977b.

365. **Viart, P.,** Hemodynamic findings during treatment of protein-calorie malnutrition, *Am. J. Clin. Nutr.,* 31, 911, 1978.

366. **Vierordt, K.,** *Physiologie des Kindesalters,* Verlag der H. Laupp'schen Buchhandlung, Tübingen, 1877.

367. **Viteri, F. E., Torún, B., et al.,** Protein energy requirements under conditions prevailing in developing countries: current knowledge and research needs, Tokyo, United Nations University, WHTR-1-/UNUP-18, *Food and Nutrition Bulletin* (Suppl. 1), 1979.

368. **Viteri, F. E. and Torún, B.,** Estudios sobre dieta-actividad fisica-crecimiento I–III. Décimo Sexto Congreso Nacional de Pediatría, Ciudad de Guatemala, Seccion de Resumenes de Travajos del Programa, 1973, 36.

369. **Vobecky, J. S. and Vobecky, J.,** Biochemical indices of nutritional status in maternal, cord and early neonatal blood, *Am. J. Clin. Nutr.,* 36, 630, 1982.

370. **Vobecky, J. S., David, P., and Vobecky, J.,** Dietary habits in relation to tracking of cholesterol level in young adolescents: a nine-year follow-up, *Ann. Nutr. Metab.,* 32, 312, 1988.

371. **Vobecky, J. S., Grant, A. M., Laplante, P., David, P., and Vobecky, J.,** Hypercholesterolemia in childhood: repercussions in adulthood, *Eur. J. Clin. Nutr.,* 47 (Suppl. 1), S47, 193.

372. **Wachtlová, M. and Pařízková, J.,** Comparison of capillary density in skeletal muscles of animals differing in respects of their physical activity — the hare *(Lepus aeropeus),* the domestic rabbit *(Oryctolagus domesticus),* the brown rat *(Rattus norvegicus)* and the trained and untrained rat, *Physiol. Bohemoslov.,* 21, 489, 1972.

373. **Wallace, J.,** *Our Kids are not OK,* TV program, BBC 1994.

374. **Walravens, P. A. and Hambidge, K. M.,** Growth of infants fed a zinc supplemented formula, *Am. J. Clin. Nutr.,* 29, 1114, 1976.

375. **Wang, ZiMiang, Heschka, S., Pierson, R. N., and Heymsfield, S. B.,** Systematic organization of body-composition methodology: an overview with emphasis on component-based methods, *Am. J. Clin. Nutr.,* 61, 457, 1995.

376. **Waterlow, J. C.,** Observations on FAO's methodology for estimating the incidence of malnutrition, *Food Nutr. Bull. (UNU),* 11, 8, 1989.

377. **Waterlow, J. C.,** Childhood malnutrition in developing nations: looking back and looking forward, *Annu. Rev. Nutr.,* 14, 1, 1994.

378. **Waterlow, J. C., with the contribution of Tomkins, A. M., and Grantham-McGregor, S. M.,** *Protein and Energy Malnutrition,* London, 1992.

379. **Waterlow, J. C., Buzina, R., et al.,** The presentation and use of height and weight data for comparing the nutritional status of groups of children under the age of 10 years, *Bull. World Hlth. Org.,* 55, 489, 1977.

380. **Waterlow, J. C. and Schürch, B., Eds.,** *Causes and Mechanisms of Linear Growth Retardation.* International Dietary Energy Consultancy Group, Proc. I/D/E/C/G Workshop, London, 1993, The University Press, Cambridge, 1993.

381. **Weststrate, J. A. and Duerenberg, P.,** Body composition in children: proposal for a method for calculating body fat percentage from total body density or skinfold thickness measurement, *Am. J. Clin. Nutr.,* 50, 1104, 1989.

382. **Wetzel, N. V.,** Growth, in *Medical Physics,* Year Book Medical Publishers, 1942, 513.

383. **Widdowson, E. M.,** Nutritional individuality, *Proc. Nutr. Soc.,* 21, 121, 1962.

384. **Widdowson, E. M.,** Rate of growth, mature weight and life span, *Proc. R. Soc. London Ser. B,* 156, 96, 1962.

385. **Widdowson, E. M.,** Intrauterine growth retardation in the pig. I. Organ size and cellular development at birth and after growth to maturity, *Biol. Neonate,* 19, 329, 1971.

386. **Widdowson, E. M.,** The demands of the fetal and maternal tissues for nutrients, and the bearing of these on the needs of the mother to "eat for two", in *Maternal Nutrition During Pregnancy. Eating for Two?,* Dobbing J., Ed., Academic Press, New York, 1981, 1.

387. **Widdowson, E. M.,** How much food does man require? An evaluation of human energy needs, *Experientia,* 44, 11, 1983.

388. **Widdowson, E. M. and McCance, R. A.,** Some effects of accelerating growth. I. General somatic Somatic Development. *Proc. Roy. Soc. B.,* 152, 188, 1960.

389. **Widdowson, E. M. and McCance, R. A.,** The effect of finite periods of undernutrition at different ages on the composition and subsequent development of the rat, *Proc. R. Soc. London Ser. B,* 158, 329, 1963.

390. **Wilson, D. M., Killen, J. D., Hammer, L. D., Litt, I. F., Vosti, C., Miner, C., Hayward, C., and Taylor, C. B.,** Insulin-like growth factor-I as a reflection of body composition, nutrition, and puberty in sixth and seventh grade girls, *J. Clin. Endocrinol. Metab.,* 73, 907, 1991.

391. **Wolanski, N. and Pařízkóvá, J.,** *Physical Fitness and the Development of Man,* Wydawnictwo Naukowe, Warszava, 1976 (in Polish).

392. **Wolanski, N. and Siniarska, A., et al.,** The effect of culture and genotype on motor development of parents and their children, *Stud. Hum. Ecol.,* 10, 243, 1992 (in Polish).

393. World Health Organization, *Energy and Protein Requirements,* Report of a Joint FAO/WHO/UNU Meeting, World Health Organization, Tech. Rep. Ser. 724, Geneva, 1985.

394. World Health Organization, *Diet, Nutrition and the Prevention of Chronic Diseases,* Tech. Rep. Ser. No. 797, World Health Organization, Geneva, 1990.

395. World Health Organization, *Prevention in Childhood and Youth of Adult Cardiovascular Diseases: Time for Action,* Report of a WHO Expert Committee, Tech. Rep. Ser. 792, WHO, Geneva, 1990.

396. World Health Organization, *Food and Health Data, Their Use in Nutrition Policy Making,* Becker, W. and Helsing, Eds., WHO Regional Publications, European Series, No. 34, WHO, 1991.

397. *Recommended Dietary Allowances,* 10th ed., National Research Council, National Academy Press, Washington, D.C., 1989.

398. *Nutrient and Energy Intakes for the European Community,* Report of the Scientific Committee for Food (31st Series), Directorate-General, Industry, Office for Official Publications, Luxemburg, 1993.

399. *Our Global Neighbourhood. The Report of The Commission on Global Governance,* Oxford University Press, 1995.

400. *Convention Relative aux Droits de l'Enfant.* United Nations, New York, 1991.

401. Update on the nutritional situation, ACC/SCN's summary, *SCN News, United Nations,* No. 12, 1995, 6.

402. Principles for evaluating health risks from chemicals during infancy and early childhood: the need for special approach, International Program on Chemical Safety (IPCS) and Commission of the European Communities (CEC), Environmental Health Criteria 59, United Nations Environ. Progr., Int. Labour Organization, World Health Organization (WHO), Geneva, 1986.

INDEX